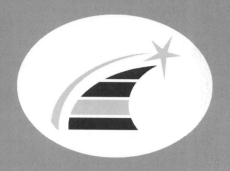
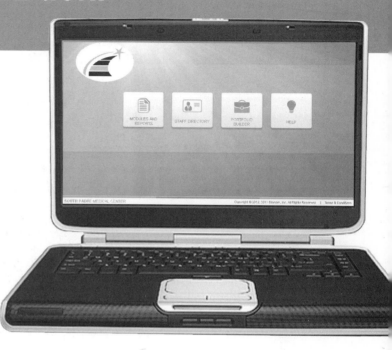
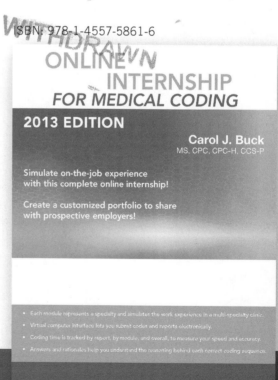

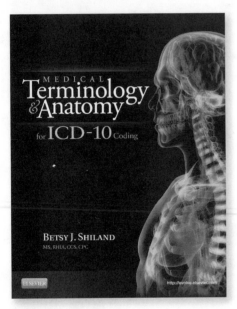
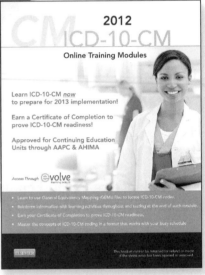
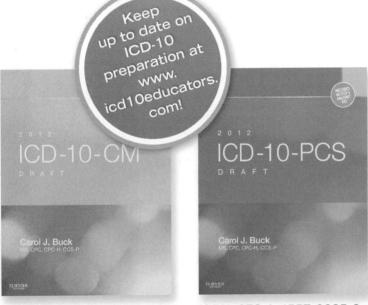
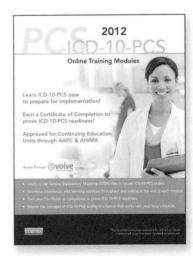

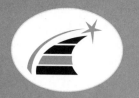

E/M AUDITING STEP

Third Edition

CAROL J. BUCK
MS, CPC, CPC-H, CCS-P
Former Program Director
Medical Secretary Programs
Northwest Technical College
East Grand Forks, Minnesota

SEVIER

3251 Riverport Lane
St. Louis, Missouri 63043

E/M AUDITING STEP, THIRD EDITION

ISBN: 978-1-4557-5199-0

Notices

Knowledge and best practice in this field are constantly changing. As new research and experience broaden our understanding, changes in research methods, professional practices, or medical treatment may become necessary.

Practitioners and researchers must always rely on their own experience and knowledge in evaluating and using any information, methods, compounds, or experiments described herein. In using such information or methods they should be mindful of their own safety and the safety of others, including parties for whom they have a professional responsibility.

With respect to any drug or pharmaceutical products identified, readers are advised to check the most current information provided (i) on procedures featured or (ii) by the manufacturer of each product to be administered, to verify the recommended dose or formula, the method and duration of administration, and contraindications. It is the responsibility of practitioners, relying on their own experience and knowledge of their patients, to make diagnoses, to determine dosages and the best treatment for each individual patient, and to take all appropriate safety precautions.

To the fullest extent of the law, neither the Publisher nor the authors, contributors, or editors, assume any liability for any injury and/or damage to persons or property as a matter of products liability, negligence or otherwise, or from any use or operation of any methods, products, instructions, or ideas contained in the material herein.

ISBN 978-1-4557-5199-0

Content Strategy Director: Jeanne R. Olson
Senior Content Development Specialist: Joshua S. Rapplean
Publishing Services Manager: Pat Joiner-Myers
Project Manager: Marlene Weeks
Senior Designer: Amy Buxton

Printed in the United States of America

Last digit is the print number: 9 8 7 6 5 4 3 2 1

Dedication

*To my fellow coders, who endeavor each day to
report services with the greatest precision.
Your dedication
is amazing to behold and is the financial foundation
of our health care system.
Thank you for all you do.*

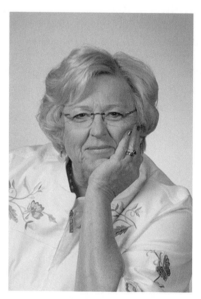

Carol J. Buck

Acknowledgments

There are so many, many people who participated in the development of this text, and only through the effort of all the team members has it been possible to publish this text. **Sheri Poe Bernard,** who has generously lent her tremendous talent to the efforts of this text and others. She possesses the knowledge and integrity that define an exemplary teacher, coder, and individual. The Village is very fortunate to have her on our team. **Nancy Maguire,** who worked diligently in the preparation of the text. She brings her guidance and knowledge to all she does, and this project is so much better because of her assistance.

Sally Schrefer, executive vice president, Nursing/Health Sciences, who possesses great listening skills and the ability to ensure the publication of high-quality educational materials. **Andrew Allen,** Vice President and Publisher, Health Professions, who sees the bigger picture and shares the vision. **Jeanne R. Olson,** Content Strategy Director, who has proven to be a tremendous asset to the team and a guiding presence in the development of this text. **Josh Rapplean,** Senior Content Development Specialist, who has taken on this task with his usual methodical approach that ensures we all stay on track and on task. **Mallory Skinner,** Project Manager, and **Jill Norath,** Senior Producer, who both ensured that we all completed our work on time. The employees of Elsevier have participated in the publication of this text and demonstrated the highest levels of professionalism and competence and have my admiration and gratitude for their never-ending patience and desire to produce the highest quality text possible.

Preface

Thank you for purchasing *E/M Auditing Step,* the latest resource for evaluation and management coding. This edition has been carefully reviewed and updated with the latest content available. The author and publishers have made every effort to equip you with skills and tools you will need to succeed. To this end, this text presents essential information about the E/M codes. No other tool on the market brings together such thorough coverage of the E/M section of the *CPT*® manual in one source.

ORGANIZATION OF THIS TEXTBOOK

Following a basic outline format, *E/M Auditing Step* takes a practical approach to assisting you with your E/M education. The text is divided into three units— E/M, Examination, and Resources—and there are five appendices for your reference.

Unit 1, Evaluation and Management
Provides a review of the categories of the E/M section of the CPT manual

Unit 2, Examination
Examination

Unit 3, Resources
1995 Documentation Guidelines for E/M Services
1997 Documentation Guidelines for Evaluation and Management Services
Internet Only Manual (IOM) 104, 30.6

Appendices
Appendix A   Unit 1, Evaluation and Management Practice Answers
Appendix B   Examination Answers
Appendix C   E/M Audit Form
Appendix D   Abbreviations
Appendix E   Further Text Resources

Development of This Edition

This book would not have been possible without a team of educators and professionals, including practicing coders and technical consultants. The combined efforts of the team members have made this text an incredible learning tool.

SENIOR TECHNICAL COLLABORATOR

Sheri Poe Bernard, CPC, CPC-H, CPC-I
Coding Education Specialist
Salt Lake City, Utah

QUERY MANAGER

Patricia Cordy Henricksen, MS, CHCA, CPC-I, CPC, CCP-P, ACS-PCS
Auditing and Coding Educator
Soterion Medical Services
Lexington, Kentucky

SENIOR COLLABORATOR AND ICD-10-CM CONSULTANT

Nancy Maguire, ACS, CRT, PCS, FCS, HCS-D, APC, AFC
Physician Consultant for Auditing and Education
Universal City, Texas

QUERY TEAM

Debra Kroll, RHIT
Denial and Billing Compliance Supervisor
Altru Health System
Grand Forks, North Dakota

Contents

Some of the 2013 CPT code descriptions for physician services now include physician extender services. Physician extenders, such as nurse practitioners, physician assistants, and nurse anesthetists, etc., provide medical services typically performed by a physician. Within this educational material the term "physician" may include "and other qualified health care professionals" depending on the code. Refer to the official CPT® code descriptions and guidelines to determine codes that are appropriate to report services provided by non-physician practitioners.

UNIT 1

Evaluation and Management

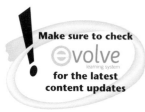
Make sure to check **evolve** *learning system* **for the latest content updates**

INTRODUCTION

E/M AUDIT FORM

E/M services may be accessed using an audit form

Figure 1-1 illustrates an audit form

Designed based on 1995 Guidelines for E/M Services (Documentation Guidelines, DG)

    Located in Unit 3 of text

    May also use 1997 Guidelines for E/M Services (located in Unit 3)

Blank audit forms located in Appendix C of this text

You are to complete an audit form for cases assigned CPT codes based on key components and 1995 Examination Guidelines.

Report in Example 1-1 (page 5) will be used to explain the audit form elements

E/M LEVELS

Components that define levels of E/M services

    History (key component)

    Examination (key component)

    Medical decision making (key component)

    Counseling

    Coordination of care

    Nature of presenting problem

    Time

Key components

    History

    Examination

    Medical decision making

HISTORY ELEMENTS	Documented
HISTORY OF PRESENT ILLNESS (HPI)	
1. Location (site on body)	
2. Quality (characteristic: throbbing, sharp)	
3. Severity (1/10 or how intense)	
4. Duration* (how long for problem or episode)	
5. Timing (when it occurs)	
6. Context (under what circumstances does it occur)	
7. Modifying factors (what makes it better or worse)	
8. Associated signs and symptoms (what else is happening when it occurs)	
*Duration not in CPT as HPI Element TOTAL	
LEVEL	

REVIEW OF SYSTEMS (ROS)	Documented
1. Constitutional (e.g., weight loss, fever)	
2. Ophthalmologic (eyes)	
3. Otolaryngologic (ears, nose, mouth, throat)	
4. Cardiovascular	
5. Respiratory	
6. Gastrointestinal	
7. Genitourinary	
8. Musculoskeletal	
9. Integumentary (skin and/or breasts)	
10. Neurological	
11. Psychiatric	
12. Endocrine	
13. Hematologic/Lymphatic	
14. Allergic/Immunologic	
TOTAL	
LEVEL	

PAST, FAMILY, AND/OR SOCIAL HISTORY (PFSH)	Documented
1. Past illness, operations, injuries, treatments, and current medications	
2. Family medical history for heredity and risk	
3. Social activities, both past and present	
TOTAL	
LEVEL	

History Level	1	2	3	4
	Problem Focused	Expanded Problem Focused	Detailed	Comprehensive
HPI	Brief 1-3	Brief 1-3	Extended 4+	Extended 4+
ROS	None	Problem Pertinent 1	Extended 2-9	Complete 10+
PFSH	None	None	Pertinent 1	Complete 2-3
				HISTORY LEVEL

EXAMINATION ELEMENTS	Documented
CONSTITUTIONAL (OS)	
• Blood pressure, sitting	
• Blood pressure, lying	
• Pulse	
• Respirations	
• Temperature	
• Height	
• Weight	
• General appearance	
(Counts as only 1) NUMBER	

BODY AREAS (BA)	Documented
1. Head (including face)	
2. Neck	
3. Chest (including breasts and axillae)	
4. Abdomen	
5. Genitalia, groin, buttocks	
6. Back (including spine)	
7. Each extremity	
NUMBER	

ORGAN SYSTEMS (OS)	Documented
1. Ophthalmologic (eyes)	
2. Otolaryngologic (ears, nose, mouth, throat)	
3. Cardiovascular	
4. Respiratory	
5. Gastrointestinal	
6. Genitourinary	
7. Musculoskeletal	
8. Integumentary (skin)	
9. Neurologic	
10. Psychiatric	
11. Hematologic/Lymphatic/Immunologic	
NUMBER	
TOTAL BA/OS	

Exam Level	1	2	3	4
	Problem Focused	Expanded Problem Focused	Detailed	Comprehensive
	Limited to affected BA/OS	Limited to affected BA/OS & other related OS(s)	Extended of affected BA(s) & other related OS(s)	General multi-system (OSs only)
# of OS or BA	1	2-7 limited	2-7 extended	8+
			EXAMINATION LEVEL	

MDM ELEMENTS	Documented
# OF DIAGNOSIS/MANAGEMENT OPTIONS	
1. Minimal	
2. Limited	
3. Multiple	
4. Extensive	
LEVEL	

AMOUNT AND/OR COMPLEXITY OF DATA TO REVIEW	Documented
1. Minimal/None	
2. Limited	
3. Moderate	
4. Extensive	
LEVEL	

RISK OF COMPLICATION OR DEATH IF NOT TREATED	Documented
1. Minimal	
2. Low	
3. Moderate	
4. High	
LEVEL	

MDM*	1	2	3	4
	Straightforward	Low	Moderate	High
Number of DX or management options	Minimal	Limited	Multiple	Extensive
Amount and/or complexity of data	Minimal/None	Limited	Moderate	Extensive
Risks	Minimal	Low	Moderate	High
			MDM LEVEL	

*To qualify for a given type of MDM complexity, 2 of 3 elements in the table must be met or exceeded.

History:

Examination:

MDM:

Number of Key Components:

Code:

Figure **1-1.** E/M audit form based on 1995 Guidelines for E/M Services.

HISTORY

Complete history has four components

Chief Complaint (CC)

Brief summary describing reason for encounter

Usually in patient's own words

Required at all E/M levels

Includes

Symptom

Problem

Condition

Diagnosis

Physician's recommendations

Any other significant factors

In Example 1-1 (page 5)

CC is obstruction of intestine (chronic bowel obstruction)

History of the Present Illness (HPI)

Description of current problem

Described in order in which symptoms occurred or have occurred since a previous encounter

Must be documented in medical record

HPI elements

Location

Site on body (e.g., arm, leg, neck)

Quality

Patient's description of problem (e.g., dull, constant, throbbing), a sensation or feeling

Severity

Patient's description concerning pain caliber (1-10 scale or how intense)

Duration*

Length of time patient has experienced symptom or episode to present time

Timing

When problem is experienced (e.g., morning, noon, when lying down), when started, if a pattern

Context

Under what circumstances does it occur (e.g., bending, standing)

---

*Although duration is not in the CPT description of the HPI, duration is in both the 1995 and 1997 Documentation Guidelines for E/M Service as an element on the HPI.

Modifying factors

Actions patient used to treat symptoms (e.g., aspirin, antacids, heat)

Associated signs and symptoms

What else is happening when it occurs (e.g., stress or incontinence), significantly related to main complaint

Levels of HPI

Brief, 1-3 elements

Problem focused (level 1) and extended problem focused (level 2)

Extended, 4+ elements

Detailed (level 3) and comprehensive (level 4)

In Example 1-1, the HPI elements checked in **Figure 1-2** are:
  Location (abdomen)
  Duration (4 weeks)
  Modifying factors (tracheostomy, feeding tube)
  Associated signs and symptoms (renal failure, respiratory failure)
  Level: 4 elements = extended (comprehensive level 4)

The level is the same whether using either the 1995 or 1997 Documentation Guidelines

---

HISTORY ELEMENTS	Documented
HISTORY OF PRESENT ILLNESS (HPI)	
1. Location (site on body)	X
2. Quality (characteristic: throbbing, sharp)	
3. Severity (1/10 or how intense)	
4. Duration* (how long for problem or episode)	X
5. Timing (when it occurs)	
6. Context (under what circumstances does it occur)	
7. Modifying factors (what makes it better or worse)	X
8. Associated signs and symptoms (what else is happening when it occurs)	X
*Duration not in CPT as HPI Element TOTAL	4
LEVEL	4

Figure **1-2.** HPI Elements.

Review of Systems (ROS)

Used to identify subjective symptoms that the patient

Deemed unimportant

Neglected to mention

May be obtained from

Questionnaire completed by patient or ancillary staff

To qualify, physician or other qualified health care professional must evaluate and document in medical record

ROS aids in

Defining problem(s)

Clarifying differential diagnoses

EXAMPLE 1-1

SURGICAL CONSULTATION

(Note: The patient had a gastrointestinal operation 4 weeks ago, but the report does not clearly indicate that the current obstruction is due to the surgical procedure, therefore, a "complication of surgery" code would not be appropriate in this case.)

LOCATION: Inpatient Hospital
PATIENT: Martin Newwell
PHYSICIAN: Alma Naraquist, MD
CONSULTANT: Daniel Olanka, MD

HISTORY OF PRESENT ILLNESS: This patient was operated on by Dr. Sanchez approximately 4 weeks ago for a misdiagnosis of appendicitis. He underwent ileocecal resection. He has had a variety of problems in the postoperative period, including renal failure, respiratory failure, tracheostomy, etc. He is currently under the care of Dr. Naraquist and is off the ventilator and breathing through the tracheostomy. He has been intermittently fed through small bowel Cor-Flo tube, but this has the appearance of a bowel obstruction. The patient has some chest discomfort, but this is due to existing hiatal hernia. Dr. Naraquist has asked me to evaluate the patient for suspected bowel obstruction, and the family has requested that another surgeon get involved in his care. I have been asked to review his case and give recommendations.

PHYSICAL EXAMINATION: On examination, the patient is resting comfortably in bed. No distress. He does have a tracheostomy in place. He is alert and does respond. Oriented to time and place. The chest is clear to auscultation. There is a catheter in place for dialysis, although the patient is not currently on dialysis. The abdomen is markedly distended. It is tympanitic. Tinkling bowel sounds are heard. There are no rushes. The midline scar is well healed. There is no particular focal tenderness, and no hernias are appreciated.

Review of the patient's films shows marked dilatation of the small bowel. Review of the CT scan shows marked dilatation of the small bowel with what appears to be a transition zone in the distal ileum. The colon is deflated.

DISCUSSION: By physical examination, this patient has chronic bowel obstruction, at least partial in nature. Certainly his x-rays support that there is a major problem intra-abdominally. My recommendation would be that the patient should be considered for re-exploration for bowel obstruction. I do not know whether the problem is at the anastomosis or near the anastomosis. I think patient would benefit from some total parenteral nutrition (TPN) and aggressive hydration over the next few days, and then we will plan to take him to the operating room next week.

Dr. Olanka, MD

Identifying tests useful for diagnosis

Providing broader knowledge of patient

Assisting in decision regarding management options

Levels of ROS

None (level 1)

Problem Pertinent (level 2)

Inquiry about system directly identified in HPI

Patient's positive/negative responses must be documented in medical record

Extended (level 3)

Inquiry about system directly related to problems identified in HPI, 2-9 related body systems

Patient's positive/negative responses must be documented in medical record

Complete (level 4)

Inquiry about the system identified in HPI and all other systems as medically necessary

CPT recognizes the following for an ROS

Constitutional symptoms (fever, weight loss, etc.)

Ophthalmologic (eyes)

Otolaryngologic (ears, nose, mouth, throat)

Cardiovascular

Respiratory

Gastrointestinal

Genitourinary

Musculoskeletal

Integumentary (skin and/or breast)

Neurological

Psychiatric

Endocrine

Hematologic/Lymphatic

Allergic/Immunologic

In Example 1-1, there are two ROS elements
Respiratory (off the ventilator and breathing through tracheostomy)
Gastrointestinal (chest discomfort due to hiatal hernia)
With two elements, this is an extended ROS (level 3, detailed)
See **Figure 1-3** for completed ROS portion of audit form

Note: The level of ROS is the same whether using the 1995 or 1997 DGs

---

REVIEW OF SYSTEMS (ROS)	Documented
1. Constitutional (e.g., weight loss, fever)	
2. Ophthalmologic (eyes)	
3. Otolaryngologic (ears, nose, mouth, throat)	
4. Cardiovascular	
5. Respiratory	X
6. Gastrointestinal	X
7. Genitourinary	
8. Musculoskeletal	
9. Integumentary (skin and/or breasts)	
10. Neurological	
11. Psychiatric	
12. Endocrine	
13. Hematologic/Lymphatic	
14. Allergic/Immunologic	
TOTAL	2
LEVEL	3

Figure **1-3.** ROS Elements.

Past, Family, and/or Social History (PFSH)

Past History

    Catalogues patient's medical history

    All-inclusive record of

        Past illnesses

        Operations

        Injuries

        Treatments

    Specific information

        Prior

            Major illnesses

            Injuries

            Operations

            Hospitalizations

        Current medication(s)

        Allergies (e.g., related to drug or food)

        Age-appropriate

            Immunization

            Feeding status

            Dietary status

Family History

    Identifies significant medical events within patient's family

        Focuses on health issues of

            Parents

            Siblings

            Children

Specific information

    Causes and age of death

        Parents

        Siblings

        Children

    Specific diseases shared by family members pertaining to

        CC

        HPI

        System review

    Potential risk factors for the patient

        Commonly identified with hereditary diseases

Social History

    Focuses on vital age-appropriate relevant information

    Specific information

        Marital status

        Current living arrangements

        Current employment and occupational history

        Use of drugs, alcohol, tobacco

        Sexual history

        Level of education

        Any other socially relevant factors

Levels of PFSH

    None (level 1 and 2)

    Pertinent (level 3)

        Review of the history area(s) directly related to HPI

            At least one item from any of the PFSH areas

    Complete (level 4)

        Documentation of at least two or three of the PFSH areas

            Sufficient for established patient in the office or other outpatient services; emergency department; subsequent nursing facility care; established patient receiving home care or domiciliary services

        Documentation of at least one item from each of the PFSH areas

            Required for new patient in the office or other outpatient services; hospital observation services; hospital inpatient services, initial care; consultations; comprehensive nursing facility assessments; new patients in the domiciliary and home care setting

---

In Example 1-1, there was one PFSH element as the ileocecal resection would count as one element of the past history

    This is a pertinent PFSH (level 3, detailed)

    See **Figure 1-4** for the audit form with the PFSH portion completed

Note: The level of PFSH is the same whether using the 1995 or 1997 Documentation Guidelines

---

PAST, FAMILY, AND/OR SOCIAL HISTORY (PFSH)		Documented
1. Past illness, operations, injuries, treatments, and current medications		X
2. Family medical history for heredity and risk		
3. Social activities, both past and present		
	TOTAL	1
	LEVEL	3

Figure **1-4.** PFSH Elements.

Four History Levels

Based on amount of data gathered

Clinical judgment and nature of presenting problem determines extent of history

Problem Focused (level 1)

Centers on CC

Brief history of present illness/problem (1-3 elements)

> Reviews pertinent information of CC in terms of
>> Severity
>>
>> Duration
>>
>> Symptoms

Does not include a PFSH or ROS

Expanded Problem Focused (level 2)

Focused on CC

Brief history of present illness/problem (1-3 elements)

Review of organ system associated with CC

Detailed (level 3)

CC

Extended HPI

Pertinent system review (4+ elements)

Related systems reviewed

> Documentation shows positive and negative responses regarding multiple organ systems (total of 2-9 systems reviewed)

Pertinent PFSH

> Related to CC

Comprehensive (level 4)

CC

Extended HPI (4+ elements)

Review of all body systems (at least 10)

Complete PFSH (2 or 3 dependent on the type of service)

In Example 1-1, the following elements were present for the history:
HPI: Extended (comprehensive level 4)
ROS: Extended (detailed level 3)
PFSH: Pertinent (detailed, level 3)
Level: Detailed, level 3

See **Figure 1-5** for the audit form with the History level assigned

History Level	1	2	3	4
	Problem Focused	Expanded Problem Focused	Detailed	Comprehensive
HPI	Brief 1-3	Brief 1-3	Extended 4+	Extended 4+
ROS	None	Problem Pertinent 1	Extended 2-9	Complete 10+
PFSH	None	None	Pertinent 1	Complete 2-3
			HISTORY LEVEL	3

Figure **1-5.** History level assigned.

Requirements for History Levels

Problem-Focused History (level 1)

1-3 HPI elements

No ROS

No PFSH

Expanded Problem-Focused History (level 2)

1-3 HPI elements

Problem-pertinent ROS (1 system)

No PFSH

Detailed History (level 3)

4+ HPI elements

Extended ROS

   2-9 ROS systems

Problem-pertinent PFSH

   1 history element

Comprehensive History (level 4)

4+ HPI elements

Comprehensive ROS (10+ systems)

Complete PFSH (established patients, 2 of 3)

To qualify for a given level of history, all elements must be met

Additional Guidelines for Documenting History

CC, ROS, and PFSH may be listed separately or included in HPI

If during a previous encounter a ROS and/or PFSH has been recorded, the provider must note the date and location of the earlier ROS

The ROS and/or PFSH does not need to be re-recorded

Physician must indicate review of ROS and/or PFSH and any updates

Questionnaire completed by ancillary staff or patient considered valid for ROS and/or PFSH if

Physician review is documented in medical record

If patient or other source is unable to provide history

Medical record must describe patient's condition or circumstance

Document the reason for patient/other source not providing HPI

Another Example of History Level

CC: Right elbow pain

HPI: The patient is a 44-year-old female who states she has had worsening pain in her right elbow (location) for 2 weeks (duration). The pain is described as stabbing (quality) and is worse after knitting (context). She experiences some relief with ice and acetaminophen (modifying factors).

ROS: Constitutional: No fevers or weight change within the past 3 months

Musculoskeletal: Negative for muscle or joint pain

Skin: No rashes, complains of mild dryness

PFSH: Positive for hyperthyroidism (past history) which is controlled with Synthroid (medication)

History Level of Example Above

HPI elements: 4+ meets requirements of an extended HPI (comprehensive level 4)

Location (right elbow)

Duration (2 weeks)

Quality (stabbing)

Context (knitting)

Modifying factors (ice, acetaminophen)

ROS: 3 meets the requirements of a detailed ROS (detailed level 3)

Constitutional symptoms

Musculoskeletal

Integumentary (skin and/or breasts)

PFSH: 1 meets pertinent PFSH (detailed level 3)

Past history of a thyroid condition controlled with medication

No mention of a family or social history

Detailed history includes

Extended HPI

4+ elements

Or status of 3 or more chronic and/or inactive conditions (1997 Guidelines)

Extended ROS

2-9 systems

Pertinent PFSH

1 element

Example report meets requirements of a detailed history with

Extended HPI, comprehensive, level 4

Extended ROS, detailed, level 3

Pertinent PFSH, detailed, level 3

> Note: The level of History level is the same whether using the 1995 or 1997 Documentation Guidelines

EXAMINATION

Objective portion of the encounter

Performed by physician or other qualified health care professional

Level of examination based on clinical judgment and nature of the presenting problem(s)

Examination Levels

Problem Focused (level 1)

Limited to affected body area (BA)/organ system (OS) identified by CC

1 BA/OS

Expanded Problem Focused (level 2)

Limited examination of BA(s) or OS(s) identified by CC and other related BA(s)/OS(s)

2-7 BA/OS

Detailed (level 3)

Extended examination of affected BA(s) or OS(s) and other symptomatic or related OS(s)

2-7 BA/OS

Comprehensive (level 4)

General multisystem examination OR complete examination of single organ system

8+ OS

The 1995 Guidelines state that the comprehensive examination must include at least 8 organ systems. Body areas and organ systems can only be combined for lower levels of examination.

The 1995 Documentation Guidelines (DGs) recognize the following body areas:

Head, including the face

Neck

Chest, including breasts and axillae

Abdomen

Genitalia, groin, buttocks

Back, including spine

Each extremity (Note "each")

For purposes of examination the following organ systems are recognized:

Constitutional (e.g., vital signs, general appearance)

> Note: The CPT guidelines do not recognize constitutional as an OS but both 1995 and 1997 DGs do

Eyes

Ears, nose, mouth and throat

Cardiovascular

Respiratory

Gastrointestinal

Hematologic/lymphatic/immunologic

Genitourinary

Musculoskeletal

Skin

Neurologic

Psychiatric

FROM EXAMPLE 1-1

PHYSICAL EXAMINATION: On examination, the patient is resting comfortably in bed. No distress. He does have a tracheostomy in place. He is alert and does respond. Oriented to time and place. The chest is clear to auscultation. There is a catheter in place for dialysis, although the patient is not currently on dialysis. The abdomen is markedly distended. It is tympanitic. Tinkling bowel sounds are heard. There are no rushes. The midline scar is well healed. There is no particular focal tenderness, and no hernias are appreciated.

Review of the patient's films shows marked dilatation of the small bowel. Review of the CT scan shows marked dilatation of the small bowel with what appears to be a transition zone in the distal ileum. The colon is deflated.

In Example 1-1, using the 1995 Documentation Guidelines, the physical examination includes 5 OSs examined: constitutional element (general appearance, resting comfortably, tracheostomy in place), respiratory (clear to auscultation), gastrointestinal (tympanitic, tinkling bowel sounds, marked distension), skin (midline scar is well-healed), and psychiatric (he is alert and does respond. Oriented to time and place.). There were no BAs reviewed. There is a total of 5 BAs/OSs. This is a level 3 or detailed examination. See **Figure 1-6** for completed audit form for the examination portion of the audit form.

When counting BAs/OSs for the examination, note that the DGs indicate that only **OSs** count for a comprehensive level 4 examination. For example, 1 OS in constitutional, 2 BAs, and 6 OSs equals 9 BAs/OSs, which is a level 4 comprehensive; however, for a comprehensive exam, deduct the BAs (2) for a total of 7 OSs or a level 3 detailed examination.

MEDICAL DECISION MAKING (MDM)

Complexity of MDM addresses the complications involved in

Establishing a diagnosis and/or

Selecting a management option(s)

Risk of potential complications associated with the patient's presenting problem

Factors in MDM Process

Number of possible diagnoses and/or management options

Information from medical records, diagnostic tests, and other relevant information must be

Obtained

Reviewed

Analyzed

Factors associated with patient's presenting problem, the diagnostic procedures, and the possible management options

Risk of significant complications

Morbidity

Mortality

Comorbidities

Four Types of MDM

2 of 3 elements must be met or exceeded to assign the level

Straightforward decision making involves (level 1)

Minimal number of diagnoses or management options

Amount and/or complexity of data is minimal or none

The risk of complications and/or morbidity or mortality is minimal

Low-complexity decision making involves (level 2)

Limited number of diagnosis or management options

Amount of data limited in scope and complexity

Low risk of complications and/or morbidity or mortality

Moderate-complexity decision making involves (level 3)

Multiple diagnoses and management options available

Moderate amount of data and complexities

Moderate risk of complications and/or morbidity

EXAMINATION ELEMENTS				Documented
CONSTITUTIONAL (OS)				
• Blood pressure, sitting				
• Blood pressure, lying				
• Pulse				
• Respirations				
• Temperature				
• Height				
• Weight				
• General appearance				X
(Counts as only 1) NUMBER				I
BODY AREAS (BA)				Documented
1. Head (including face)				
2. Neck				
3. Chest (including breasts and axillae)				
4. Abdomen				
5. Genitalia, groin, buttocks				
6. Back (including spine)				
7. Each extremity				
NUMBER				0
ORGAN SYSTEMS (OS)				Documented
1. Ophthalmologic (eyes)				
2. Otolaryngologic (ears, nose, mouth, throat)				
3. Cardiovascular				
4. Respiratory				X
5. Gastrointestinal				X
6. Genitourinary				
7. Musculoskeletal				
8. Integumentary (skin)				X
9. Neurologic				
10. Psychiatric				X
11. Hematologic/Lymphatic/Immunologic				
NUMBER				4
TOTAL BA/OS				5 OS

Exam Level	1	2	3	4
	Problem Focused	Expanded Problem Focused	Detailed	Comprehensive
	Limited to affected BA/OS	Limited to affected BA/OS & other related OS(s)	Extended of affected BA(s) & other related OS(s)	General multi-system (OSs only)
# of OS or BA	I	2-7 limited	2-7 extended	8+
EXAMINATION LEVEL				3

Figure **1-6.** Examination portion of audit form.

High-complexity decision making involves (level 4)

Extensive management options and diagnoses

Extensive amount and complexity of data

High risk of complications and/or morbidity

Guidelines used to document management options

Each encounter requires documentation that is explicitly stated or implied, and describes an assessment, clinical impression, or diagnoses

For a presenting problem **WITH** an established diagnosis, the documentation should indicate the problem is either

Improved, well controlled, resolving, or resolved

OR

Inadequately controlled, worsening or failing to change

For a presenting problem **WITHOUT** an established diagnosis, the assessment is recorded in the context of a differential diagnosis

Commonly used terms are

Possible

Probable

Rule out

Any initiation of or change in a treatment should be documented

Changes in management options include those in

Either patient or nursing care instructions

Any therapies

Medication usage changes

When a referral is made, documentation should have recorded the following

Consultation(s) requested or advice that has been sought

To whom or where the request has been made

The origination of the request

MDM ELEMENTS				Documented
# OF DIAGNOSIS/MANAGEMENT OPTIONS				
1. Minimal				
2. Limited				
3. Multiple				X
4. Extensive				
			LEVEL	3
AMOUNT AND/OR COMPLEXITY OF DATA TO REVIEW				Documented
1. Minimal/None				
2. Limited				X
3. Moderate				
4. Extensive				
			LEVEL	2
RISK OF COMPLICATION OR DEATH IF NOT TREATED				Documented
1. Minimal				
2. Low				
3. Moderate				
4. High				X
			LEVEL	4

MDM*	1	2	3	4
	Straightforward	Low	Moderate	High
Number of DX or management options	Minimal	Limited	Multiple	Extensive
Amount and/or complexity of data	Minimal/None	Limited	Moderate	Extensive
Risks	Minimal	Low	Moderate	High
			MDM LEVEL	3

*To qualify for a given type of MDM complexity, 2 of 3 elements in the table must be met or exceeded.

Figure **1-7.** Medical decision making portion of audit form.

In Example 1-1, using the 1995 Documentation Guidelines, the MDM includes multiple diagnosis and management options, limited data (review of the patient's films and CT scan), and high risk to the patient. The patient does have a chronic condition (chronic bowel obstruction), is breathing through a tracheostomy, and is going to have another major surgery at a time when he is not yet recovered from his prior surgery. This indicates a high risk.

See **Figure 1-7** with the Medical Decision Making portion of the audit form completed.

When considering all levels on this case, using the 1995 Documentation Guidelines, (See **Figure 1-8** for completed form), the level of the E/M service is 99253.

SPRING CREEK CAMPUS

History Elements

HISTORY ELEMENTS	Documented
HISTORY OF PRESENT ILLNESS (HPI)	
1. Location (site on body)	X
2. Quality (characteristic: throbbing, sharp)	
3. Severity (1/10 or how intense)	
4. Duration* (how long for problem or episode)	X
5. Timing (when it occurs)	
6. Context (under what circumstances does it occur)	
7. Modifying factors (what makes it better or worse)	X
8. Associated signs and symptoms (what else is happening when it occurs)	X
*Duration not in CPT as HPI Element TOTAL	4
LEVEL	4

REVIEW OF SYSTEMS (ROS)	Documented
1. Constitutional (e.g., weight loss, fever)	
2. Ophthalmologic (eyes)	
3. Otolaryngologic (ears, nose, mouth, throat)	
4. Cardiovascular	
5. Respiratory	X
6. Gastrointestinal	X
7. Genitourinary	
8. Musculoskeletal	
9. Integumentary (skin and/or breasts)	
10. Neurological	
11. Psychiatric	
12. Endocrine	
13. Hematologic/Lymphatic	
14. Allergic/Immunologic	
TOTAL	2
LEVEL	3

PAST, FAMILY, AND/OR SOCIAL HISTORY (PFSH)	Documented
1. Past illness, operations, injuries, treatments, and current medications	X
2. Family medical history for heredity and risk	
3. Social activities, both past and present	
TOTAL	1
LEVEL	3

History Level	1 Problem Focused	2 Expanded Problem Focused	3 Detailed	4 Comprehensive
HPI	Brief 1-3	Brief 1-3	Extended 4+	Extended 4+
ROS	None	Problem Pertinent 1	Extended 2-9	Complete 10+
PFSH	None	None	Pertinent 1	Complete 2-3
			HISTORY LEVEL	3

Examination Elements

EXAMINATION ELEMENTS	Documented
CONSTITUTIONAL (OS)	
• Blood pressure, sitting	
• Blood pressure, lying	
• Pulse	
• Respirations	
• Temperature	
• Height	
• Weight	
• General appearance	X
(Counts as only 1) NUMBER	1

BODY AREAS (BA)	Documented
1. Head (including face)	
2. Neck	
3. Chest (including breasts and axillae)	
4. Abdomen	
5. Genitalia, groin, buttocks	
6. Back (including spine)	
7. Each extremity	
NUMBER	0

ORGAN SYSTEMS (OS)	Documented
1. Ophthalmologic (eyes)	
2. Otolaryngologic (ears, nose, mouth, throat)	
3. Cardiovascular	
4. Respiratory	X
5. Gastrointestinal	X
6. Genitourinary	
7. Musculoskeletal	
8. Integumentary (skin)	X
9. Neurologic	
10. Psychiatric	X
11. Hematologic/Lymphatic/Immunologic	
NUMBER	4
TOTAL BA/OS	5 OS

Exam Level	1 Problem Focused	2 Expanded Problem Focused	3 Detailed	4 Comprehensive
	Limited to affected BA/OS	Limited to affected BA/OS & other related OS(s)	Extended of affected BA(s) & other related OS(s)	General multi-system (OSs only)
# of OS or BA	1	2-7 limited	2-7 extended	8+
			EXAMINATION LEVEL	3

MDM Elements

MDM ELEMENTS	Documented
# OF DIAGNOSIS/MANAGEMENT OPTIONS	
1. Minimal	
2. Limited	
3. Multiple	X
4. Extensive	
LEVEL	3
AMOUNT AND/OR COMPLEXITY OF DATA TO REVIEW	Documented
1. Minimal/None	
2. Limited	X
3. Moderate	
4. Extensive	
LEVEL	2
RISK OF COMPLICATION OR DEATH IF NOT TREATED	Documented
1. Minimal	
2. Low	
3. Moderate	
4. High	X
LEVEL	4

MDM*	1 Straightforward	2 Low	3 Moderate	4 High
Number of DX or management options	Minimal	Limited	Multiple	Extensive
Amount and/or complexity of data	Minimal/None	Limited	Moderate	Extensive
Risks	Minimal	Low	Moderate	High
			MDM LEVEL	3

*To qualify for a given type of MDM complexity, 2 of 3 elements in the table must be met or exceeded.

History: Detailed
Examination: Detailed
MDM: Moderate
Number of Key Components: 3 of 3
Code: 99253

Figure 1-8. Completed audit form for Example 1-1.

COUNSELING

Some aspect of counseling will usually take place during physician-patient encounters

One or more of following items are present in discussion with patient, family members, and/or caregivers

Diagnostic results, impressions, and/or recommended diagnostic studies

Prognosis of CC

Management options presented with

Potential risks and/or benefits

Instructions given for

Treatment of the CC

Follow-up directions

Communication explaining importance of patient following through with management/treatment option(s)

Discussion of risk factor reduction

Education (patient and/or family) regarding the clinical judgment(s)

COORDINATION OF CARE

Physician makes arrangements to provide the patient with additional services from other agencies or healthcare providers

NATURE OF THE PRESENTING PROBLEM (FOUNDATION)

The CC or situation for which clinical judgment is made concerning appropriate level of care to diagnose and treat patient

Medical record should include physician's observations regarding the level of care determined necessary to diagnose and treat patient

CPT describes the present problem by using the following terms

Disease

Condition

Illness

Injury

Symptom

Sign

Finding

Complaint

Or other reason for the encounter

A diagnosis need not be made during the face-to-face encounter for these terms to be used

TYPES OF PRESENTING PROBLEMS

Minimal

May/may not require the presence of physician

Service provided must be provided under the physician's supervision

> Example: Blood pressure readings, dressing changes

Self-Limited

Also known as minor presenting problem

Problem

> Follows definite course
>
> Is transient
>
> Does not permanently alter patient's health status

Good prognosis possible with proper management and compliance

Low Severity

Risk of morbidity without treatment is minimal

Full recovery is likely

No indication of future health impairment

Moderate Severity

Risk of morbidity/mortality without treatment is moderate

Prognosis uncertain

Possibility of future impairment exists

High Severity

Risk of morbidity without treatment is very high/extremely likely

Moderate to high risk/morbidity

Presenting problem in which severe, prolonged, and functional impairment is highly probable

TIME

"Time" in E/M code description is not meant to be precise measurement tool

Estimated amount of time based on the average physician-patient encounter

Used in determining level of service when 50% or more of the time involves counseling and/or coordination of care

Three Measures of Time

Direct Face-to-Face Time

Describes office visits, outpatient visits, and office consultations

Refers to the time the physician actually spends in the presence of patient and/or family and/or other caregivers

Typical face-to-face time includes obtaining history and performing examination of patient and counseling

Non Face-to-Face Time

Time spent by physician before/after encounter

While this information is not specifically addressed with E/M codes, it is factored in calculations of time based E/M codes upon surveys

Face-to-face time stated in E/M codes reflects the physician's work before, during, and after encounter

Non-face-to-face time is not calculated for code selection of face-to-face time in outpatient setting

Unit/Floor Time

Time spent at the hospital unit

Time providing direct bedside services to patient

Further Time

Intra-service time is face-to-face time during which the physician

Reviews the patient chart

Conducts the examination

Engages in discussion with other professionals concerning patient

Communicates with patient's family and/or caregivers

Time is not a descriptive element to be used when evaluating emergency department services due to the difficulties involving the physician's multiple encounters with a variety of patients. The emergency department codes do not have "time" in code descriptors. Time is not considered in the selection of E/M codes unless it specifically addresses counseling/coordinating care. The amount of time spent face-to-face between the provider and the patient must be documented in addition to the amount of time spent in counseling and/or coordination.

Most important question to answer with time in E/M codes:

Did the counseling and/or coordination of care comprise more than 50% of the visit?

If counseling and/or coordination of care did not comprise 50% or more of the visit, then the level of service selected would be based on the level of history, examination, and MDM

E/M CODES

1. OFFICE OR OTHER OUTPATIENT SERVICES (99201-99215)

Two subcategories of patients

New patient:

One who has not received any professional services from the physician/ qualified health care professional or another physician/qualified health care professional of the exact same specialty and subspecialty who belongs to the same group practice within the past three years

Established patient:

One who has received any professional services from the physician/ qualified health care professional or another physician/qualified health care professional of the exact same specialty and subspecialty who belongs to the same group practice within the past three years

Criteria that must be documented in the medical record as having been met or exceeded

New patient

3 of 3 key components must be met or exceeded

Established patient

2 of 3 key components must be met or exceeded

Note: These codes should never be used to report "annual asymptomatic physicals" or "well-child" visits

Patients receiving care are considered to be outpatients unless admitted to a health care inpatient facility

If admitted to a health care facility during the course of physician/patient encounter

Services performed by physician are considered part of initial hospital care service when all records have same date

Initial office visit or outpatient encounter would not be reported

Bundled into initial hospital care code

Admitting physician must record all services related to admission

Including those that occurred prior to admission when services were same date as the admission

---

Some of the 2013 CPT code descriptions for physician services now include physician extender services. Physician extenders, such as nurse practitioners, physician assistants, and nurse anesthetists, etc., provide medical services typically performed by a physician. Within this educational material the term "physician" may include "and other qualified health care professionals" depending on the code. Refer to the official CPT® code descriptions and guidelines to determine codes that are appropriate to report services provided by non-physician practitioners.

PRACTICE 1, OFFICE OR OTHER OUTPATIENT SERVICES

Now it is time to put this information to practice by coding two reports. The first report is multiple choice and you are to select the correct choice to report the services provided and diagnosis(es) documented in the report.

The second report is fill-in-the-blank in which you assign the CPT service and ICD-9-CM diagnosis codes. Be certain to complete an audit form for each of the fill-in-the-blank reports in which the code selection is based on key components.

Once you have coded the two cases, check your answers in Appendix A.

Practice 1, Report A

LOCATION: Outpatient Clinic

Brooke is a 7-year-old established patient who presents to the clinic today with a cough that she has had for more than a week. It is definitely worse at night; however, it is there all the time. It is quite harsh and she is having productive green sputum. She has had a low-grade temperature and has not really felt very well.

PHYSICAL EXAMINATION reveals both tympanic membranes are normal. Her nose is clear. Throat is clear. Lungs are really coarse in both bases. There is an occasional wheeze. Heart has a normal sinus rhythm without murmur.

IMPRESSION: Acute Bronchitis.

We gave her a prescription for Zithromax Z-Pak liquid 200 mg/5 cc 2 teaspoons today and then 1 teaspoon daily for the following 4 days. We will see how she does. If she has difficulty next week, we will recheck her.

ICD-9-CM:

A. 99212; 466.0

B. 99213; 466.0, 786.2

C. 99213; 466.0

D. 99202; 466.0

ICD-10-CM:

A. 99212; J20.9

B. 99213; J20.9, R05

C. 99213; J20.9

D. 99202; J20.9

Practice 1, Report B

LOCATION: Outpatient, Clinic

NOTE: Start Augmentin. Stat CT of abd/pelvis.

This is a woman well known to me 4 months status post open cholecystectomy for gallstone pancreatitis. She had some fevers and gastrointestinal pain. Presents today with GI pain (abdomen) generalized. CT scan of the abdomen shows a persistent pseudocyst. No hydronephrosis gross abscess. She looks better today. Her abdomen is soft.

ASSESSMENT AND PLAN: A 44-year-old woman presents with acute recurrent pancreatitis and generalized abdominal pain. CT scan showing pseudocysts, but no frank abscess. I will have her continue her Augmentin and I would like to see her again in 1 week.

Codes:_____

2. HOSPITAL OBSERVATION SERVICES (99217-99226) OUTPATIENT CARE

Purpose of patient observation is to determine the severity of patient's condition

Patient's illness does not meet acute inpatient criteria

Codes apply to either new or established patients

Observation discharge service (99217)

Reports all services provided to patient being discharged from observation status

Must be on day other than initial day of observation status

Same day admission and discharge reported with 99234-99236

When patient status changes from observation status to inpatient status on the same date, the observation is not reported separately

Rather bundled into initial hospital admission service

Codes do not apply to post-surgery care (RPPR = Routine post procedure recovery)

That care is part of surgical package and not reported separately

Subcategories of codes are

Observation Care Discharge Services

Initial Observation Care

Subsequent Observation Care

PRACTICE 2, HOSPITAL OBSERVATION SERVICES

Once you have coded the two cases, check your answers in Appendix A.

Practice 2, Report A

LOCATION: Outpatient, Hospital

REASON FOR ADMISSION: Hyperglycemia, diabetic renal disease

HISTORY OF PRESENT ILLNESS: The patient is well-known to me. He has end-stage renal disease and is on CAPD. I was called by his daughter last night informing me that a couple of days ago he was driving in bad weather and he went in the ditch. There have been lots of problems at his home with his wife and the daughter was worried about him and was wondering if he needs to be admitted. His wife states the patient's father struggled with depression in his later years.

I was called by the emergency room staff for guidance. His son-in-law brought him to the emergency room. At that time, the patient was seen by the emergency physician and myself. He seemed to have been oriented ×3 without any focal neurological deficits and vital signs were stable. He had some edema in the lower extremities but he was walking and talking. His STATs were maintained. His PO2 was 65. His chest x-ray showed bilateral infiltrates which seemed to be getting better. His blood sugar was 895 and a couple of hours later went up to 1,468. Magnesium was 1.3 and phosphorus was 6.2.

His white count was only 11,000. Hemoglobin was 9.5. He had some metamyelocytes and myelocytes in his differential with eosinophilia.

After long discussions with the patient and his son-in-law, we convinced him to be admitted for observation to control his blood glucose at least and be discharged the next morning. I also found out yesterday that he had a prior M-spike on serum protein electrophoresis suggestive of a multiple myeloma. This was ordered because of elevated protein and low albumin in addition to a prior episode of hypercalcemia.

He has not been compliant with his medications and probably more ignorant of how to manage insulin rather than compliance issues for his type II diabetes. He had some personality changes over the past 2 months.

The patient expressed sorrow and he was depressed and cried a couple of times in the emergency room and was concerned about the situation at home. He was not suicidal at the time I saw him in the emergency room. Obviously, his sugar was elevated because he did not take his insulin all day and was eating cookies and candy all day, in addition to his peritoneal dialysis fluid.

Finally, the patient agreed to be admitted for observation. His blood sugar will be controlled with 20 units of regular insulin IV and insulin drip and he will be discharged in the morning. The patient has uncontrolled D.M. with renal complication on dialysis.

Because of chronic cough and the infiltrates, he is scheduled to have CT scan next week. I will have to also schedule him to see our hematologist/oncologist to do a bone marrow aspiration and biopsy.

ICD-9-CM:

A. 99220; 250.82, 585.6, 786.2, 793.19, 790.99, V45.11

B. 99218; 99354, 99355×3, 250.82, 585.6, 786.2, 793.19, 790.99, V45.11

C. 99218; 250.42, 585.6, 790.99, V45.11

D. 99218; 250.42, 583.81, 786.2, 793.19, 790.99, V45.11

ICD-10-CM:

A. 99220; E11.65, N18.6, R05, R91.8, R78.9, Z99.2, Z79.4

B. 99218; 99354, 99355 ×3, E11.65, N18.6, R05, R91.8, R78.9, Z99.2

C. 99218; E11.21, N18.6, R78.9, Z99.2

D. 99218; E11.21, E11.65, N18.6, R05, R91.8, R78.9, R77.0, Z99.2, Z79.4

Practice 2, Report B

LOCATION: Outpatient, Hospital (Observation status)

DIAGNOSES:
1. Chronic renal failure secondary to hypertensive renovascular disease.
2. Renovascular disease.
3. Right-sided renal artery stent re-stenosis post angioplasty and placement of new stent by interventional radiology.
4. Anemia secondary to acute peri-procedure bleeding without evidence of hematomas.
5. Longstanding renovascular hypertension.
6. Hypotension secondary to angioplasty and stent placement of the right renal artery and peri-procedure bleeding.

HOSPITAL COURSE: The patient is an 87-year-old female known to have chronic renal failure and renovascular disease with right-sided renal artery stenosis with previous in-stent restenosis. She had her procedure done on the day of admission. She had blood pressure of 70 systolic afterwards with some peri-procedure bleeding at the site in the right inguinal area but she did not seem to have any hematoma. She was asymptomatic with her low blood pressure. Her antihypertensive medications were held. The patient was given IV fluids. Her hemoglobin was monitored. She was around 8.8 to 9.3 grams.

On the day of discharge her hemoglobin was 8.8. Her creatinine has come down to 1.4 with a BUN of 31, sodium of 143, chloride of 117, bicarb of 21.1, and glucose of 94.

The patient was asymptomatic on this day of discharge and she was discharged in good general condition.

DISCHARGE PLAN:
1. The patient will not be on any antihypertensive medications at least until I see her again next week. Altace and Toprol both will be on hold.
2. Return to clinic next week with basic panel and CBC before her appointment.
3. I have advised her to contact me immediately if she has dizzy spells or if she has any questions or any problems. She knows how to contact me.

Codes:_____

3. HOSPITAL INPATIENT SERVICES (99221-99239)

Attending is one who is

Qualified on the basis of education and training and has staff membership/appointment and is therefore

Qualified to oversee patient care

Authorized to order/perform therapeutic/diagnostic procedures

Codes apply to patients officially admitted into the hospital

Key components of history, examination, and MDM determine code assignment

Subcategories

Initial Hospital Care

Must match the admission date listed by the hospital

Codes only used by admitting individual

Any service performed by physician in a setting other than the hospital on the day the patient was admitted is considered when assigning admission code

Requires 3 of 3 key components

Subsequent Hospital Care

Codes apply to services rendered to patient after admission date

Requires 2 of 3 key components

History component in this subcategory reflects any new information that has been recorded in interval since most recent physician/patient encounter

Three levels of service are recognized

When the patient is stable or demonstrates improvement (99231)

When the patient has experienced a relatively minor complication or is not responding to current therapy as desired (99232)

When patient is significantly unstable or has developed either serious complications or new problem(s) (99233)

These codes can be used by physicians other than admitting physicians when physicians provide different services from the admitting physician on the same day

Hospital Discharge Services

Reports time spent by attending when discharging the patient

Time based codes

Two levels

30 minutes or less, and more than 30 minutes

Time must be documented to report 99239

Include following services when applicable

Final patient examination

Discussion about patient's hospital stay

Discussion with the family and/or caregiver regarding continuing care

Paperwork for discharge records

Prescriptions

Referral forms

Patient is deceased and the above-mentioned services were provided

PRACTICE 3, HOSPITAL INPATIENT SERVICES

Once you have coded the two cases, check your answers in Appendix A.

Practice 3, Report A

LOCATION: Inpatient, Hospital

CHIEF COMPLAINT: Extreme shortness of breath for the last 8-10 days.

HISTORY OF PRESENT ILLNESS: Lewis is a 33-year-old white male, well known to me, who came to the office this morning and was sent directly to the hospital with a complaint of progressively worsening shortness of breath for the last 10 days. It has gotten to the point he cannot even walk from the house to the mailbox without having to stop to catch his breath. He even gets short of breath while changing his clothes or during routine activities inside the house. He even gets short of breath while just sitting and talking. He denies any productive cough, fever, chest pains, or any other problems. His symptoms are mainly located in the chest, all the time. He describes it as tightness around his chest and he has difficulty breathing. Exertion makes it worse, rest makes it feel better. He rates it as a 8-9/10. It has been going on for the last 10 days and the only associated signs and symptoms are decreased exercise tolerance and some dry cough.

REVIEW OF SYSTEMS: CONSTITUTIONAL: As noted above, no fever. Also denies change of weight. HEENT: He denies any blurry vision or discharge. He denies any earaches, runny nose, or sore throat. HEMATOLOGY: He denies any bleeding from any site. Denies unusual bruising. CARDIAC: He denies any chest pain or palpitations. RESPIRATORY: He is complaining of severe shortness of breath and dry cough. GI: He denies any abdominal pain, nausea, vomiting, diarrhea, constipation, melena, hematochezia. GENITOURNINARY: He denies any burning micturition. DERMATOLOGICAL: He denies any jaundice or rash. NEUROLOGICAL: He denies any loss of consciousness, light-headedness, dizziness or any weakness on any one side. PSYCHIATRIC: He denies feeling depressed or anxious.

PAST MEDICAL HISTORY:
1. Nodular sclerosing Hodgkin's disease, abdomen only, diagnosed in 08/1991, status post Adriamycin, bleomycin, viblastine and decarbazine therapy.
2. Post radiation hypothyroidism.
3. Gastroesophageal reflux disease, hiatal hernia with subsequent stricture formation requiring repeated balloon dilation of the esophagus.
4. Possible Gilbert's syndrome.
5. Relative lymphocytosis persistent since chemotherapy.
6. Hemorrhoids.

PAST SURGICAL HISTORY:
1. Neck/groin lymph node biopsy.
2. Exploratory laparotomy with splenectomy in 1983.
3. Right subclavian Port-A-Cath insertion and removal.
4. Multiple esophagogastroduodenoscopies with esophageal balloon dilations. The last esophagogastroduodenoscopy was in 2002.

CURRENT MEDICATIONS: Synthroid 75 mcg qam, Prilosec 20 mg qam, Anusol HC cream prn.

ALLERGIES: No known drug allergies.

SOCIAL HISTORY: He denies any history of smoking, alcohol, or drug abuse. He is single and has no children.

FAMILY HISTORY: His mother had hypertension, hyperlipidemia, and multiple ventral hernias.

LABORATORY STUDIES: White blood count 10, hemoglobin 15.9, hematocrit 48.7, platelets 701, glucose 118, BUN 9, creatinine 1.1, calcium 10.1, albumin 4.7, alkaline phosphatase 142, sodium 137, potassium 4.5, CO2 30, PT 13.6, INR 1.14, PTT 26.8.

RADIOLOGY STUDIES: Chest x-ray shows complete whitening of the left lung field. CT Scan of the chest shows complete fluid accumulation on the left side with complete collapse of the left lung. It also shows some lymphadenopathy.

PHYSICAL EXAMINATION:
VITAL SIGNS: blood pressure 120/88, pulse 104 regular, respirations 18, temperature 97.7, weight 168.4 pounds, oxygen saturation 98% on room air. GENERAL: He is alert, awake, in mild to moderate respiratory distress at this time. EYES: Pink conjunctiva, anicteric sclera. Pupils are equal, round, and reactive to light. Extraocular movements are intact. NECK/LYMPH: Neck is supple. No jugular venous distention or cervical lymphadenopathy. LUNGS: He has absent breath sounds on the left side. Good air entry on the right side. No wheeze or rhonchi. HEART: Regular rate and rhythm. Tachycardia. Normal S1 and S2. No murmurs. ABDOMEN: Soft, non-tender, nondistended. No hepatosplenomegaly. Normoactive bowel sounds. MUSCULOSKELETAL: No CVA tenderness. EXTREMITIES: No cyanosis, clubbing or edema. Good distal pulses. NEUROLOGICALLY: There is no evidence of any focal neurological deficits. PSYCHOLOGICALLY: Alert and oriented times three.

ASSESSMENT:
1. Huge left sided pleural effusion with shortness of breath.
2. History of nodular sclerosing Hodgkin's disease, status post Adriamycin, bleomycin, viblastine, and decarbazine therapy and status post node irradiation and splenectomy.
3. Gastroesophageal reflux disease.
4. Post radiation hypothyroidism.
5. Hemorrhoids.

PLAN: The patient was sent directly from the office to radiology to get a chest x-ray. I reviewed the chest x-ray showing there is a complete opacification of the left lung, subsequently we immediately got a CT scan of the chest which showed complete collapse of the left lung and the left side is full of fluid. It also showed some lymphadenopathy. At that time, the decision was made to admit the patient as a direct admit. He was sent to the third floor. We will start oxygen 2 liters nasal cannula. We will have Dr. Green on consult for a left sided thoracocentesis. We will give him a regular diet. IV Heplock. Synthroid 75 mcg qam, Prilosec 20 mg qam. We will repeat a complete blood count and basic metabolic profile tomorrow morning. All of the above findings and plan were discussed with the patient. He seems to understand and agree. The patient has a guarded prognosis.

A. 99205

B. 99223

C. 99215

D. 99221

Practice 3, Report B

LOCATION: Inpatient, Hospital
Discharge Summary

FINAL DIAGNOSIS:
1. Acute gastrointestinal bleed with anemia, stable.
2. Coronary artery disease/stents/angioplasty.
3. Severe peripheral vascular disease.
4. Moderate to severe chronic obstructive pulmonary disease.

HOSPITAL COURSE: He is a 63-year-old white male with a known history of native coronary artery disease, status post PTCA with stents, peripheral vascular disease, chronic obstructive pulmonary disease who was admitted to the general medical floor on the 5th of August as a direct admit because of persistently low hemoglobin level and persistent melena. An esophagogastroduodenoscopy was performed yesterday, which did not show any source of active bleeding. He was transfused two units of packed red blood cells and his hemoglobin has been stable around 11.4. He denies any complaints and wishes to go home.

DISCHARGE MEDICATIONS: He has been instructed to resume all his home medications as before.

PLAN: He is scheduled for a colonoscopy as an outpatient with Dr. Blue on the 9th of August at 6:30 AM. All instructions and the preparatory material have been given to the patient. If his colonoscopy does not show any source of bleeding we will get a capsule endoscopy done. We will get a hemoglobin level one day prior to his visit. He is scheduled for a follow-up visit with me in the office in one week.

Codes: _____

4. CONSULTATIONS (99241-99255)

Requesting physician or other appropriate source is the one asking for opinion/advice of another physician

Individual who gives the opinion/advice is consultant

Consultation codes reflect inquiries between physicians or other qualified health care professionals

Written or verbal request for consultation must be documented in medical record

Consultant must provide documentation of

> Examination

> Clinical judgment(s)

> Treatment(s) prescribed/recommended

Consultant is authorized to order all medically necessary tests/services to render an opinion

According to CPT and CMS, only one consultation code should be reported per inpatient stay/per consultant

Same individual may be consulted more than once regarding same patient provided there is documentation in the medical record indicating a change in patient's status to support another consultation or a new condition in office setting

> This varies by payer

Requires 3 of 3 key components be met

Types of consultations

> Office or other outpatient consultations

>> Applies to both new and established patients

>> Reflects consultations occurring in one of the following sites

>>> Physician office

>>> Hospital observation services

>>> Home services

>>> Nursing facility

>>> Rest home or custodial care

>>> Emergency department

>>> Any other ambulatory facility

> Inpatient consultation

>> Reported for both new and established patients, no separate designation

>> Documentation on all three key components must either be met or exceeded

>> Limited to one initial inpatient consultation per patient/hospitalization by a consultant

PRACTICE 4, CONSULTATIONS

Once you have coded the two cases, check your answers in Appendix A.

Practice 4, Report A

LOCATION: Outpatient, Office

Dear Dr. Green:

Thank you for asking me to evaluate Ms. N., a 50-year-old female for fever, rash, and mouth sores occurring after a trip.

The patient and her husband tell me that they traveled to Hawaii in November. They flew into San Diego and took a bus to the ship in Ensenada, Mexico. The cruise ship then went to the islands of Hawaii. While in Hawaii, they took tours by bus to volcanoes. She did shopping in the towns they stopped in. The patient did no swimming while there and had no fresh water exposure. She was not around any animals. There were no ill contacts on the cruise ship. She did not eat any food while in Mexico, but did drink bottled water.

The patient and her husband returned to town on December 6. The patient notes that 2 weeks ago she began feeling fatigued and "not good." Twelve days ago she developed a fever to 103.8, as well as "sores" along the side of her tongue and her throat. Since then, she notes that she has developed both gingival and buccal lesions. She did have severe odynophagia and reports trouble drinking water. She denies any lesions on her lips.

Eight days ago, due to ongoing oral pain as well as pain that had developed in the neck and on the right side of her face and ear, she was seen as an outpatient. She tells me that she was given Prednisone because of oral swelling. She does not know the dosage of her Prednisone, but states that it was given for 5 days.

Six to seven days ago, the patient developed a cough. She tells me that this was nonproductive until this morning, when she began having "phlegmy, yucky stuff." She had a chest x-ray done three days ago and tells me that it was "free of pneumonia."

Three to four days ago, the patient began developing lesions on her neck and scalp. They are non pruritic, but are associated with sharp "nerve pain" which the patient describes as "intense."

The patient's fevers have decreased since her initial illness. She tells me that she is still having maximum temperatures of 101, and is taking Advil and Tylenol around the clock.

Past medical history is well known to you, and will not be reiterated here. Social history includes that the patient is married. She has three dogs and three cats, all of which are full grown. The cats are declawed on all four paws. She has had no nips or bites. The patient does not work outside the home. She was taking care of her 18-month-old granddaughter 2 days per week, up until the time that the patient became ill. The patient notes that the granddaughter has not been ill throughout this time.

On physical examination in my clinic, temperature was 99.0. Her pulse was 78 and her blood pressure was 118/86. Her weight was 168 pounds (decreased 15 pounds from October). The exam was significant only for skin, head, and neck exam. The mouth had multiple small punctate ulcers, all of which were on a white base. These were all between 1 and 3 mm and were on the buccal mucosa and in the oropharynx. There were labial lesions and no palatal lesions. There was mild anterior cervical lymphadenopathy, which was mildly to moderately tender. This all measured less than 2 cm and there was no associated erythema or fluctuance. Skin exam revealed several small pustular lesions located on the scalp and neck.

I suspect that the patient has a Coxsackie virus infection with predominance of oral lesions. With no exposure to animals or fresh water while in Hawaii, more unusual infections such as Leptospirosis would be exceedingly unusual. Additionally, her symptom complex (and particularly her oral ulcers) is not suggestive of either Typhus or Leptospirosis. Also in the differential diagnosis would be an adverse drug reaction to her chronic Augmentin. The patient was due to complete this in one week with a planned total duration of Augmentin of 6 months. I recommended that the patient stop her Augmentin 1 week early. I think that it would safe to re-challenge her with Augmentin into the future, if she required antibiotics. However, if she redeveloped oral ulcers with re-challenge of Augmentin, she would then need to be labeled as allergic to Augmentin.

Follow up will be on an as-needed basis in our clinic.

A. 99243

B. 99244

C. 99203

D. 99215

Practice 4, Report B, DOS - 5/20/xx

LOCATION: Inpatient, Hospital

CONSULT REQUESTED BY: Dr. Sutter, attending physician

REASON FOR CONSULTATION: Nausea, vomiting, and abdominal pain.

HISTORY OF PRESENT ILLNESS: The patient is a 33-year-old woman with a past medical history of diabetes, diabetic gastroparesis, status post J-tube placement in 2010, who now presents with an approximately 2-day history of nausea and vomiting. According to old records, the patient had been made n.p.o. with strict J-tube feedings; however, the patient has been noncompliant with this therapy and admits to taking moderate p.o. intake. The patient also complains of diffuse abdominal pain that does not radiate. The patient states that she has had this pain in the past. It is not specific and is not localized to any one point. The patient denies any chest pain, shortness of breath, fevers, or chills. She denies any change in her bowel movements. She states that she has been somewhat more constipated lately with her last formed bowel movement approximately 1 day prior. The patient states that she had diarrhea this morning. She denies any hematochezia or melena. She denies any dysuria or symptoms related to gastroesophageal reflux disease.

PAST MEDICAL HISTORY:
1. Diabetes, Type II.
2. Hypertension.
3. Diabetic gastroparesis.

PAST SURGICAL HISTORY:
1. Cholecystectomy.
2. Tubal ligation.
3. J-tube placement.

MEDICATIONS: Duragesic patch, Diflucan, insulin, Prevacid, Phenergan, Reglan, lisinopril, Lexapro, methadone.

ALLERGIES: No known medical allergies.

SOCIAL/FAMILY HISTORY: The patient does not smoke or drink alcohol. No family history of GI problems.

REVIEW OF SYSTEMS: The patient has a detailed review of systems per history and physical examination of 3 days prior to admission to hospital (5/17/XX).

PHYSICAL EXAMINATION:
GENERAL: The patient is a 33-year-old woman who appears older than her stated age. She is in no acute distress. She closes her eyes easily during questioning and responds only to repeated questions. VITAL SIGNS: Temperature 97.4 degrees, heart rate 91, blood pressure 106/57, oxygen saturation 97% on room air. HEENT: Pupils equal, round, reactive to light and accommodation and extraocular motions intact. Sclerae are anicteric. Oropharynx is benign. Mucous membranes are dry. NECK: Soft, supple, and nontender. No masses were felt.

LUNGS: Clear to auscultation, bilaterally. There are no rhonchi, rales, or wheezes. The patient is not in respiratory distress. HEART: Regular rate and rhythm, normal S1 and S2, no S3, murmurs, or rubs heard. ABDOMEN: Shows a well-healing midline scar, as well a J-tube. Abdomen is soft and slightly distended. There is no focal tenderness. There are hypoactive bowel sounds. There is no guarding, hepatosplenomegaly, or masses felt. The patient does not have any growing hernias. EXTREMITIES: Non-tender without edema. NEUROLOGIC: The patient is intact.

LABORATORY STUDIES: Electrolytes are within normal limits. Alkaline phosphatase is 119, ALT 583, AST 679, bilirubin 0.4, albumin 2.8, white blood count 6.6, and hemoglobin 12.1.

RADIOLOGY STUDIES: Upright abdominal x-ray showed minimal distention of the small bowel. There were some small associated air fluid levels. There is a small amount of gas and stool in the colon. There are no signs of free air or free fluid. CT scan of abdomen and pelvis is pending at this time.

IMPRESSION/RECOMMENDATIONS: The patient is a 33-year-old woman with a history of diabetic gastroparesis who presents now with nausea, vomiting, and abdominal pain.

1. These symptoms could represent diabetic gastroparesis. The patient will need a nasogastric tube placed. We will keep the patient n.p.o., as well as hold her J-tube feeding for now. We will review the CT scan findings with the radiologist. Otherwise, we will continue to treat this conservatively with intravenous fluids. In addition to her past medical history, the patient is on methadone for pain control, as well as Duragesic patch, which could cause significant ileus. The patient may need further small bowel imaging if the CT scan is inconclusive and her symptoms persist. However, the CT scan is a good modality for evaluating partial small-bowel obstructions.

2. Elevated transaminase. The patient was admitted with normal ALT and AST; however, on admission the patient developed AST and ALT elevations. This could be due to multiple causes; however, drug induced is likely given that the patient was started on Diflucan and Zosyn, both with known hepatic toxicity profiles. We will defer changing these antibiotics per the primary service. Bilirubin is within normal limits and the patient is not clinically jaundiced or complaining of any upper quadrant pain suggestive of biliary obstruction. We will discuss this case with the general surgeon who is on call for general surgery today.

Codes:_____

5. EMERGENCY DEPARTMENT SERVICES (99281-99288)

ED services may also be billed by physicians who are not assigned to the ED

No distinction is made between new and established patients

Requires 3 of 3 key components be met

No "time" component

Any physician who provides services in the ED may use these codes to report the service

If the physician asks the patient to meet him/her in ED as an alternative to the physician's office and the patient is not registered as an ED patient

Report the service with appropriate office/outpatient visit codes (99201-99215)

Facilities qualifying as EDs must be

Open and available 24 hours a day

Located in organized hospital-based facility

Exist to provide immediate medical attention to persons without the constraints of prior scheduled appointments

Code assignment determined by severity of patient's condition as reported by physician in medical record and complexity of medical decision making

Facilities may use acuity sheet "as guidance," such as that in **Figure 1-9** to assign level of ED service

Level 1—99281	Level 2—99282	Level 3—99283
1. Initial (triage) assessment 2. Suture removal 3. Wound recheck 4. Note for work or school 5. Simple discharge information	Interventions from previous level plus any of the following: 1. OTC med administration 2. Tetanus booster 3. Bedside diagnostic tests (stool hemoccult, glucometer) 4. Visual acuity 5. Orthostatic vital signs 6. Simple trauma not requiring x-ray 7. Simple discharge information	Interventions from previous level plus any of the following: 1. Heparin/saline lock 2. Crystalloid IV therapy 3. X-ray, one area 4. RX med administration 5. Fluorescein stain 6. Quick cath 7. Foley cath 8. Receipt of ambulance patient 9. Mental health emergencies (mild) not requiring parenteral medications or admission 10. Moderate complexity discharge instructions 11. Intermediate layered and complex laceration repair
Level 4—99284	**Level 5—99285**	**Critical Care 99291, 99292**
Interventions from previous level plus any of the following: 1. X-ray, multiple areas 2. Special imaging studies (CT, MRI, ultrasound) 3. Cardiac monitoring 4. Multiple reassessments of patient 5. Parenteral[1] medications (including insulin) 6. Nebulizer treatment (1 or 2) 7. NG placement 8. Pelvic exam 9. Mental health emergencies (moderate). May require parenteral medications but not admission 10. Administration of IV medications [1] *not through the alimentary canal but rather by injection through some other route, such as subcutaneous, intramuscular, intraorbital, intracapsular, intraspinal, intrasternal, or intravenous*	Interventions from previous level plus any of the following: 1. Monitor/stabilize patient during in hospital transport and/or testing (CT, MRI, ultrasound) 2. Vasoactive medication 3. Administration (dopamine, dobutamine, multiple) nebulizer treatments (3 or more) 4. Conscious sedation 5. Lumbar puncture 6. Thoracentesis 7. Sexual assault exam 8. Admission to hospital 9. Mental health emergency (severe) psychotic and/or agitated/combative 10. Requires admission 11. Fracture/dislocation reduction 12. Suicide precautions 13. Gastric lavage 14. Complex discharge instructions	Interventions from any previous level plus any of the following: 1. Multiple parenteral medications 2. Continuous monitoring 3. Major trauma care 4. Chest tube insertion 5. CPR 6. Defibrillation/cardioversion 7. Delivery of baby 8. Control of major hemorrhage 9. Administration of blood or blood products

Figure **1-9.** Example of an acuity sheet used to determine level of emergency department services.

PRACTICE 5, EMERGENCY DEPARTMENT SERVICES

*Using the acuity sheet (**Figure 1-9**), code the following two cases and then check your answers in Appendix A.*

Practice 5, Report A

CHIEF COMPLAINT: Abdominal pain.

HISTORY OF PRESENT ILLNESS
This is a 34-year-old female who presents to the ED and has had upper abdominal pain, nausea, and diarrhea today not associated with fevers, pain with urination, urgency, or frequency. The patient had similar problems about a month ago, and that workup was negative. It is not associated with food, melena, hematochezia, and no sick contacts that she is aware of.

PAST MEDICAL HISTORY: Asthma, hypertension, depression, migraines, esophageal reflux, and arthritis.

MEDICATIONS/ALLERGIES: (Reviewed. See nursing notes on Lisinopril for HTN.)

PAST SURGICAL HISTORY: She has had a tubal ligation.

FAMILY HISTORY: Unremarkable for present condition, but a history of hypertension.

SOCIAL HISTORY: Denies alcohol, drug, or tobacco use.

REVIEW OF SYSTEMS: Positive for abdominal pain, nausea, and diarrhea. Remainder of 10-point review of system performed is negative.

PHYSICAL EXAMINATION
General—the patient is a 34-year-old female who does not appear toxic or in distress. Vital signs—she has stable vitals blood pressure 140/84 and afebrile. HEENT—nonicteric sclerae. Oropharynx does not appear significantly dry. Neck—supple. Lungs—clear. Heart—regular rate and rhythm without murmur. Abdomen—she has some diffuse upper abdominal pain, but no peritoneal signs nor flank discomfort. Skin—exam is unremarkable. Neurological—she is awake, alert, appropriate, and ambulates normally.

EMERGENCY DEPARTMENT COURSE
The patient was given pain medication and IV fluids. She had an ultrasound performed 1 month ago and was essentially negative. All her lab work was normal. Her pain was controlled. I felt she probably was coming down with some type of viral syndrome.

PROVISIONAL DIAGNOSIS/DIAGNOSES: Evaluation of upper abdominal pain, etiology undetermined.

PLAN(S)
1. The patient was given abdominal pain instruction sheet.
2. Sent home with a prescription for Bentyl.
3. I recommend that she follow up with her primary care physician if she has persistent problems.
   Condition at discharge was stable.

ICD-9-CM:

A. 99284; 789.09, 787.02, 787.91, 401.9

B. 99285; 789.00, 079.99, 401.9

C. 99283; 789.00, 401.9

D. 99284; 789.09, 079.99, 401.9

ICD-10-CM:

A. 99284; R10.10, R11.0, R19.7, I10

B. 99285; R10.9, B97.89, I10

C. 99283; R10.9, I10

D. 99284; R10.10, B97.89, I10

Practice 5, Report B

CHIEF COMPLAINT: Ankle injury.

HISTORY OF PRESENT ILLNESS

The patient is a 16-year-old male who was skateboarding today and had an inversion injury of his left ankle. He is ambulatory but complains of pain and swelling. No other complaints or injuries at this time. See nurse's notes for medications and allergies.

ROS

Patient states no dizziness prior to or after the fall. No recent muscle or joint problems. No broken skin.

HISTORY

No past surgeries. The patient is a junior in school and does play sports.

PHYSICAL EXAMINATION

Height 68", weight 185, BP 120/58. He is an alert and pleasant male in no acute distress. Examination of the left lower extremity shows a soft tissue swelling of the lateral malleolus. He has no base of the 5th metatarsal tenderness. He has no proximal tibial tenderness. Neurovascularly intact distally.

EMERGENCY DEPARTMENT COURSE

Plain films were performed and showed no evidence of acute fracture or malalignment and told this represented sprain. I recommend symptomatic care, air cast, ice, crutches, and Motrin. Follow up with primary care physician. Return for any problems. He is agreeable to this plan. He was discharged home in stable condition.

PROVISIONAL DIAGNOSIS/DIAGNOSES: Left ankle sprain.

Codes:_____

6. CRITICAL CARE SERVICES (99291, 99292)

Critical care is provided for

Outpatient (ED or office) neonates and pediatric patients up to 71 months

Outpatient and inpatient services for patients over 71 months

Infants or young children ages 2 through 5 years receiving inpatient critical care assign 99475, 99476

Infants 29 days through 24 months receiving inpatient critical care assign 99471, 99472

Infants 28 days or younger assign 99468, 99469

One or more of the vital organ(s) is in/has high probability for being in a life threatening state

A high complexity of MDM is required for treating vital organ(s) failure and/or prevention of further deterioration in the patient's condition

Examples of vital organ failure

Central nervous system

Circulatory failure

Presence of shock

Renal failure

Hepatic failure

Metabolic failure

Respiratory failure

Threats to vital organs are not limited to the above list

Most (but not all) critical care involves an interpretation of either advanced technology and/or multiple interpretations with physiologic parameters

Codes may also be assigned for critical care services for

Postoperative patient

Patient with a deteriorating condition

Type of physician time and location are important keys in assigning these codes

Time spent on critical care may include time

On medical unit reviewing patient care with or without other medical staff

Spent documenting patient's status into medical record

Spent with the patient's family or caregivers compiling a history and/or discussing medical management if patient is clinically incompetent

Time spent in a face-to-face encounter may be accumulated over course of day

Example: Three 30-minute encounters result in 90 minutes of time

Time spent must be documented in the medical record

PRACTICE 6, CRITICAL CARE SERVICES

These are time-based codes, so no audit form is required. Once you have coded the two cases, check your answers in Appendix A.

Practice 6, Report A

CHIEF COMPLAINT: Syncope, neck pain.

HISTORY OF PRESENT ILLNESS

An 88-year-old male who presents to the ED after he apparently had a syncopal episode at home. Unfortunately, the patient does not remember the episode. He was found by his wife, he was able to stand on his own. He complained of some neck pain and was placed on a backboard and transported via EMS. The patient does not remember walking around the house this morning and does not know what he was feeling, does not remember if he had any symptoms prior to the collapse. Vital signs documented per supplemental sheet. I do not believe the patient is a reliable historian.

Per the family, he has had a history of cancer, COPD, atrial fibrillation.

PSH: Left carotid endarterectomy and a Nissen. The patient quit smoking 40 years ago.

FH: Positive for coronary disease.

MEDICATIONS/ALLERGIES: A full 10-point review of systems is otherwise negative. (Some Medicare carriers require systems to be noted).

PHYSICAL EXAMINATION

The patient was afebrile, vital signs notable for a pulse of 116, otherwise normal. In general, a pleasant male on a backboard, wearing a C-collar, in no acute distress. HEENT: Pupils equal, round and reactive, extraocular movements intact. There are no signs of trauma about the face or scalp. Neck is examined with in-line stabilization, in a C-collar. The patient had some tenderness over the upper cervical spine and was kept in a C-collar. CV tachy and irregular but no murmur. Lungs are clear. Abdomen is soft, nontender. Extremities unremarkable with no rash, no focal tenderness. Back exam revealed no tenderness. Neurologically the patient was oriented to person and place.

EMERGENCY DEPARTMENT COURSE

The patient was carefully log-rolled off the backboard. Did have an EKG which showed atrial fibrillation with some lateral ST depression consistent with digitalis effect. Patient did have a metabolic panel which showed the glucose of 114, otherwise normal. CBC showed a white count of 10.9, hemoglobin 12.1. Troponin 0.04, myoglobin 611, thought to be elevated secondary to his syncope. Urinalysis was negative. CT of the head was unremarkable except for possible left basal ganglia lacunar infarct. CT of the C-spine did show fracture of the C4 left pedicle and left transverse foramina. With this finding, the patient was kept in a C-collar, was seen by orthopedics. Discussed with primary care physician. The patient will be admitted in guarded condition.

PROVISIONAL DIAGNOSIS/DIAGNOSES

1. C4 fracture displaced.
2. Syncope of uncertain cause.

The patient is neurologically intact. Total critical care time did exceed 30 minutes.

ICD-9-CM:

A. 99291; 806.00, 780.09

B. 99221; 805.04, 780.2, E888.8

C. 99291; 805.04, 780.2

D. 99221; 99291, 806.00, 780.2

ICD-10-CM:

A. 99291; S12.300A, S14.104A, R40.0

B. 99221; 99291, S12.300A, R55

C. 99291; S12.300A, R55

D. 99221; 99291, S12.300A, R55

Practice 6, Report B

CHIEF COMPLAINT: Altered level of mental status.

HISTORY OF PRESENT ILLNESS

This is an 84-year-old male who was found by his son to be somewhat unresponsive and seeming to have difficulty with gasping for air. This was at his group home where he is in assisted living. The son had the staff check an oxygen level and it was 70%, so EMS was called and the patient was brought here. The patient has responded to verbal stimuli, but has not indicated any pain. The son is not aware of any fever or vomiting, although the patient has not been eating well for the last week or so. PAST MEDICAL HISTORY: There is a history of bladder cancer. There is also a history of pulmonary embolism and deep venous thrombosis and the patient is on Coumadin. He has also had a history of stroke. SOCIAL HISTORY: The patient is here with his son. There is a "do not resuscitate order" within his advance directive that indicates he does not want intubation or CPR according to the son. The son does want to see the patient get necessary medication or fluids. As noted above, he lives in assisted living. ROS: I was not able to do a review of systems on the patient because of his lethargy. The son stated he did not know of any recent fever or cough. He did not know of any vomiting or urinary difficulties.

PHYSICAL EXAMINATION

Vital signs show a low blood pressure of 89/48 with a normal pulse of 90 and regular. Increased respiratory rate of 28, but not labored. Now that the patient is on oxygen he is not using accessory muscles respiration or gasping. The pharynx shows no inflammation or exudate, but is very dry. There is no cervical adenopathy and his neck is supple. Pupils equal, round, and reactive to light.

Cranial nerves II-XII are intact. The patient is able to cooperate enough to squeeze my fingers or to lift his arms and legs, and he does this in a symmetrical way in all 4 extremities. The heart has normal S1-S2 without murmur. Lungs are clear to auscultation and percussion. The abdomen is soft and nontender throughout without mass, guarding or rebound tenderness. Lower extremities show no swelling, tenderness, or cords. Skin is clear of significant rashes.

DIAGNOSTIC STUDIES

LABORATORY/PATHOLOGY: Pulse oximetry is adequate at 96% on an oxygen mask by nonrebreather. CBC shows low hemoglobin of 11.1 and elevated white count of 14,300. Electrolytes show high potassium of 5.1, high chloride of 114 and low CO2 of 19. BUN is high at 50 and creatinine high at 3.3. These are significant elevations since a previous level done 8 days ago when he had a BUN of 17 and creatinine of 1.3. Glucose is high at 154, albumin is low at 2.7. Liver studies are basically normal. Urinalysis is positive for probable infection with 11 white cells and small leukocyte esterase.
Troponin I is normal at less than 0.03.

IMAGING: Chest x-ray shows no active infiltrate.

EKG: A 12-lead electrocardiogram was done for the indication of lethargy and hypotension, and the computer interpretation was reviewed. The tracing shows normal sinus rhythm with frequent premature atrial contractions. There is nonspecific T-wave flattening present in the inferior and lateral leads. There are Q waves in leads III and aVF consistent with old inferior MI. There are no acute ischemic changes.

EMERGENCY DEPARTMENT COURSE

I gave the patient a liter of IV fluids in the emergency department over a couple of hours and this with the oxygen resulted in definite improvement of his mental status. He was alert and easily responsive after the first 700 mL of saline. I ordered Levaquin 250 mg IV. I spoke with his primary physician and he is going to come over to the emergency department and admit the patient.

PROVISIONAL DIAGNOSIS/DIAGNOSES

1. Altered mental status.
2. Upper respiratory infection.
3. Urosepsis (UTI).
4. History of bladder cancer.
5. Low blood pressure reading, which has now improved.
6. History of anticoagulation for pulmonary embolism and deep venous thrombosis.

Will continue to monitor therapeutic levels.

DISPOSITION

He was admitted as noted. Condition on discharge from the emergency department is improved. Critical care time was 30 minutes on this patient.

Codes:_____

7. NURSING FACILITY SERVICES (99304-99318)

These codes are used for patients in

Nursing facilities

Intermediate care facilities

Long-term care facilities

Psychiatric residential treatment centers

Psychiatric residential treatment centers are those that

Provide a 24-hour therapeutically planned living and/or learning environment with professionally trained staff

Medical psychotherapy is not included in codes

There are four subcategories of codes in nursing facility codes

Dependent on assessment instruments used by the nursing facility to assess a resident's functional capacity

Initial Nursing Facility Care

Subsequent Nursing Facility Care

Nursing Facility Discharge Services

Other Nursing Facility Services (Annual Assessments)

Two forms are used to determine the patient's status

Resident Assessment Protocols (RAP)

Residential Assessment Instrument (RAI) with uniform Minimum Data Set requirements (MDS)

Uniform MDS for nursing facilities must include or exceed following information

Medically defined conditions and prior medical history

Medical status measurement

Physical and mental functional status

Discharge potential

Dental condition

Activities potential

Rehabilitation potential

Cognitive status

Drug therapy

MDS must contain input from physician for evaluation and formulation of multidisciplinary care

When an MDS appears incomplete or signals a need for supplementary information, RAPs are used

RAP must be used by nursing facility in following situations

At time of patient admittance to facility

When 12 months have lapsed since previous assessment

When a major permanent change in patient's status is observed

RAP is helpful in assessing potential problems and provides useful information for follow-up procedures

When a patient is admitted to a nursing care facility from another medical service site, such as a physician office or an emergency department, all services performed on date of admission are evaluated (considered) as part of initial facility care codes

Discharge day code is used when either a discharge from a hospital or observation status in a hospital occurs on same date as admission to a nursing facility, code also the nursing home admission.

Note: When a physician discharges a patient from a nursing facility, the appropriate code is based on the time spent with the patient and/or family and/or caregiver discussing both the facility stay and management options, which the physician bases on his/her final examination

---

PRACTICE 7, NURSING FACILITY SERVICES

Once you have coded the two cases, check your answers in Appendix A.

Practice 7, Report A

LOCATION: Light Hills Nursing Home, established patient
Emily is seen for a review of chronic controlled conditions listed below. The chart is reviewed along with the nursing notes. Advanced directives are in place.

S: No fevers or chills. No chest pain or shortness of breath.

0: This well-developed, well-nourished lady is sitting without distress. HEENT is normal, normocephalic, and atraumatic. Neck is supple. Lungs clear to auscultation.

A: 1. Chronic headaches
2. Bipolar disorder
3. Hypertension, primary
4. Tardive dyskinesia secondary to antidepressants
5. Urinary incontinence

P: 1. The patient has chronic headaches for which she has been taking Fioricet as needed, but I will go ahead and start her on Topamax for preventative measures, 25 mg one p.o. H.S. for 10 days and then one p.o. bid for 10 days and then one in the AM and two at H.S. for 10 days. Then we will start 50 mg p.o. bid.
2. Reassess in 4 weeks.
3. In the meantime, the case was discussed with the charge nurse and I advised that the Topamax may cause a little increased fatigue and hypersomnolence but if it is clinically significant, we might have to decrease the doses.

ICD-9-CM:

A. 99309; 784.0, 296.90, 401.9, 333.82, 788.30, E939.3

B. 99308; 784.0, 296.80, 401.9, 333.82, 788.30, E939.3

C. 99336; 784.0, 296.90, 401.9, 969.3, 788.30, E939.3

D. 99309; 784.0, 296.80, 401.1, 333.85, 788.30, E939.3

ICD-10-CM:

A. 99309; R51, F39, I10, G24.4, R32

B. 99308; R51, F31.9, I10, G24.4, R32

C. 99336; R51, F39, I10, T43.011A, R32

D. 99309; R51, F31.9, I10, G24.01, R32

Practice 7, Report B

LOCATION:
Nursing Facility
    This patient is seen for a routine visit for chronic conditions. No code in place. The chart is reviewed along with the nursing notes. Advanced directives are in place. The graphic chart is also reviewed.

S: No fevers or chills. No chest pain or shortness of breath. Nurse states patient continues to be frequently combative and wanders off.

O: This well-developed, well-nourished gentleman is sitting without distress. HEENT - normocephalic and atraumatic. Neck is supple. Lungs - clear to auscultation.

A: 1. Alzheimer dementia
2. Dementia and combative behavior

P: 1. As the patient is otherwise clinically stable; the rest of the treatment is without change.

Codes:_____

8. DOMICILIARY, REST HOME (E.G., BOARDING HOME), OR CUSTODIAL CARE SERVICES, AND DOMICILIARY, REST HOME (E.G., ASSISTED LIVING FACILITY), OR HOME CARE PLAN OVERSIGHT SERVICES (99324-99340)

Domiciliary, Rest Home (e.g., Boarding Home), or Custodial Care Services (99324-99337)

These codes are used to report services in two settings

- Facility providing room, board, and other personal assistance services on a long-term basis

- Assisted living facility without a medical component

Code choice based on whether patient is new or established patient

- For a new patient all 3 key components must be met or exceeded

- For an established patient, 2 of 3 key components must be met or exceeded

Time spent by a physician is considered a contributory factor when assigning a code for service

Domiciliary, Rest Home (e.g., Assisted Living Facility), or Home Care Plan Oversight Services (99339-99340)

Reports physician supervision of patient, when patient is not present

Patient resides in

- Own home

- Rest home or domiciliary

  - Includes assisted living facility

Codes based on time spent during calendar month

Not for patients receiving

- Home health care (99374-99375)

- Hospice care (99377-99378)

- Nursing facility services (99379-99380)

Physician or other qualified health care professonial provides the following types of services

- Reviews subsequent reports, laboratory studies, or other studies

- Integrates new data into patient's care plan

- Adjusts medical therapy

- Develops or revises care plans

- Communicates with other health care professionals

PRACTICE 8, DOMICILIARY, REST HOME (E.G., BOARDING HOME), OR CUSTODIAL CARE SERVICES, AND DOMICILIARY, REST HOME (E.G., ASSISTED LIVING FACILITY), OR HOME CARE PLAN OVERSIGHT SERVICES (99324-99340)

Once you have coded the two cases, check your answers in Appendix A.

Practice 8, Report A

LOCATION: Custodial Care Center, established patient

Patient evaluated today for a rash on her arms for the last 3 days. Nursing staff reports that lotion has been applied with no relief. Examined the patient and rash is contained to her arms. Staff also noticed that the patient has been sleeping a lot during the day. When I questioned the patient on her sleeping, she let me know that she has not been sleeping at night. Other than the rash and her sleeping habits, the patient is overall healthy.

Benadryl cream will be given prn for the patient's rash. Watch to make sure it doesn't spread. There is no change in her care plan at this time.

ICD-9-CM:

A. 99335; 782.1

B. 99307; 782.1, 307.42

C. 99347; 782.1, 307.42

D. 99325; 782.1, 780.52

ICD-10-CM:

A. 99335; R21

B. 99307; R21, F51.01

C. 99347; R21, F51.01

D. 99325; R21, G47.00

Practice 8, Report B

LOCATION: Shady Lane Rest Home

This is an 80-year-old man, who resides in a rest home, complaining of painful urination. The pain is 5 out of 10. He has a suprapubic catheter due to urinary retention. He has been treated for urinary tract infections in the past with Cipro. He is having acute abdominal pain and fever. He has been eating fair.

EXAMINATION: When I visit with him today, he denies any weight loss, SOB, or palpitations. He is mildly confused. He answers yes and no, but there is very little conversation. His color is pink. His HEART is regular without murmur. His CHEST is diminished breath sounds with mild crackles at both bases. ABDOMEN is soft and nontender with active bowel sounds. His EXTREMITIES show no edema.

PLAN: Medications and treatments have been reviewed. I will place the patient on Cipro to treat UTI. No other changes to care plan at this time.

Codes:_____

9. HOME SERVICES (99341-99350)

Reports interaction between a physician and either new or established patient within the patient's residence

"Homebound" status required by some payers

New patient visit

   3 key components must be met or exceeded

Established patient visit

   2 of 3 key components must be met or exceeded

PRACTICE 9, HOME SERVICES

Once you have coded the two cases, check your answers in Appendix A.

Practice 9, Report A

LOCATION: Patient's Home, established patient

CHIEF COMPLAINT: Cough.

HISTORY OF PRESENT ILLNESS: This 89-year-old male, who is well known to me, has been coughing somewhat more as reported by the nurse and his wife over one week but he seems to be sleeping rather well, without having to be propped up for any possible paroxysmal nocturnal dyspnea. He does not awaken through the night with difficulty breathing. His appetite appears to be normal. He is otherwise not complaining of any other discomforts, but notes ankle swelling.

EXAMINATION:
General: The patient is seen in his home. Vital signs are stable. He has some coughing and has more swelling of his right leg than the left. He is mostly bed-bound but does get up and eat his meals but gets out sometimes with help. HEENT: Head is normocephalic. Ears are clear bilaterally. Throat is slightly dry. Neck is supple. LUNGS: Lungs demonstrate rhonchi bilaterally. No wheezes are noted. HEART: Heart demonstrates a regular rate and rhythm with no murmur, click, or rub. ABDOMEN: Abdomen is protuberant. Benign with no masses or tenderness. GENITALIA: Normal, no swelling. RECTAL: Deferred. EXTREMITIES: Pitting edema localized bilaterally (LE), the right a little more than the left. He does have several decubiti (sacral, hip) which are currently being treated and appear to be healing and not getting worse.

IMPRESSION:
1. Bronchitis.
2. Severe osteoarthritis.
3. Multiple decubiti of sacrum and hip.
4. Pitting edema localized.

RECOMMENDATION:
He will be started on Zithromax Z-pak as directed.
    He will continue his cough syrup, Robitussin AC 1 tsp 4 times a day.
    Continue Lasix 40 mg a day.
    Decrease salt intake. His wife is instructed to not add any salt at the table and to make sure that he does not eat any potato chips or obviously salty foods.

ICD-9-CM:

A. 99343; 491.0, 715.90, 782.3, 707.03, 707.04

B. 99343; 490, 715.90, 782.3, 707.00

C. 99349; 490, 715.90, 707.03, 782.3, 707.04

D. 99349; 491.0, 715.90, 707.00, 782.3

ICD-10-CM:

A. 99343; J41.0, M19.90, R60.0, L89.159, L89.209

B. 99343; J40, M19.90, R60.0, L89.90

C. 99349; J40, M19.90, L89.159, R60.0, L89.209

D. 99349; J41.0, M19.90, L89.90, R60.0

Practice 9, Report B

LOCATION: Patient's Home

PATIENT: 91-year-old male

CC: Cough with underlying CHF

The 91-year-old gentleman is seen at home in bed. He has had more of a productive cough since Monday with no swelling of his ankles. He has been continuing on his usual medication including Tequin 400 mg once a day and Robitussin AC one teaspoon 4 times a day, with some relief. I have asked for his head to be elevated 30 degrees while he is in this respiratory condition. Today he is doing much better. He awakens every now and then. I believe he still recognizes me.

ROS was attempted but not obtained due to the patient's condition. The patient does suffer from CHF and Parkinson's, primary.

Vital signs: BP 130/62, R 16, T 37. Head is normocephalic, atraumatic. Lungs: few basilar rales; otherwise clear. Heart: RRR. Abdomen: benign with no mass or tenderness. He certainly does not grimace when palpating his abdomen. Extremities: 1+ edema bilaterally. Pulses are 2+ bilaterally in the lower extremities.

IMPRESSION:
1. CHF
2. Cough
3. Bronchitis
4. Osteoarthritis
5. Parkinson's primary

RECOMMENDATIONS
Finish the antibiotics.
Continue to monitor.

Codes:_____

10. PROLONGED SERVICES (99354-99360)

Under the Prolonged Services subsection there are three categories

Prolonged Service With Direct Patient Contact (99354-99357)

Prolonged Service Without Direct Patient Contact (99358, 99359)

Standby Services (99360)

Prolonged Service With or Without Patient Contact

Codes 99354-99359 are all add-on codes

Only assigned when estimated service exceeds the time listed by more than 30 minutes

First 30 minutes of prolonged services are not reported but are considered part of initial service

Used in addition to codes reported for other E/M services

Used in addition to other codes to show an extension of the service

Unusual length of service may be in inpatient or outpatient setting

Codes available for services with or without direct provider and patient contact

PRACTICE 10A, PROLONGED SERVICES WITH OR WITHOUT DIRECT PATIENT CONTACT (99354-99359)

These are time based codes; therefore, no audit form is required. Once you have coded the two cases, check your answers in Appendix A.

Practice 10A, Report A

LOCATION: Outpatient Clinic

Chief Complaint:	Chronic Renal Failure, Diabetes Mellitus and Hypertension
Hx of Present Illness:	The patient presents to the clinic today for a follow-up appointment for hypertension and chronic kidney disease. At her last visit the Norvasc was increased to 5 mg PO QD. She has been seeing a cardiologist and pulmonologist for breathing problems. The Labetalol was discontinued and she was started on Toprol XL 50 mg PO QD. She was also started on an Advair inhaler b.i.d. by the pulmonologist. Her breathing has been much better. Her BP has been higher running 150's systolic at home. She has been feeling relatively well. She does have a history of renal artery stenosis with right renal artery stent placement. Labs today include: BUN 26, sodium 140, creatinine is better at 1.2 mg/dL, CO2 28.6, K+ 4.5.
Urinary Symptoms:	Patient has no urinary symptoms.
Uremic Symptoms:	Patient has no uremic symptoms.
Cardiovascular Symptoms:	Patient has no cardiovascular symptoms.
PAST MEDICAL HISTORY:	Hypertension Proteinuria Atrial Fibrillation Osteoarthritis in lt knee Coronary Artery Disease Cataract surgery Open cholecystectomy
CURRENT MEDICATIONS:	1. Insulin 70/30 2. Insulin 3. Aspirin 4. Pravachol 5. Labetolol 6. Bumex 7. Tylenol 8. Multivitamin/Iron 9. Norvasc 10. Toprol XL 11. Advair inhaler
SOCIAL HISTORY:	Marital Status: Current Occupation: Past Occupation: Current Alcohol use: No Current Smoker: No Ex-Smoker: No Residence:

REVIEW OF SYSTEMS:	
Constitutional:	Negative
Eyes:	Wear glasses
ENT:	Negative
Cardiovascular:	Mentioned in HPI
Respiratory:	Dry cough
Gastrointestinal:	Negative
Genitourinary:	Mentioned in HPI
Musculoskeletal:	Arthritis
Skin:	Negative
Neurological:	Negative
Psychological:	Negative
Endocrine:	Diabetes Mellitus
Hematology:	Negative
PHYSICAL EXAMINATION:	
	Patient does not appear in any respiratory, cardiac, or neurological distress. No pallor, jaundice, or cyanosis.
	Temperature: 97.9° F, Respiration 28/min, Pulse 72/min and regular
	Height: Weight: 155 lbs.
Blood Pressure:	Left (sitting): 166/72 mmHg Left (standing): 162/73 mmHg
Eyes:	Pupils are equal and reactive to light and accommodation. No evidence of conjunctivitis.
Fundoscopy:	Not done
ENT:	No hearing loss. Normal oropharyngeal and nasal mucosa.
Neck:	Normal jugular venous pressure. No carotid bruits.
Lungs:	Good air entry bilaterally. No wheezes or crackles.
Heart:	Regular S1, S2.
Abdomen:	Not done.
Extremities:	No edema.
Neurologic:	Patient was alert and oriented x3. Cranial nerves II through XII were intact. Motor power was 5/5 bilaterally. Normal gait.
Skin:	No lesions or rashes.
Other:	None
Diagnosis:	Hypertensive kidney disease, Renal Artery Stenosis. Direct face-to-face time spent with patient was 80 minutes. Meds reviewed and discussion about treatment and prognosis.
Plan:	1. Increase the Toprol XL to 100 mg PO QD. Script written. 2. She will continue to monitor her BP at home. 3. She knows to call with any questions or concerns. 4. Return to clinic in 3-4 week with a basic metabolic panel. 5. Continue other medications for now.

ICD-9-CM:

A. 99215; 99354, 403.90, 585.9, 250.40, 483.8, V45.89, V58.67

B. 99214; 403.90, 250.00, V45.89

C. 99214; 99358, 401.9, 585.9, 440.1

D. 99215; 99354, 401.9, 585.9, V45.89

ICD-10-CM:

A. 99215; 99354, I12.9, N18.9, E11.22, J16.8, Z98.89, Z79.4

B. 99214; I12.9, E11.9, Z98.89

C. 99214; 99358, I10, N18.9, I70.1

D. 99215; 99354, I10, N18.9, Z98.89

Practice 10A, Report B

HOSPITAL-PROGRESS NOTE

CC: Worsening Acute Renal Failure

The patient was seen and examined multiple times today. His BUN was down to 40, sodium 135. His hiccups are better. He is getting them intermittently. His potassium was 3.9. He had no shortness of breath, no chest pain. Ultrasound was done. I evaluated him later in the evening. The patient was found to have right-sided hydronephrosis and right-sided hydroureter. I had a long discussion with him and his family and I discussed the case with the consulting physicians. We proceeded with right-sided percutaneous nephrostomy tube placement. The patient had bloody urine. He tolerated that procedure well. He was evaluated afterwards again. The patient also had a PD catheter placed, without difficulty and uneventfully.

EXAMINATION: The patient had no edema and felt well. His LUNGS are clear. His VITALS remain stable, BP 138/82, Pulse 126. He is afebrile.

I spent quite a bit of time with this patient today and with his family at bedside. Had lots of discussions on the different procedures that were done. His family asked a lot of questions. They were all answered. We discussed hemodialysis and peritoneal dialysis. We discussed nephrostomy tube and distal ureteric obstruction could be related to his surgery. We have addressed all of the concerns and issues. We discussed the fact that we might end up placing a stent, either cystoscopically or antegrade. I discussed this with his surgeon and we decided to proceed again tomorrow with antegrade stent placement.

IMPRESSION:

1. Acute renal failure.
2. Obstructive uropathy.
3. Right-sided hydronephrosis.
4. Chronic renal failure.
5. Hyponatremia from fluid overload state.

PLAN:

1. Hold dialysis for now.
2. Repeat laboratories in the morning.
3. High protein boost t.i.d.
4. Will keep him n.p.o. after midnight.
5. We will proceed with antegrade stent placement.
6. Consult urologist.
7. The patient is code level 1.

   Total time spent on this patient today was 2 hours and 25 minutes.

Codes:_____

Standby Services (99360)

Used when a physician, at request of the attending is standing by in case his/her services are needed

Standby individual cannot be rendering services to another patient during standby time

Reported in increments of 30 minutes

Only reported when no service is performed and there is no face-to-face contact with the patient

> Not reported when a standby status ends, and the individual provides a service to the patient

> The service is reported as any other service would be, even though it began as a standby service

CMS does not pay for standby services

PRACTICE 10B, STANDBY SERVICES

These are time-based codes; therefore, no audit form is required. Once you have coded the two cases, check your answers in Appendix A.

Practice 10B, Report A

LOCATION: Outpatient Hospital

Surgeon is called in to be on standby for a female patient with proteinuria undergoing a biopsy of her right kidney. Specimen was sent for frozen section. Patient remains in surgery suite prepped for a procedure if diagnosis comes back malignant. Surgeon had been on standby for approximately 15 minutes when he received a call regarding another patient. Surgeon spent 6 minutes on the phone. Within 10 minutes of ending his call he was notified that his services were not needed as the biopsy came back negative for malignancy.

A. Not reportable/billable service

B. 99360

C. 50205-80

D. 99360-52

Practice 10B, Report B

LOCATION: Inpatient, Hospital

OB/GYN physician on call has asked me (pediatrician) to standby due to 19-year-old patient in labor with fetal monitoring showing increased fetal distress. Patient is at 32-weeks gestation. Possible neonatal resuscitation may be required. After 1 hour and 40 minutes of constant standby, patient delivered without my assistance to newborn.

Codes:_____

11. CASE MANAGEMENT SERVICES (99363-99368)

Anticoagulant Management (99363, 99364)

Codes used to report anticoagulant (warfarin) therapy management

  Require physician review and interpretation

Reported based initial or subsequent services

Outpatient management only

Assessments taken based on International Normalized Ratio (INR)

  A system developed to report blood coagulation (clotting)

Reported for each 90 days

  Initial service must include a minimum of 8 assessments

  Subsequent service must include at least 3 assessments

Any period less than 60 days is not reported

Medical Team Conferences (99366-99368)

Management of complex cases involving individuals, such as

  Hospice patient

  Patient who is homebound and receives majority of health care from visiting nurse

Reported when a team of at least 3 different specialists meet to discuss

  Revising care plan

  Coordinating treatment plan with other professionals

  Adjusting therapies

  Face-to-face with patient and/or family—**99366**

    Participation by nonphysician qualified health care professional

    30 minutes or more

  Without patient and/or family—**99367**

    Participation by physician

    30 minutes or more

  Without patient and/or family—**99368**

    Participation by nonphysician qualified health care professional

    30 minutes or more

PRACTICE 11A, CASE MANAGEMENT SERVICES (99363-99368)

These are time- and complexity-based codes, so no audit form is required. Once you have coded the two cases, check your answers in Appendix A.

Practice 11A, Report A

PHONE CALL

I spoke to the family today in conference. Present were 2 sons, 1 daughter and the patient's husband. The interdisciplinary team of 5 was present for the conference. We spoke in great detail about the prognosis of the patient and that the ongoing chemotherapy is not working and that decisions had to be made on behalf of the patient as far as code status. Besides the patient's stomach cancer with mets to the lungs, she is also deteriorating in regards to chronic interstitial pneumonia along with CHF. We explained to the family that the patient should be put on comfort measures, maybe bringing in hospice.

We will meet in my office next week to discuss this further.

The patient's prognosis is very grim, but we have left the decision to family to decide the care of their mother/wife. The conference lasted 45 minutes.

ICD-9-CM:

A. 99366; V66.7, 151.9, 197.0, 428.0, 515

B. 99367; V65.49, 151.9, 197.0, 428.1, 515

C. 99368; V66.7, 151.9, 197.0, 428.0, 515

D. 99366; V65.49, 151.9, 197.0, 428.0, 515

ICD-10-CM:

A. 99366; Z51.5, C16.9, C78.00, I50.9, J84.10

B. 99367; Z71.89, C16.9, C78.00, I50.1, J84.10

C. 99368; Z51.5, C16.9, C78.00, I50.9, J84.10

D. 99366; Z71.89, C16.9, C78.00, I50.9, J84.10

Practice 11A, Report B

TEAM CONFERENCE

This is an 87-year-old female who was discharged from the Rehabilitation Center to the Lilly Basic Care Facility. She was admitted with the diagnosis of nephritis and previous right below-the-knee amputation acquired. An interdisciplinary team of 4 met to discuss the best plan for this patient. No family was in attendance during the conference.

The patient's goal was to improve with her strength and overall health status. The patient has shown improvement with both her health status cares and mobility. At this time, she is ambulatory with the wheeled walker and her prosthesis and moderately independent. She is managing well enough at this time with mobility, transfers, and toileting to be a candidate for transition to a basic care facility. The basic care facility will provide assistance with bathing, meals, housekeeping, and medication monitoring. A physical therapy exercise program is planned. The patient does receive renal dialysis 3 days a week for her ESRD and will continue dialysis on Tuesday, Thursday, and Saturdays. She will receive her IV antibiotic dosing during her dialysis treatments under the direction of pharmacy. Dial-A-Ride has been arranged for transport for her Tuesday and Thursday appointments at dialysis and family will assist with transport for Saturday dialysis appointments. A referral has been made through County Social Service to assess eligibility for vouchers for the Saturday Dial-A-Ride. Referral information was faxed to the basic care facility on the day of discharge as requested. Family did provide transport at discharge. Time spent on conference was 60 minutes.

Codes:_____

PRACTICE 11B, ANTICOAGULANT MANAGEMENT

These are time- and complexity-based codes, so no audit form is required. Once you have coded the two cases, check your answers in Appendix A.

Practice 11B, Report A

LOCATION: Outpatient

Patient was initially seen in the office to establish an anticoagulant regimen. The patient had some high risk of clot formation, so the initial INR needed to be higher and he was started at 3.3. The tests and instruction were discussed with the patient. He returned for INR measurements and adjustment of his medications 9 times during the initial 3 months of therapy.

A. 99363

B. 99363, 99364

C. 99364

D. 99364, 99363

Practice 11B, Report B

LOCATION: Outpatient

The patient has been responding well to the initial 3 months of therapy and his dosage of warfarin was reduced significantly to 2.5 at the end of the initial 3-month treatment period. He was then seen once a month for the next 3 months for 3 INR measurements. He responded well to treatment and his coagulation rates were within normal limits.

Codes:_____

The patient presented for warfarin therapy due to acute deep vein thrombosis of the lower legs.

12. CARE PLAN OVERSIGHT SERVICES (99374-99380)

Codes are divided according to the supervision provided to the patient being cared for by

Home health agency

Hospice

Nursing facility

Time-based codes

15-29 minutes

30 minutes or more

Reporting is by time over a month

One individual may report the code per month

Reports physician or other qualified health care professional supervision of patient for a 30 day period, when patient is not present

Patient resides in

Own home

Rest home or domiciliary

Includes assisted living facility or hospice

For patients under

Home health care (99374-99375)

Hospice (99377-99378)

Nursing facility services (99379-99380)

Qualified health care professional provides the following types of services

Reviews subsequent reports, laboratory studies, or other studies

Integrates new data into patient's care plan

Adjusts medical therapy

Develops or revises care plans

Communicates with other health care professionals

PRACTICE 12, CARE PLAN OVERSIGHT SERVICES (99374-99380)

Once you have coded the two cases, check your answers in Appendix A.

Practice 12, Report A

Care plan review of 77-year-old female in the local nursing facility. Patient suffers from advanced ovarian cancer and is currently receiving chemotherapy. Spoke with gynecologist and patient seems to be doing well with current treatments, although has increased pain. Per nurse's remarks in chart, patient seems to have increased edema in the lower extremities. Plan includes continuing with current dose of chemotherapy per gynecologist, IV morphine infusion for pain, and IV diuretics for edema. After reviewing her labs, I have ordered Aranesp 100 mcg if her hemoglobin drops below 12, currently it is 12.4. Documentation includes review of chart, nurse's remarks noted and medication adjustments of patient's care plan. Total time spent this month formulating care plan was 40 minutes.

ICD-9-CM:

A. 99367, 99380; 183.0, 338.3, 782.3

B. 99380; 183.0, 338.3, 782.3

C. 99308; V58.11, 183.0, 338.3, 782.3

D. 99380; V58.11, 183.0

ICD-10-CM:

A. 99367, 99380; C56.9, G89.3, R60.0

B. 99380; C56.9, G89.3, R60.0

C. 99308; Z51.11, C56.9, G89.3, R60.0

D. 99380; Z51.11, C56.9

Practice 12, Report B

CARE PLAN OVERSIGHT

Care plan oversight for terminal care of a 78-year-old male hospice patient with advanced lower lobe lung cancer. Plan includes continuous oxygen and pain control management involving IV morphine infusion. Have had contact with nurses, family members, and patient's social worker. Phone conference with patient's family to discuss concerns of continuing supportive care that the patient wishes to discontinue. Documentation includes review and modification of patient's care plan and orders to pharmacy. Total time spent this month formulating care plan was 45 minutes.

Codes:_____

13. PREVENTIVE MEDICINE SERVICES (99381-99429)

There are two categories under Preventive Medicine Services

Preventive Medicine Services (99381-99397)

Counseling Risk Factor Reduction and Behavior Change Intervention (99401-99429)

Preventive Medicine Services (99381-99397)

Reports routine E/M for patient who is healthy and has no complaints

Used to identify comprehensive services, not a single-system examination

Such as an annual gynecologic examination

Codes based on age and if new or established patient

If physician encounters a problem or abnormality that requires significant additional service during preventative service

Report appropriate level office visit code with modifier -25

Code descriptions indicate terms "comprehensive history" and "comprehensive examination" are used

Not same definition as in 99201-99350

Comprehensive means a complete history and a complete examination appropriate for age/gender

Examination is a multi-system examination

Extent of examination is determined by age of patient and risk factors for patient

Counseling Risk Factor Reduction and Behavior Change Intervention (99401-99429)

Both new and established healthy patients

Based on whether individual or group counseling is provided and time spent in service

Used to report professional services to a patient for risk factor interventional counseling

Codes used to report services focused on promoting health and preventing illness/injury

Patient does NOT have symptoms or an established illness

If patient does have symptoms or an established illness, report service with appropriate E/M code

Examples

Diet and exercise program

Smoking cessation

Contraceptive management

PRACTICE 13, PREVENTIVE MEDICINE SERVICES

These are age-based codes, so no audit form is required. Once you have coded the two cases, check your answers in Appendix A.

Practice 13, Report A

SUBJECTIVE: This is an established 43-year-old white female, four previous pregnancies, two children, in today for a GYN exam and Pap smear with her annual physical exam. Her only concern is weight gain over the last couple of years. She had tried switching her antidepressant medicine from Zoloft to Wellbutrin and reacted very severely to the Wellbutrin. She is now back on Zoloft which she is aware can increase appetite. She has never tried portion control and increased exercise. She has generalized body aches.

CURRENT BIRTH CONTROL METHOD: She had a hysterectomy.

OTHER MEDICATIONS: 1. Protonix. 2. Lipitor. 3. Zoloft

ALLERGIES: Poppy seeds.

IMMUNIZATIONS: Tetanus and flu shot are up to date.

MENSTRUAL HISTORY: Hysterectomy for a bicornuate uterus. The cervix was adhesed on to the bladder so the cervical stub was left. Last Pap smear was August 2 years ago. Pap smears are being done every 2 to 4 years.

MEDICAL HISTORY, SOCIAL HISTORY, AND FAMILY HISTORY are unchanged since her last appointment. Please refer to consultation.

REVIEW OF SYSTEMS: No current HEENT, respiratory, cardiovascular, or breast problems. Irritable bowel symptoms are relieved by diet and Protonix. Multiple musculoskeletal problems related to bursitis and hip and back pain. No neurological, endocrine, or integumentary problems. Depression symptoms are well controlled by Zoloft.

PHYSICAL EXAMINATION: Declines the presence of a chaperone in the room today. Blood pressure: 106/66. Weight: 189. Height: 5 feet 5 inches. Thyroid is normal to palpation without enlargement. Cervical nodes are negative. Lungs are clear to auscultation without rates or wheezes. Heart: Regular rate and rhythm without murmurs. Breasts are normal to inspection and bilaterally symmetrical. Normal to palpation. No nipple discharge. Negative axillary nodes. Negative CVAT. Abdomen is soft without organomegaly or hernia. Vulva is normal to inspection. Normal hair distribution. Negative BUS. Negative inguinal nodes. Vagina has a scant amount of creamy discharge. Cervix is normal. A Pap smear was obtained. Bimanual exam shows no masses. Skin is warm and dry. Distal pulses are equal. No edema of the extremities.

ASSESSMENT:
1. Gynecologic examination with Pap.
2. Health maintenance issues.

PLAN:
1. We will notify her of her Pap within 2 weeks.
2. She will schedule a mammogram in the near future. Fasting lab work has all been done within the last 2 years.
3. Return to the clinic p.r.n. and for GYN care.

ICD-9-CM:

A. 99396; V70.0, V72.31, V76.47

B. 99213; V70.0, 783.1

C. 99386; 783.1, 311

D. 99395; V70.0

ICD-10-CM:

A. 99396; Z00.00, Z01.419, Z12.72

B. 99213; Z00.00, R63.5

C. 99386; R63.5, F32.9

D. 99395; Z00.00

Practice 13, Report B

Patient is a 44-year-old white female who comes to our office this afternoon for a yearly physical. She denies any active complaints. She is established with our clinic.

PMH: None.

PSH: Tubal ligation in 1982.

MEDICATIONS: None.

ALLERGIES: NKA.

SOCIAL HISTORY: She has smoked one pack of cigarettes per day for the last 20 years. She denies any history of alcohol or drug abuse. She is married and has three adult children. Her husband is currently in the service. She lives alone at home.

FAMILY HISTORY: Her father died at age 62 from unknown reasons. Her mother died at age 35 from unknown reasons. She has three brothers and one sister who are in good health.

PE: Declines the presence of a chaperone in the room today. Blood pressure: 108/78. Weight: 228 pounds. Height: 5 feet 5 inches. Thyroid is normal to palpation without enlargement. Cervical nodes are negative. Lungs are clear to auscultation without rates or wheezes. Heart: Regular rate and rhythm without murmurs. Breasts are normal to inspection and bilaterally symmetrical. Normal to palpation.

No nipple discharge. Negative axillary nodes. Abdomen is soft without organomegaly or hernia. Vulva is normal to inspection. Normal hair distribution. Negative BUS. Negative inguinal nodes. Vagina is clean with a scant amount of creamy discharge. On opening of the speculum to visualize the cervix, the patient complains of some discomfort and there is a slight amount of oozing at the posterior aspect of the cervical apex under the cervical stump. A Pap smear was obtained. Bimanual exam shows tenderness with deep penetration into the vagina and tenderness with cervical stump movement anteriorly. No masses palpated in the cul-de-sac or with bimanual exam. Skin is warm and dry. Distal pulses are equal. No edema of the extremities.

ASSESSMENT/PLAN:
1. Yearly physical done today with GYN examination.
2. Smoking cessation, tobacco dependence.

I talked to the patient about quitting smoking and she told me she has been thinking about it and will try. We will get a CBC, fasting CMP, fasting lipid panel, TSH, UA, EKG, chest x-ray, mammogram and stool occult cards ×3. The patient is scheduled for a follow-up visit in 1 month.

Codes:_____

14. NON-FACE-TO-FACE SERVICES (99441-99444); SPECIAL E/M SERVICES (99450-99456); AND OTHER E/M SERVICES (99499)

Non-Face-to-Face Services (99441-99444)

Report physician E/M services using the telephone or internet

99441-99443 used to report telephone E/M services

Provided to an established patient, family member of the patient, or a guardian

Cannot originate from an E/M service within the previous 7 days

Cannot lead to an E/M service within the next 24 hours or the next available urgent appointment

Reported based on the time documented in the medical record

99444 reports online E/M services

Provided to an established patient, family member of the patient, or a guardian

Cannot originate from an E/M service within the previous 7 days

Cannot lead to an E/M service within the next 24 hours or the next available appointment

Special E/M Services (99450-99456)

Reports examination for life, work, or disability insurance

Establishes patient health baseline information

Provided in office or other setting

Reported for both new and established patients

If other E/M services provided the same day

Report additional service with appropriate E/M code(s)

99455 reports examination by treating physician

99456 reports examination by other than treating physician

Other E/M Services (99499)

99499 reports unlisted E/M services

Accompanied by a special report

PRACTICE 14, NON-FACE-TO-FACE SERVICES; SPECIAL E/M SERVICES; AND OTHER E/M SERVICES

No audit form is required for these codes. Once you have coded the two cases, check your answers in Appendix A.

Practice 14, Report A

DISABILITY ASSESSMENT

This patient has suffered neck and low back injuries from an automobile accident. We determined from her Spinal Disability Evaluation that she has a Spinal Disability Rating of 50%.

Lost Pre-Injury Capacity: Disability precluding heavy lifting, repeated bending, stooping, and crawling. This individual has also lost approximately HALF of her pre-injury capacity of lifting, bending, stooping, and crawling.

Patient will continue with the prescribed chronic pain management regimen and ongoing physical therapy 3 times a week.

ICD-9-CM:

A. 99455; 723.1, 724.2, 846.8, E819.9

B. 99456; 723.1, 724.2, 905.7, E920.0

C. 99456; 723.1, 724.2, 846.8, E819.9

D. 99455; 723.1, 724.2, 338.21, 905.7, E929.0

ICD-10-CM:

A. 99455; M54.2, M54.5, S33.8XXA, V89.2XXA

B. 99456; M54.2, M54.5, S33.8XXS, W28.XXXS

C. 99456; M54.2, M54.5, S338XXA, V89.2XXA

D. 99455; M54.2, M54.5, G89.21, S33.8XXS, X58.XXXS

Practice 14, Report B

DISABILITY ASSESSMENT

This is a 42-year-old man who has been disabled due to work-related trauma injury for about 6 months now. He is unable to use his hands or arms in any type of lifting due to carpal tunnel syndrome. Patient still has pain status post surgery.

The patient's pain level today is 7 out of 10. He will continue with his prescribed medication at the current dosage. I will also consult physical therapy to strengthen his arms. I will see this patient back after his first treatment in therapy.

Completion of performance examination has been completed.

Codes:_____

15. NEWBORN CARE SERVICES (99460-99465)

99460-99463 reports initial and subsequent care in or in other than hospital/birthing center

> For normal newborn infant, birth through 28 days

> Reported per day

99463 reports initial hospital/birthing center when admission and discharge are same day

Newborn assessment includes Apgar assessment at 1 minute and 5 minutes after delivery

> Physician assesses

> Muscle tone (activity)

> Heart rate (pulse)

> Reflex response (grimace)

> Color (appearance)

> Breathing (respiration)

Each assessment area is assigned a rating of 0 to 2

Recorded on the newborn's medical record

Delivery/Birthing Room Attendance and Resuscitation Services (99464-99465)

99464 reports attendance at delivery

> Requested by delivering physician

> Request for attendance must be documented in medical record

> Provides initial stabilization

99465, resuscitation and ventilation

Attendance and resuscitation codes are not reported together

PRACTICE 15, NEWBORN CARE SERVICES

Once you have coded the two cases, check your answers in Appendix A.

Practice 15, Report A

36-week male born at 1:27 AM by vaginal delivery. APGAR 8/9. Disorganized suck, but once eating, takes 10-20 cc per feeding. Patient has (+) urine and stool output. Patient is discharged from the hospital the same day at 7:30 PM.

ICD-9-CM:

A. 99463; V30.1, 779.31

B. 99234; V30.1

C. 99234; V30.00, 779.31

D. 99463; V30.00

ICD-10-CM:

A. 99463; Z38.1, P92.2

B. 99234; Z38.1

C. 99234; Z38.00, P92.2

D. 99463; Z38.00

Practice 15, Report B

	Normal	Abnormal	NEWBORN EXAM RECORD ADMISSION EXAM Comments Date: 07/28/XX	Normal	Abnormal	DISCHARGE EXAM Comments Date:
Head/Fontanels		✓	Scalp bruised due to birth injury			
Eyes	✓					
Ears/Nose/Throat	✓					
Heart	✓					
Lungs	✓					
Abdomen	✓					
Trunk/Spine	✓					
Anus	✓					
Genitalia	✓					
Negative Barlow Test	✓					
Negative Ortolani Test	✓					
Extremities/Clavicles	✓					
Skin	✓					
Neurological/Tone	✓					

PROGRESS NOTES: 07/29/XX

Day two: Vitals stable, afebrile. Exam is unchanged.	
(+) urine and stool. Weight is up 2.3%.	
Continue normal newborn care.	

Codes:_____

16. OTHER

Neonatal and Pediatric Critical Care Services (99466-99480)

Pediatric Critical Care Patient Transport (99466, 99467 and 99485, 99486)

- 99466, 99467
- First 30-74 minutes
- Each additional 30 minutes
- 99485, 99486
- First 30 minutes and each additional 30 minutes
- Supervision by a control physician of transport

Reports interfacility transport (this is transport from one facility to another and not a step down unit)

- Critically ill or injured patient

Patients that are 24 months or less

Services provided face-to-face with the patient

Inpatient Neonatal Critical Care (99468, 99469)

Divided by
- Initial day
- Subsequent day

Critically ill neonate

Age 28 days or younger

Inpatient Pediatric Critical Care (99471-99476)

Inpatient services

Divided by age
- 29 days-24 months
- 2-5 years

Subdivided on day
- Initial
- Subsequent

Initial and Continuing Intensive Care Services (99477-99480)

Hospital Care

Divided on
- Age
  - 28 days or younger
- Birth weight
  - Very low birth weight (VLBW) ≤1500 grams (≤3.3 pounds)
  - Low birth weight (LBW) 1500-2500 grams (3.31-5.5 pounds)
  - Normal birth weight 2501-5000 grams (5.51-11.01 pounds)

Subdivided on day

   Initial

   Subsequent

Complex Chronic Care Coordination

- Codes 99487-99489 report complex chronic care coordination

   Based on if face-to-face

   Reported for first hour of service and each additional 30 minutes

Transitional Care Management Services

- Codes 99495 and 99496 report transitional management codes

   Based on:

     ○ Number of days after discharge from a medical facility

     ○ Medical decision making complexity (moderate or high)

PRACTICE 16, OTHER

These are time-based codes, so no audit form is required. Once you have coded the two cases, check your answers in Appendix A.

Practice 16A, Report A

The physician accompanies a 13-month-old critical-care patient during transport from one hospital to another. The documented time spent was 1 ½ hours with the patient in the first hospital, 2 hours transporting the patient to the second hospital.

A. 99479, 99467 ×2

B. 99466, 99467 ×5

C. 99466, 99467 ×2

D. 99291, 99292, 99466, 99467

Practice 16A, Report B

Total of 2 hours, 40 minutes spent with 18-month-old burn patient burned by hot liquid that went into shock. Patient was being transported to The Children's Burn Center by air flight.

Codes:_____

Practice 16B, Report A

NICU INPATIENT PROGRESS NOTE

S: No acute events overnight, brief cardiac bradycardia arrhythmia, sleep study overnight

O: Resp: Rate: 32-76   Exam: Upper airway congestion
          CV: Rate: 94-154   Map: 50-69
                        Exam: RRR, good perfusion
          FEN/GI: I: 630   TF: 134   Wt: 4696 grams
          O: 345
                        Exam: Soft NT ND with +BS
          HEME: none
          GU: Within normal limits.
          ID: Temp Max: 36.7
          Cultures: none
          NEURO:
                        Exam: warm, no edema. Alert and appropriate, good tone

A/P: 2 month 1 wk old male was admitted for a unilateral, incarcerated inguinal hernia and subsequently developed acute pneumonia. Sleep study done yesterday. Continue to monitor perfusion. Continue with 22 kcal feedings.

ICD-9-CM:

A. No code; post-operative global period

B. 99231; 764.09, V45.89, 550.10

C. 99480; 550.10, 486, 427.89

D. 99480; 550.10, 486, V45.89

ICD-10-CM:

A. No code; post-operative global period

B. 99231; Z98.89, K40.30

C. 99480; K40.30, J18.9, R00.1

D. 99480; K40.30, J18.9, Z98.89

Practice 16B, Report B

NICU INPATIENT

S: Quiet night

O: Resp: Rate: 26-73   Exam: Lungs clear
CV: Rate: 131-174   Map: 44-51
Exam:
FEN/GI: I: 250   TF: Wt: 2100 grams
O: 138
Exam: Abd soft with +BS
HEME:
ID: Temp Max: 37
Cultures: 0
NEURO:
Exam: AF soft, ext: good tone

A/P: 55 day old, 27 week premature, resp stable, PE benign. Occ desats monitor. Follow up echo this week to look at coronary arteries. Monitor weight.

Codes:_____

UNIT 2

Examination

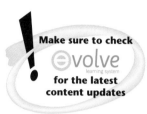

Make sure to check
evolve *learning system*
for the latest
content updates

EXAMINATION, REPORT 1

LOCATION: Shady Lane Nursing Facility
Nursing Facility Admission

HISTORY
Chief Complaint: Dementia, Primary, Parkinson's disease, and inability to care for self.

HISTORY OF CHIEF COMPLAINT: (Obtained mostly from the patient's guardian and wife of 27 years, Margaret.) The patient's wife relates that the patient was diagnosed in 2001 at Community General with Alzheimer's dementia that has progressively worsened. In addition, he has also had a 10-year history of Parkinson's disease. He is very unsteady on his feet and has recurrent falls. He is also Type II insulin-requiring diabetic. He also has urinary incontinence.

The wife, until recently, had been having an aide come in twice a week to assist with showering and activities of daily living of the patient. An RN was also coming in twice a week to check on his medications and diabetic status. Unfortunately, the falls have progressively worsened and the wife is becoming overwhelmed by the need now for 24-hr-care. He has also become more assaultive and is exhibiting inappropriate behaviors. It should be noted he was placed on Prozac and the wife indicates he responded well in terms of his inappropriate behaviors. In addition to his other signs and symptoms, he has now developed some sundowning. All of these have culminated in the need for admission to this nursing facility.

CURRENT MEDICATIONS: Bumex 0.5 mg daily, Celexa 20 mg daily, Sinemet 25 -100 mg tid, Humulin 70/30 insulin 30 units in AM.

MEDICAL HISTORY: Surgeries—myocardial infarction 6 years ago with stenting at Community General.

ILLNESSES: Myocardial infarction 6 years ago, diabetes mellitus type II—approximately 15 years, Parkinson's disease—approximately 15 years.

ALLERGIES: NO KNOWN DRUG ALLERGIES.

FAMILY HISTORY: Mother and father both died in their 70's. The remainder of the family history is not really known by the patient or the wife.

SOCIAL HISTORY: He has a 10th grade education. He served in the US Navy in World War II. A previous marriage ended in divorce. His current marriage, as noted, has been for 27 years. There are no biologic children from either of the marriages.

REVIEW OF SYSTEMS

Gastrointestinal: Good appetite; no reported nausea, vomiting, melena, fecal incontinence, or hematochezia. Genitourinary: He had long-standing incontinence but no reported dysuria or gross hematuria. Cardiovascular: As noted above; sleeps on 1 pillow. No paroxysmal nocturnal dyspnea. He has intermittent dependent edema. Neuromuscular: As noted above; he has severely impaired balance and has had frequent falls. No fractures. Respiratory: As noted above. Habits: Cigarettes—20 to 30 pack-a-year history of nicotine abuse; stopped about 20 years ago. Alcohol—history of abuse that he also stopped about 20 years ago.

PHYSICAL EXAMINATION

General: This is a very pleasant, well-nourished, well-developed Caucasian male who appears his stated age. He's reasonably alert. His speech is clear and fairly fluent. He knows the year, but doesn't know his exact birth date. He's a somewhat inconsistent historian. He recalls remote events more easily than any short-term memories.

HEENT: Head—normocephalic with male pattern baldness. Eyes—pupils are slightly myotic but reactive. Extraocular movements are intact. Sclerae are non-icteric. Conjunctivae are non-injected. Fundi suggest arteriolar narrowing without any obvious hemorrhages or exudates. No papilledema. Ears—otic canals are cerumen-filled bilaterally. Face is symmetrical. There's evidence of some actinic keratoses. Mouth/Throat—lips, tongue, and mucous membranes are moist. Tongue is in the midline. He has multiple indigenous teeth, but there are many absent teeth. There's a suggestion of halitosis. Neck: Supple; thyroid gland is not palpable. Carotid upstrokes are satisfactory. No overt delays or bruits noted. Lymphadenopathy is not evident in the neck and supraclavicular region. Cervical neck veins are non-distended. Chest/Lung: Symmetrical and moves symmetrically with inspiration and expiration. No thrills or heaves. Rate and rhythm are regular. There's a faint grade 2/6 aortic ejection murmur radiating along the left sternal border without any concomitant 53 or 54 gallops. Lungs reveal some dry crackles in the right lower lobe. Abdomen: Round, non-distended, and non-tender. No scars visible. No inguinal hernias noted. Liver, spleen, kidneys, and urinary bladder are not palpably enlarged. Normal bowel sounds. No abdominal or flank bruits. Genitalia: External- penis is uncircumcised with normal scrotal contents. Rectal: Digital exam—anal sphincter is tonic. The prostate gland is slightly atrophic and smooth. There's a moderate amount of semi-solid, light brown stool in the rectal vault. Hemoccult is obtained. Extremities: There is +1/+4 bilateral pitting pretibial and ankle edema. Dorsalis pedis and posterior tibial pulses are not palpable. Popliteals are trace/+4 on the right and +1/+4 on the left. Neurologic: Deep tendon reflexes are hypoactive but symmetrical. He's not exhibiting any drooling or tremor at this time. He has positive cogwheel rigidity.

MINI-MENTAL STATE: He can only recall 2 out of 3 objects within one minute. He is unable to spell the word "world" backwards. He cannot do any simple arithmetic problems. It is obvious that this gentleman is not capable of making decisions regarding his personal, medical, or financial affairs.

IMPRESSIONS:
1. Alzheimer's dementia.
2. Parkinson's disease.
3. Diabetes mellitus type II.
4. Arteriosclerotic heart disease, native arteries
    a. History of myocardial infarction—stented 7 years ago at Community General.
5. Urinary incontinence.
6. Seborrhea.
7. Actinic keratoses.
8. Peripheral vascular disease.
He is now being admitted to this nursing facility due to DM.

PLAN: The patient is to have a Do Not Resuscitate code status. The patient will be assessed by the doctor in the Musculoskeletal Clinic for PT/OT evaluation. Glucoscan monitors will be instituted. We'll monitor renal function and serum electrolytes in light of the diuretic therapy. It certainly appears he's, possibly, exhibiting increased signs of left ventricular failure and we'll certainly increase the Bumex dosage.

The goals for this gentleman are to provide a reasonably safe and secure environment and maximize his comfort in life. He's functioning at a fairly high level for a dementia individual and may very well integrate pretty well into the unit and facility with participation in those activities for which he's capable of appreciating and enjoying, as well as interacting with his peers and members of the staff. General medical status is fair at this time. Unfortunately, the overall prognosis in this gentleman with irreversible neurologic disorders superimposed on significant comorbidities, certainly, doesn't portend well for long-term life expectancy.

Codes:_____

EXAMINATION, REPORT 2

LOCATION: Outpatient, Hospital
Patient clearance for left heart catheterization.

INDICATION: Abnormal stress test with exercise intolerance. Pre-op consultation requested by Dr. Cardiologist for medical clearance.

HISTORY OF PRESENT ILLNESS: The patient is a very pleasant 61-year-old gentleman, past medical history significant for unstable angina, multivessel coronary disease. After identifying multivessel coronary disease at cardiac catheterization, the patient went on to 5-vessel coronary artery bypass grafting surgery. Surgery performed in June included LIMA to LAD, saphenous vein graft to OM-1, reverse saphenous vein graft to PDA at junction of PDA and PLV with extension to the main body of the right coronary artery. Utilization of PADCAB (perfusion assisted direct coronary artery bypass) for infusion of graft during the off pump coronary bypass grafting surgery and utilization of VasoView for harvesting leg vein for saphenous vein graft was performed.

Shortly thereafter the patient underwent exercise treadmill stress testing with complaints of exercise intolerance. The patient underwent exercise treadmill stress testing in August where he was found to have functional capacity class II/III under modified Bruce protocol.

Double product (this is the systolic blood pressure times the heart rate) was 26,280, disproportionately elevated from a minimal amount of physical exertion and provocation, challenged the patient by modified Bruce protocol stress test.

The patient did exercise 9 minutes at 1.7 miles per hour, 10% grade maximum, METs 4. Initial heart rate 74 beats per minute, reached a maximum of 147 beats per minute, 98% maximum predicted heart rate for age with initial blood pressure of 150/86 and a maximum of 180/82. There was appropriate heart rate and blood pressure response to exercise and the treadmill stress test was discontinued once maximum heart rate achieved. There was clear evidence of disproportionate amount of fatigue, exercise intolerance to the minimal amount of stress challenge given patient. There was no chest pain. No significant electrocardiogram changes were found.

He went on to imaging which showed ejection fraction of 54%, no significant regional wall motion abnormalities, mixed largely reversible perfusion defect at the lateral wall involving the base and reversible perfusion defect, apex extending to the inferior wall and a mild anterior wall perfusion defect.

The patient now presents for consideration of a left heart catheterization.

REVIEW OF SYSTEMS: The patient has had intermittent chest pain and some dyspnea on exertion.

PHYSICAL EXAMINATION: Well-developed, well-nourished gentleman, alert and oriented to time, place, and person. Mood congruent, affect appropriate, goal oriented speech. VITAL SIGNS: Reveal BLOOD PRESSURE of 140/80, HEART RATE 80, RESPIRATIONS 14 per minute. The patient is afebrile. HEAD, EYES, EARS, NOSE, AND THROAT: Unremarkable. HEART: Reveals regular rate and rhythm. LUNGS: Clear. ABDOMEN: Benign.

LABORATORY STUDIES: CBC shows a white count of 4.3, hemoglobin of 9.6, chronically anemic. Hematocrit is 31.1, platelets 198,000. The patient has microcytic, hypochromic anemia with an MCV of 76, MCH of 23, MCHC of 31. Basic metabolic profile shows sodium of 138, potassium of 4.1, chloride of 105, bicarb 26, BUN 13, creatinine 1.2, glucose 133, calcium 8.4, GFR greater than 60. PT, INR is 10.4, 1.0 respectively. PTT is 23.1 baseline. Normal differential and CBC.

IMPRESSION: 61-year-old gentleman status post multivessel coronary artery bypass grafting surgery after coronary disease identified, now with exercise intolerance on cardiolite stress testing, evaluated for left heart catheterization. Has medical clearance for left heart catheterization, cardiologist notified.

Codes:_____

EXAMINATION, REPORT 3

LOCATION: Outpatient, Office

I was asked to see Mr. W. for consultation by Dr. Jones for treatment recommendations for continuing right knee pain. The following is a summary of my findings and recommendations.

SUBJECTIVE: The patient is a 71-year-old white male, new patient, who presents complaining of right knee pain. This has been ongoing for a few months. When he goes to pivot on his knee he is having buckling and giving way. He was coming out of his pickup truck a couple of weeks ago when his knee did give way and he felt a "pop." He is not having any swelling to speak of, but he has the same problems stair climbing and he does feel unstable. He denies any paresthesias.

PAST MEDICAL HISTORY: Significant for coronary artery disease, cardiac arrhythmia, hypercholesterolemia, hypertension, reflux, right inguinal hernia, Dupuytren's disease.

His current medications are:
1. Atenolol 50 mg three tablets daily
2. Coumadin 2 mg daily
3. Cozaar 50 mg daily
4. Prilosec 20 mg daily
5. Aspirin 81 mg daily
6. Pravachol 80 mg daily
7. Lopid 600 mg bid
8. IMDUR daily, dose unknown
9. Nitro sublingual on a prn basis

PAST SURGICAL HISTORY: Significant for coronary artery bypass grafting, coronary stenting ×3, right inguinal herniorrhaphy repair, and bilateral Dupuytren's contracture release.

REVIEW OF SYSTEMS: The history form was reviewed. Neurologic: denies any history of seizure disorder, tinnitus, and vertigo. Cardiovascular: positive for coronary disease, occasional chest pain, positive for essential hypertension, controlled. No lower extremity edema. GI: positive for gastroesophageal reflux disease, but no change in bowel habits, weight loss or gain. GU: no frequency, dysuria, hematuria, but does complain of nocturia ×2. Constitutional, ophthalmologic, otolaryngologic, respiratory, musculoskeletal, integumentary, psychiatric, endocrine, hematologic, and immunologic were negative.

PHYSICAL EXAM: Well developed, well-nourished white male 5′ 8″ in height and 200 pounds. BP: 176/86, pulse: 60, respiratory rate: 24, temperature: 97.3. He has a genu varus deformity of the right knee with atrophy of his right quadriceps, which is mild. He has a positive McMurray's medially, equivocal anterior drawer, negative posterior drawer, medial joint line tenderness, no lateral joint line tenderness is noted. The left knee has 5/5 quadriceps strength, very minimal Grade I valgus deformity, no varus instability. Negative McMurray's medially or laterally.

X-RAYS: Standing AP, as well as sunrise, notch, and lateral views of the right knee. There is a mild genu varus deformity of the right knee of about 5 to 10 degrees with total loss of joint space in the medial femoral compartment. Lateral view shows spurring on the superior and inferior poles of the patella with decreased joint space in the patellofemoral compartment. The notch view shows chondromalacia and varus deformity of the right knee, chondromalacia in the lateral femoral compartment. Primary osteoarthrosis of right knee.

Review of the MRI, which is accompanying the patient, reveals a very large tear of the posterior horn of the medial meniscus as well as chondromalacia in the patellofemoral compartment, large medial plica, and cysts noted in the anterior and posterior horns of the lateral meniscus.

ASSESSMENT:
1. Degenerative joint disease.
2. Meniscal tears medial and lateral femoral compartments with associated genu varus deformity, injury a couple of weeks ago.
3. Coronary artery disease.
4. Pure hypercholesterolemia.

PLAN: The patient will need arthroscopic intervention in the hopes of saving the knee. I did explain to him that we would not be able to give him 100% relief, probably because of the chronicity of the problem and the medial femoral compartment is pretty much at this point Grade IV chondromalacia in several spots with bare bone "kissing lesions" noted. He will need medical clearance/

consultation prior to any surgical intervention and will probably have to get a preoperative INR level and stop the Coumadin 1 to 2 days prior to surgical intervention and repeat the PT INR the day of surgery. This will be under general anesthetic and he will be placed back on Coumadin postoperatively. We also gave him Celebrex samples 200 mg once daily, which he can take while taking Coumadin. He can take his Tylenol with this. Continue his regular medication.

Thank you for allowing me to evaluate your patient. If you have any questions don't hesitate to call.

Dr. Jones notified of findings and recommendations.

Codes:_____

EXAMINATION, REPORT 4

LOCATION: Emergency Department

CHIEF COMPLAINT: Sore throat.

HISTORY OF PRESENT ILLNESS
This is a 53-year-old female with history of bipolar disorder who has had 5-7 days of sore throat, constitutional symptoms, generalized aches and some fatigue. She has had no fever. Some slight cough but no shortness of breath. No abdominal pain. No other complaints at this time. She comes for evaluation today.

Please see nursing notes for medications and allergies.

ROS
The patient has had no fever or weight loss. Has had some fullness of the ears. No SOB. No rashes.

SOCIAL HISTORY
The patient does not smoke and only consumes occasional alcohol.

PHYSICAL EXAMINATION
Blood pressure 128/68, respirations 20, afebrile. She is an alert, pleasant female in no apparent distress. HEENT—clear tympanic membranes bilaterally. Oropharynx has some slight posterior oropharyngeal erythema. There is no exudate. There is no mass or asymmetry. She has nasopharynx and oropharynx cobblestoning with postnasal drip. Neck supple. Cervical lymphadenopathy. Heart regular. Lungs clear to auscultation bilaterally.

EMERGENCY DEPARTMENT COURSE
It was felt that this represented a viral pharyngitis. Recommended continued symptomatic care. Motrin, warm salt water gargles. Administered 200 mg oral Motrin. Return for any problems. Follow up with primary care physician. She is agreeable with this plan. Discharged home in stable condition.

PROVISIONAL DIAGNOSIS/DIAGNOSES: Pharyngitis.

Codes:_____

EXAMINATION, REPORT 5

LOCATION: ED (Critical Care Service)

CHIEF COMPLAINT: Weakness, fever, mental status changes.

HISTORY OF PRESENT ILLNESS

The patient is an 83-year-old male with multiple medical problems who presents to the ED accompanied by his wife. Apparently has had increased lethargy and decreased level of consciousness for the last 3 days. Wife states it has been progressively worse, especially over the last 24 hours. She did notice several days ago that he would occasionally choke and cough on some food. He has had very little food over the last 24 hours. States he has been trying to up his fluid intake. She denies any recent trauma, other than falling and hitting his buttocks up against the countertop. Denies chest pain. Has had no cough or abdominal pain or vomiting. He was brought to the ED for further evaluation and treatment.

ROS/SH/FH/PMH: Not able to obtain due to patient status. Please see supplemental sheet from what I could get from the chart.

MEDICATIONS/ALLERGIES: Please see nursing notes.

PHYSICAL EXAMINATION

Oral temperature 100.7F°, vitals as charted. General—this is an elderly male, ill-appearing. HEENT—mucous membranes appear dry. Neck is supple. Cardiac exam is regular. Chest—there is apparent asymmetry of the rales, best heard in the right base. No extra accessory muscle use. Chest wall is nontender. Pacemaker in place. Abdomen is soft, flat, and nontender. Neurologic—the patient does move all 4 extremities spontaneously. Appears somewhat fatigued. He is able to answer a few questions and converse. Integumentary—skin warm and dry. He has abrasions by the left lower extremity as well as the right buttock from a recent fall. Please see supplemental sheet for exam findings.

EMERGENCY DEPARTMENT COURSE

The patient was seen and evaluated by myself. IV access was established. He was given supplemental oxygen to keep his saturations in the mid-90 percents. He was placed on continuous cardiac monitor. A 12-lead EKG was obtained. This revealed a ventricularly paced rhythm, STEMI. His CMP reveals BUN 76, creatinine 3.1, total bilirubin 2.1, AST 43, and ALT 39. WBC 6.8, hemoglobin 10.0 (previous hemoglobins were in the 9 to 10 range), and he has had previous renal insufficiency. His INR is 3.2. Troponin is 7.64. BNP 1457. Digoxin level 2.0. Urinalysis does not reveal any white blood cells, negative leukocyte esterase and nitrite. He was given IV fluids. CT scan of the head was obtained and pending at time of this dictation. Blood and urine cultures were sent. Single-view chest radiograph has an apparent right-sided infiltrate. Administered IV Claforan and clindamycin, given his history of possible aspiration. Discussed the findings with the patient as well as his family members present, including his wife. Reviewed his labs and condition here. They did re-affirm he is a DNR/DNI (do not resuscitate/do not intubate). They understand that he has multiple organs that are failing at this point and that he is very sick, and that his condition very well could be terminal. He was admitted to monitored bed in guarded condition.

Cultures are pending, blood and urine.

PROVISIONAL DIAGNOSIS/DIAGNOSES

1. Acute febrile illness/acute mental status changes.
2. Pneumonia.
3. Acute renal failure.
4. Elevated troponin/myocardial infarction, acute.
5. Elevated BNP (elevated in cardiac disease).
6. Evaluation of dyspnea/hypoxemia.
   Critical care time 90 minutes.

Codes:_____

EXAMINATION, REPORT 6

LOCATION: Patient's Home

PATIENT: 89-year-old male

SUBJECTIVE: The patient is an 89-year-old gentleman who is cared for at home by his wife and attendant along with home health nurses. He has COPD and Parkinson's and has gotten over an episode of pneumonia. He has occasional anxiety episodes for which he takes Xanax with good relief. He sits up in a chair several times a week and is doing relatively well. He has minimal edema and his appetite is good. He has occasional coughing spells for which he uses a nebulizer with good results.

OBJECTIVE: He is afebrile. Pulse is 68 per minute and regular, respiratory rate is 18 per minute and unlabored. He is in no acute distress. He is somewhat lethargic today. Lungs are clear with no wheezes, rales or rhonchi. Heart demonstrates a regular rate and rhythm. Abdomen is soft, benign with no masses or tenderness. Extremities demonstrate no edema.

ASSESSMENT:
1. COPD.
2. Parkinson's.
3. Primary, osteoarthritis, severe, bilateral knees.

PLAN:
He will continue his current therapy. He has had excellent care with no break down or pressure sores at this point.

He will be seen again in 1 month.

Codes:_____

EXAMINATION, REPORT 7

LOCATION: Hospital, Inpatient

NEPHROLOGY/PROLONGED SERVICE PROGRESS NOTE:
CC: Pericardial Effusion

The patient was seen, examined, and evaluated multiple times. Discussions were held with him and his wife.

The patient did well overnight. He was making adequate amounts of urine. His blood pressure was maintained in the 130 range. Saturations were maintained in the high 90s on 3 liters per nasal cannula. I gave him 6 units of fresh frozen plasma and it brought his INR down to 1.7 this morning.

PHYSICAL EXAMINATION: He feels tired and weak. He has some chest pressure but no chest pain. He does not seem to be in any distress. He has good air entry bilaterally. He has a few crackles, if any, in the bases. ABDOMEN: Nontender. He has right IJ tunneled dialysis catheter. He does have slight generalized edema all over.

LABS TODAY: Phosphorus is 3.7, ionized calcium 4.2, INR 1.7. White count is 18.9, hemoglobin 8.9 grams and platelets 361,000. His BUN is 58, creatinine down to 1.5, sodium 131, potassium 4.1, chloride 97, glucose 151, albumin 3, alkaline phosphatase up to 190, total bilirubin 2.2, AST 279, ALT 350, bicarb 21.

IMPRESSION:
1. Pericardial effusion non-inflammatory, without tamponade yet.
2. Acute renal failure, improved.
3. Hyponatremia, improving.

4. Hypocalcemia secondary to blood transfusion.
5. Leukocytosis, improving.
6. Urinary tract infection.
7. Anemia chronic, secondary to subcutaneous bleeding and multiple blood draws in addition to the pericardial effusion.
8. Elevated liver function tests secondary to pericardial effusion most likely.

PLAN:

1. I attempted to contact his cardiologist twice this morning but I have been unsuccessful. I have talked to his nurse practitioner; she informed me that Cardiothoracic Surgery probably should be involved in the case. I have discussed the case with the patient's surgeon, and he indicated to me that the procedure could be done in our facility without any problems and the patient could be drained percutaneously.
2. I will have 2 units packed red blood cells ready to be transfused on-call to the cardiac catheterization laboratory.
3. Repeat labs in the morning.
4. Will hold on any IV fluids unless his blood pressure drops.
5. Replace his calcium with calcium gluconate 2 grams IV q.2.h. for 3 doses.
6. Expect liver function tests to improve once his pericardial effusion is drained.
7. Hold Coumadin for the time being.
8. Continue with Cipro.
9. Will keep NPO.

I discussed the case with cardiology and I appreciate his help on the case. We will await the patient's cardiologist's recommendations.

I discussed the case with the patient and his family. They were in agreement with our approach and they were satisfied with the service today. All their questions were answered. I discussed the case with the patient's primary care physician, who was here this morning, as well. I have discussed my entire plan with the nursing staff.

Total time spent on this patient this morning was 1 hour and 55 minutes (bedside and unit).

Codes:_____

EXAMINATION, REPORT 8

LOCATION: Hospital

Surgery operator paged me to be on standby for Neurosurgery. The patient is a 67-year-old male who was having a hemilaminectomy due to stenosis of the lumbar region without neurogenic claudication. I arrived to the operative suite at 8:45 AM. I stayed in the suite until I was notified by one of the surgical team members that I was not needed at 9:25 AM.

Codes:_____

EXAMINATION, REPORT 9

CASE MANAGEMENT SERVICES

LOCATION: Office

I called Mrs. Johnson at home regarding the results of her chest x-ray that she had at our facility this morning for a chronic cough. I met with the radiologist and the pulmonary specialist and his nurse practitioner in conference for

35 minutes to discuss the case. I discussed with her that there was a very small shadow in the lower lobe of the left lung. I told her that there wasn't anything to be concerned about after my conference with the team members and that we are going to follow-up in 3 months with another chest x-ray. I called in a prescription to her pharmacy for Robitussin with codeine to help her with her cough at nighttime. I notified her that if she worsens or has any questions to call our office immediately. Will follow-up with her in 3 months.

Codes:_____

EXAMINATION, REPORT 10

LOCATION: Office

ANNUAL PHYSICAL EXAM

SUBJECTIVE: This patient is a 39-year-old white female, Gravida 4, Para2, in today for a GYN exam and Pap smear. She has some concerns about some occasional right lower quadrant pain and some vaginal bleeding that she has had off and on for the last couple of weeks. She did have a urinalysis done that showed no blood in the urine. She states the discharge is very minimal and she has not found any contributing factors.

CURRENT HORMONE THERAPY: Nothing.

MENSTRUAL HISTORY: She had a hysterectomy for a bicornuate uterus and menorrhagia. The cervix was adhered to the bladder so a cervical stump has been left. She has no hot flashes or sleep disturbances. Last Pap was March 30. She has never had a previous abnormal pap.

MEDICAL HISTORY: Chronic illnesses include gastroesophageal reflux disease, high cholesterol, anxiety, history of one kidney, and history of irritable bowel.

SURGERIES:
1. Hysterectomy.
2. Two cesarean sections.

HOSPITALIZATIONS: For surgery only.

SOCIAL HISTORY: She is married and has no concerns of STD risks or abuse in this 23-year relationship. She works in an office. She feels that her diet has been fairly healthy. She is down over 15 pounds with healthy eating over the last few months and hoping to lose a lot more. She has two to three servings of calcium a day and no caffeine. She does continue to smoke rarely and has minimal secondhand smoke exposure. She has no alcohol intake. She is trying to walk consistently for exercise. She does wear a seatbelt, does use a sunscreen, and does do a breast exam.

FAMILY HISTORY: Father has high blood pressure, high cholesterol, coronary artery disease. Maternal grandmother had breast cancer. No ovarian or colon cancer history. Father is diabetic. No family history of thyroid disorders or osteoporosis. No depression or mental health issues.

REVIEW OF SYSTEMS: No current HEENT, respiratory, cardiovascular, breast, or GI problems. Lower abdominal pain and vaginal bleeding as noted above on a couple of instances. No pain during intercourse. No neurological, endocrine, or integumentary problems. No further depression symptoms.

PHYSICAL EXAMINATION: Declines the presence of a chaperone in the room today. Blood pressure 108/78. Weight 168 pounds. Height: 5 feet 4 inches.

Thyroid is normal to palpation without enlargement. Cervical nodes are negative. Lungs are clear to auscultation without rales or wheezes. Heart: Regular rate and rhythm without murmurs. Breasts are normal to inspection and bilaterally symmetrical. Normal to palpation.

No nipple discharge. Negative axillary nodes. Negative CVAT. Abdomen is soft without organomegally or hernia. Vulva is normal to inspection. Normal hair distribution. Negative BUS. Negative inguinal nodes. Vagina is clean with a scant amount of creamy discharge. On opening of the speculum to visualize the cervix, the patient complains of some discomfort and there is a slight amount of oozing at the posterior aspect of the cervical apex under the cervical stump. A Pap smear was obtained. Bimanual exam shows tenderness with deep penetration into the vagina and tenderness with cervical stump movement anteriorly. No masses palpated in the cul-de-sac or with bimanual exam. Skin is warm and dry. Distal pulses are equal. No edema of the extremities.

ASSESSMENT:
1. Gynecologic examination with Pap and general health check-up.
2. Vaginal tenderness and slight abnormal vaginal bleeding, post hysterectomy.
3. Health maintenance issues.

PLAN:
1. We will notify her of her Pap results within 2 weeks. Pending results.
2. I did give the patient two samples of vaginal Premarin cream and advised that she apply weekly to thicken the vaginal skin to decrease vaginal bleeding.
3. Mammogram will be scheduled in the near future.
4. Reinforced that she does a monthly breast exam, maintain an adequate calcium intake, and encouraged her efforts towards resuming a Weight Watcher's food plan and consistent exercise regimen.
5. Return to the clinic p.r.n. and for gynecologic care.

Codes: _____

EXAMINATION, REPORT 11

LOCATION: Office

This 58-year-old woman comes in for a life insurance examination. She currently has no complaints.

EXAM: Ht: 5' 4", Wt: 171, BP: 130/72. The patient's lungs are clear, heart regular with no murmur present. Abdomen is soft with bowel sounds. Extremities show no edema.

The patient is a healthy 58-year-old female with no complaints. I will send her to the lab for a basic metabolic panel and UA. I will contact her with the results. At that time I will complete the insurance form and forward a copy to the insurance company as well as the patient.

Codes: _____

EXAMINATION, REPORT 12

LOCATION: NICU INPATIENT

S: No events overnight

O: Resp: Rate: 38-73   Exam: upper airway congestion
    CV: Rate: 110-150   Map: 50-63

Exam: RRR and well perfused

FEN/GI: I: 710   TF: 150   Wt: 4725

O: 490

Exam: Soft NT ND with +BS

HEME: none

GU: Right side of scrotal sac enlarged and unable to reduce hernia, nontender.

ID: Temp Max: 36

Cultures:

NEURO:

Exam: Alert, no edema.

A/P: 2 month 1 wk old male status post incarcerated hernia repair (left inguinal region) who is also status post supraglottoplasty now working on increasing weight. Continues to PO well, formula had mistakenly been formulated to 18 kcal vs. 22 kcal, mistake fixed and subsequently we should see much better weight gain.

Codes:_____

EXAMINATION, REPORT 13

LOCATION: Office

CARE PLAN OVERSIGHT

Six-month care plan for a 90-year-old Alzheimer's patient in SNF. Patient also has COPD and ESRD, currently on peritoneal dialysis. Plan includes review of current medications, oxygen prn and to continue dialysis daily. Patient is to see nephrologist in dialysis center for monthly service and labs next Monday. Documentation includes review, nurse's remarks noted and modification of patient's care plan. Total time spent this month formulating care plan was 20 minutes.

Codes:_____

EXAMINATION, REPORT 14

LOCATION: Office

Home Care Plan Oversight

Gladys is a 92-year-old woman that I have had the pleasure of seeing within the past 6 months. She now resides in a rest home about 30 miles from here. The purpose of this note is to go over her monthly care plan. Gladys has severe primary osteoarthritis in her knees and uses a walker. She also has emphysema from years of smoking, for which she is on oxygen prn. I have gone over her latest labs, which show hemoglobin of 9.2. I have a standing order of Aranesp 60 mcg if her hemoglobin drops below 11, in which case she will receive this in the clinic. This will be increased to 100 mcg every two weeks. Per conversations with family members, Gladys seems in good spirits when they visit. The order for Aranesp 100 mcg will be sent to the clinic. She will continue with her current dose of medication and current dose of oxygen prn. Total time spent this month formulating care plan was 45 minutes, plus 38 minutes conversing with family via telephone.

Codes:_____

EXAMINATION, REPORT 15

LOCATION: Outpatient, Clinic

SUBJECTIVE: This is a 42-year-old Caucasian female who presents to the clinic today to establish with me as her primary care provider. At this particular service she is complaining of right hip pain and would also like to be weaned off her Zoloft because she is thinking that this is contributing to her increase in weight. She also complains of a nagging dry cough and would like to find out what might possibly be causing that. Her right hip pain has been going on for about three months now, which is constant and is aggravated by standing up from sitting. She does not feel the pain as much when walking and she says that this pain sometimes radiates to the buttocks and all the way down to her heel area. She occasionally feels a tingling sensation at the lateral aspect of the thigh, particularly at night. She has been treating this with over-the-counter pain medication but that is not found to be helpful. In terms of her cough, she noticed that she usually gets this whenever she has heartburn. She also thought that it might be related to her smoking as well.

PAST MEDICAL HISTORY is remarkable for:
1. Gastroesophageal reflux disease and has been taking medication for this but she cannot recall the name of that medication right now.
2. She also was found to have only one kidney and this was thought to be congenital.
3. Obesity, BMI, 34.

PAST SURGICAL HISTORY is remarkable for a hysterectomy due to a bicornuate uterus.

PSYCHIATRIC HISTORY: She suffered from a major depressive disorder and anxiety.

SCREENINGS: She gets a Pap smear and mammogram every year. Last time was last year, which were normal.

CURRENT MEDICATIONS:
1. Aspirin 81 mg daily.
2. Tums as needed.
3. Zoloft 100 mg daily.

ALLERGIES: She otherwise has no known drug allergies.

FAMILY MEDICAL HISTORY: Her father died at the age of 70 from a myocardial infarction. Mother is presently having high blood pressure and is taking medication for her heart. She also has high blood cholesterol. She is presently 67 years old. There is one brother who has ankylosing spondylitis and she has a total of three sisters. One sister has a benign breast tumor.

PERSONAL AND SOCIAL HISTORY: She is married. She has been doing her job for about 11 years now. She smokes and currently one pack will last her about two weeks. She denies alcohol use. I have established a quitting date of smoking with her and that would be May 1. She has a total of two children. One is 18 years old and one is 6 years old. She had a miscarriage and one stillbirth. She does not particularly exercise but has been watching her diet, drinking Slim-Fast once a day, and following Weight Watchers.

REVIEW OF SYSTEMS: Constitutional, eyes, head, mouth, chest and lungs, cardiovascular, gastrointestinal, genitourinary, and extremities reviewed and are otherwise negative other than what is already mentioned above.

OBJECTIVE FINDINGS: Vital signs: Blood pressure is 110/70. Pulse rate of 88. Weight is 201 pounds. General survey: She is an obese middle-aged lady who is pleasant, in no acute distress. Head and neck: Normocephalic and atraumatic. Pink conjunctivae and anicteric sclerae. Pupils are equal, round, and reactive to light and accommodation. Extraocular movements are intact. Neck is supple. No jugular venous distention. No carotid bruit. No thyromegaly. No cervical lymphadenopathy. Chest and lungs: Symmetrical expansion. Clear breath sounds. No rales or wheezes. Cardiovascular: Normal rate and regular rhythm. No murmur and no gallop. Abdomen is obese, soft; normoactive bowel sounds; non-tender. No organomegaly. Skin, warm and dry. Extremities: She has no edema, cyanosis, or clubbing. Palpable distal pulses. Straight-leg testing on both lower extremities is essentially negative. She has pain on internal rotation of the right hip joint. No pain on external rotation. On the left side internal and external rotation of the hip joints are negative.

ASSESSMENT/PLAN:

1. Hip pain, exact etiology is uncertain but this could be most likely secondary to degenerative joint disease of the hip versus mild bursitis. Superficial femoral nerve syndrome is also a consideration but not very likely. Discussed management with patient and we will just continue to observe for now. I advised her to give us a call when she develops progression of symptoms and referral to orthopedics might be appropriate if that happens.
2. Cough, dry, probably related to heartburn symptoms. Advised her to elevate her bed at night and continue to take a proton pump inhibitor for heartburn and also to quit smoking at the established quitting day.
3. Major depressive disorder, presently stable. She wants to be weaned off Zoloft and we are therefore decreasing her dose to 50 mg in the next two weeks and 25 mg after that. Then we will just discontinue it after one month. She agrees to this plan. She does not need to come to the clinic unless there is a new concern.

Codes:_____

EXAMINATION, REPORT 16

LOCATION: Hospital Inpatient

PROGRESS NOTE

SUBJECTIVE: Patient feels better. He was up and around yesterday and he felt very much better. Shortness of breath has improved. He has no orthopnea but some apparent dyspnea.

REVIEW OF SYSTEMS: Constitutional, ophthalmologic, otolaryngologic, cardiovascular, respiratory, GI, GU, musculoskeletal, integumentary, neurologic, psychiatric, endocrine, hematologic, immunologic negative other than what I have mentioned.

OBJECTIVE: He looks okay, in no acute distress. VITALS are stable. He is afebrile. HEAD, EYES, EARS, NOSE, and THROAT unremarkable. NECK supple, no JVD. The ABDOMEN is benign. EXTREMITIES: The swelling has gone down but he still has some swelling on the feet. NEUROLOGIC examination is grossly intact and nonfocal. His WEIGHT today is 194 pounds.

LABORATORY: Basic metabolic panel: BUN 43, creatinine 1.8, glucose 122. During the day his glucose has come up to around 200. Platelet count today is 128.

ASSESSMENT:
1. Congestive heart failure.
2. Aortic stenosis, non rheumatic.
3. Chronic renal failure, currently on hemodialysis.
4. Fluid overload state, improving.

RECOMMENDATIONS:
1. We will resume Amaryl 2 mg p.o. qd, watch his Accu-Cheks.
2. Follow up kidney function.
3. Increase activity and discharge.

Codes:_____

EXAMINATION, REPORT 17

LOCATION: Hospital

Ten-month-old male is admitted straight to NICU after going into cardiac arrest due to electrical shock when he chewed on an electrical cord. Patient also has second degree burns to lower face, lips and oral cavity (9% body surface). Patient was prepped for transport to The Children's Hospital and stabilized for air flight. During the air flight I personally spoke to the transport team, via two-way radio, instructing them on pulmonary and cardiac resuscitation when the patient again went into cardiac arrest. Total direct face-to-face time spent trying to stabilize the patient for air flight was 70 minutes.

Codes:_____

EXAMINATION, REPORT 18

LOCATION: Domiciliary Facility, new patient

I am evaluating the patient today, in the domiciliary care setting, for complaints of moderate cough and wheezing. The nursing staff reports that the patient started coughing yesterday afternoon. He denies feeling short of breath. There is no peripheral edema and his weight has been stable.

Today, he is alert and oriented. He denies any complaints other than he feels he has a sore throat. He says his glands in his neck have also been swollen. He is very pleasant. His vitals are stable.

EXAMINATION: BLOOD PRESSURE is 105/61. PULSE is 73. RESPIRATIONS are 20. TEMPERATURE is 97.4 degrees. He is lying flat in his bed and gets very upset when I attempt to elevate his head. His LUNGS have wheezes throughout, more accentuated in the upper airway. His abdomen is soft and nontender. EXTREMITIES ×4 show no edema.

PLAN: He does have some DuoNebs ordered p.r.n. and I am going to schedule them for a few days and see how he does. I know that he does not like using these nebulizers, but I think it will help his breathing. We will also have the patient go to the clinic for a chest x-ray because he does have a history of pneumonia.

Codes:_____

UNIT 3

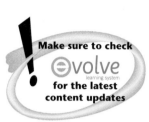

Make sure to check
evolve
learning system
for the latest
content updates

1995 Documentation Guidelines for E/M Services

I. INTRODUCTION

What Is Documentation and Why Is It Important?

Medical record documentation is required to record pertinent facts, findings, and observations about an individual's health history including past and present illnesses, examinations, tests, treatments, and outcomes. The medical record chronologically documents the care of the patient and is an important element contributing to high quality care. The medical record facilitates:

- ■ the ability of the physician and other health care professionals to evaluate and plan the patient's immediate treatment, and to monitor his/her health care over time.

- ■ communication and continuity of care among physicians and other health care professionals involved in the patient's care;

- ■ accurate and timely claims review and payment;

- ■ appropriate utilization review and quality of care evaluations; and

- ■ collection of data that may be useful for research and education.

An appropriately documented medical record can reduce many of the "hassles" associated with claims processing and may serve as a legal document to verify the care provided, if necessary.

What Do Payers Want and Why?

Because payers have a contractual obligation to enrollees, they may require reasonable documentation that services are consistent with the insurance coverage provided. They may request information to validate:

- ■ the site of service;

- ■ the medical necessity and appropriateness of the diagnostic and/or therapeutic services provided; and/or

- ■ that services provided have been accurately reported.

II. GENERAL PRINCIPLES OF MEDICAL RECORD DOCUMENTATION

The principles of documentation listed below are applicable to all types of medical and surgical services in all settings. For Evaluation and Management (E/M) services, the nature and amount of physician work and documentation varies by type of service, place of service and the patient's status. The general principles listed below may be modified to account for these variable circumstances in providing E/M services.

1. The medical record should be complete and legible.

2. The documentation of each patient encounter should include:

   ■ reason for the encounter and relevant history, physical examination findings and prior diagnostic test results;

   ■ assessment, clinical impression or diagnosis;

   ■ plan for care; and

   ■ date and legible identity of the observer.

3. If not documented, the rationale for ordering diagnostic and other ancillary services should be easily inferred.

4. Past and present diagnoses should be accessible to the treating and/or consulting physician.

5. Appropriate health risk factors should be identified.

6. The patient's progress, response to and changes in treatment, and revision of diagnosis should be documented.

7. The CPT and ICD-9-CM codes reported on the health insurance claim form or billing statement should be supported by the documentation in the medical record.

III. DOCUMENTATION OF E/M SERVICES

This publication provides definitions and documentation guidelines for the three **key** components of E/M services and for visits which consist predominately of counseling or coordination of care. The three key components—history, examination, and medical decision making—appear in the descriptors for office and other outpatient services, hospital observation services, hospital inpatient services, consultations, emergency department services, nursing facility services, domiciliary care services, and home services. While some of the text of CPT has been repeated in this publication, the reader should refer to CPT for the complete descriptors for E/M services and instructions for selecting a level of service. **Documentation guidelines are identified by the symbol •DG.**

The descriptors for the levels of E/M services recognize seven components which are used in defining the levels of E/M services. These components are:

   ■ history;

   ■ examination;

   ■ medical decision making;

   ■ counseling;

   ■ coordination of care;

   ■ nature of presenting problem; and

   ■ time.

The first three of these components (i.e., history, examination and medical decision making) are the *key* components in selecting the level of E/M services. An exception to this rule is the case of visits which consist predominantly of counseling or coordination of care; for these services time is the key or controlling factor to qualify for a particular level of E/M service.

For certain groups of patients, the recorded information may vary slightly from that described here. Specifically, the medical records of infants, children, adolescents and pregnant women may have additional or modified information recorded in each history and examination area.

As an example, newborn records may include under history of the present illness (HPI) the details of mother's pregnancy and the infant's status at birth; social history will focus on family structure; family history will focus on congenital anomalies and hereditary disorders in the family. In addition, information on growth and development and/or nutrition will be recorded. Although not specifically defined in these documentation guidelines, these patient group variations on history and examination are appropriate.

A. Documentation of History

The levels of E/M services are based on four types of history (Problem Focused, Expanded Problem Focused, Detailed, and Comprehensive.) Each type of history includes some or all of the following elements:

- Chief complaint (CC);
- History of present illness (HPI);
- Review of systems (ROS); and
- Past, family and/or social history (PFSH).

The extent of history of present illness, review of systems and past, family and/or social history that is obtained and documented is dependent upon clinical judgement and the nature of the presenting problem(s).

The chart below shows the progression of the elements required for each type of history. To qualify for a given type of history, **all three elements in the table must be met.** (A chief complaint is indicated at all levels.)

History of Present Illness (HPI)	Review of Systems (ROS)	Past, Family, and/or Social History (PFSH)	Type of History
Brief	N/A	N/A	*Problem Focused*
Brief	Problem Pertinent	N/A	*Expanded Problem Focused*
Extended	Extended	Pertinent	*Detailed*
Extended	Complete	Complete	*Comprehensive*

•*DG: The CC, ROS and PFSH may be listed as separate elements of history, or they may be included in the description of the history of the present illness.*

•*DG: A ROS and/or a PFSH obtained during an earlier encounter does not need to be re-recorded if there is evidence that the physician reviewed and updated the previous information. This may occur when a physician updates his or her own record or in an institutional setting or group practice where many physicians use a common record. The review and update may be documented by:*

- *describing any new ROS and/or PFSH information or noting there has been no change in the information; and*

- *noting the date and location of the earlier ROS and/or PFSH.*

•*DG: The ROS and/or PFSH may be recorded by ancillary staff or on a form completed by the patient. To document that the physician reviewed the information, there must be a notation supplementing or confirming the information recorded by others.*

•*DG: If the physician is unable to obtain a history from the patient or other source, the record should describe the patient's condition or other circumstance which precludes obtaining a history.*

Definitions and specific documentation guidelines for each of the elements of history are listed below.

Chief Complaint (CC)

The CC is a concise statement describing the symptom, problem, condition, diagnosis, physician recommended return, or other factor that is the reason for the encounter.

•*DG: The medical record should clearly reflect the chief complaint.*

History of Present Illness (HPI)

The HPI is a chronological description of the development of the patient's present illness from the first sign and/or symptom or from the previous encounter to the present. It includes the following elements:

- location,
- quality,
- severity,
- duration,
- timing,
- context,
- modifying factors, and
- associated signs and symptoms.

Brief and **extended** HPIs are distinguished by the amount of detail needed to accurately characterize the clinical problem(s).
   A **brief** HPI consists of one to three elements of the HPI.

•*DG: The medical record should describe one to three elements of the present illness (HPI).*

An **extended** HPI consists of four or more elements of the HPI.

•*DG: The medical record should describe four or more elements of the present illness (HPI) or associated comorbidities.*

Review of Systems (ROS)

A ROS is an inventory of body systems obtained through a series of questions seeking to identify signs and/or symptoms which the patient may be experiencing or has experienced.
   For purposes of ROS, the following systems are recognized:

- Constitutional symptoms (e.g., fever, weight loss)
- Eyes
- Ears, Nose, Mouth, Throat

96

■ Cardiovascular

■ Respiratory

■ Gastrointestinal

■ Genitourinary

■ Musculoskeletal

■ Integumentary (skin and/or breast)

■ Neurological

■ Psychiatric

■ Endocrine

■ Hematologic/Lymphatic

■ Allergic/Immunologic

A ***problem pertinent*** ROS inquires about the system directly related to the problem(s) identified in the HPI.

•*DG: The patient's positive responses and pertinent negatives for the system related to the problem should be documented.*

An ***extended*** ROS inquires about the system directly related to the problem(s) identified in the HPI and a limited number of additional systems.

•*DG: The patient's positive responses and pertinent negatives for two to nine systems should be documented.*

A ***complete*** ROS inquires about the system(s) directly related to the problem(s) identified in the HPI <u>plus</u> all additional body systems.

•*DG: At least ten organ systems must be reviewed. Those systems with positive or pertinent negative responses must be individually documented. For the remaining systems, a notation indicating all other systems are negative is permissible. In the absence of such a notation, at least ten systems must be individually documented.*

Past, Family and/or Social History (PFSH)

The PFSH consists of a review of three areas:

■ past history (the patient's past experiences with illnesses, operations, injuries and treatments);

■ family history (a review of medical events in the patient's family, including diseases which may be hereditary or place the patient at risk); and

■ social history (an age appropriate review of past and current activities).

For the categories of subsequent hospital care, follow-up inpatient consultations and subsequent nursing facility care, CPT requires only an "interval" history. It is not necessary to record information about the PFSH.

A ***pertinent*** PFSH is a review of the history area(s) directly related to the problem(s) identified in the HPI.

•*DG: At least one specific item from <u>any</u> of the three history areas must be documented for a pertinent PFSH .*

A ***complete*** PFSH is of a review of two or all three of the PFSH history areas, depending on the category of the E/M service. A review of all three history areas is required for services that by their nature include a comprehensive assessment or reassessment of the patient. A review of two of the three history areas is sufficient for other services.

•*DG: At least one specific item from two of the three history areas must be documented for a complete PFSH for the following categories of E/M services: office or other outpatient services, established patient; emergency department; subsequent nursing facility care; domiciliary care, established patient; and home care, established patient.*

•*DG: At least one specific item from each of the three history areas must be documented for a complete PFSH for the following categories of E/M services: office or other outpatient services, new patient; hospital observation services; hospital inpatient services, initial care; consultations; comprehensive nursing facility assessments; domiciliary care, new patient; and home care, new patient.*

B. Documentation of Examination

The levels of E/M services are based on four types of examination that are defined as follows:

- **Problem Focused**—a limited examination of the affected body area or organ system.

- **Expanded Problem Focused**—a limited examination of the affected body area or organ system and other symptomatic or related organ system(s).

- **Detailed**—an extended examination of the affected body area(s) and other symptomatic or related organ system(s).

- **Comprehensive**—a general multi-system examination or complete examination of a single organ system.

For purposes of examination, the following **body areas** are recognized:

- Head, including the face
- Neck
- Chest, including breasts and axillae
- Abdomen
- Genitalia, groin, buttocks
- Back, including spine
- Each extremity

For purposes of examination, the following **organ systems** are recognized:

- Constitutional (e.g., vital signs, general appearance)
- Eyes
- Ears, nose, mouth and throat
- Cardiovascular
- Respiratory
- Gastrointestinal
- Genitourinary
- Musculoskeletal
- Skin

- Neurologic
- Psychiatric
- Hematologic/lymphatic/immunologic

The extent of examinations performed and documented is dependent upon clinical judgement and the nature of the presenting problem(s). They range from limited examinations of single body areas to general multi-system or complete single organ system examinations.

•*DG: Specific abnormal and relevant negative findings of the examination of the affected or symptomatic body area(s) or organ system(s) should be documented. A notation of "abnormal" without elaboration is insufficient.*

•*DG: Abnormal or unexpected findings of the examination of the unaffected or asymptomatic body area(s) or organ system(s) should be described.*

•*DG: A brief statement or notation indicating "negative" or "normal" is sufficient to document normal findings related to unaffected area(s) or asymptomatic organ system(s).*

•*DG: The medical record for a general multi-system examination should include findings about 8 or more of the 12 organ systems.*

C. Documentation of the Complexity of Medical Decision Making

The levels of E/M services recognize four types of medical decision making (straight-forward, low complexity, moderate complexity and high complexity). Medical decision making refers to the complexity of establishing a diagnosis and/or selecting a management option as measured by:

- the number of possible diagnoses and/or the number of management options that must be considered;

- the amount and/or complexity of medical records, diagnostic tests, and/or other information that must be obtained, reviewed and analyzed; and

- the risk of significant complications, morbidity and/or mortality, as well as comorbidities, associated with the patient's presenting problem(s), the diagnostic procedure(s) and/or the possible management options.

The chart below shows the progression of the elements required for each level of medical decision making. To qualify for a given type of decision making, **two of the three elements in the table must be either met or exceeded.**

Number of Diagnoses or Management Options	Amount and/or Complexity of Data to Be Reviewed	Risk of Complications and/ or Morbidity or Mortality	Type of Decision Making
Minimal	Minimal or None	Minimal	*Straightforward*
Limited	Limited	Low	*Low Complexity*
Multiple	Moderate	Moderate	*Moderate Complexity*
Extensive	Extensive	High	*High Complexity*

Each of the elements of medical decision making is described below.

Number of Diagnoses or Management Options

The number of possible diagnoses and/or the number of management options that must be considered is based on the number and types of problems addressed during the encounter, the complexity of establishing a diagnosis and the management decisions that are made by the physician.

Generally, decision making with respect to a diagnosed problem is easier than that for an identified but undiagnosed problem. The number and type of diagnostic tests employed may be an indicator of the number of possible diagnoses. Problems which are improving or resolving are less complex than those which are worsening or failing to change as expected. The need to seek advice from others is another indicator of complexity of diagnostic or management problems.

•*DG: For each encounter, an assessment, clinical impression, or diagnosis should be documented. It may be explicitly stated or implied in documented decisions regarding management plans and/or further evaluation.*

- *For a presenting problem with an established diagnosis the record should reflect whether the problem is: a) improved, well controlled, resolving or resolved; or, b) inadequately controlled, worsening, or failing to change as expected.*

- *For a presenting problem without an established diagnosis, the assessment or clinical impression may be stated in the form of a differential diagnoses or as "possible", "probable", or "rule out" (R/O) diagnoses.*

•*DG: The initiation of, or changes in, treatment should be documented. Treatment includes a wide range of management options including patient instructions, nursing instructions, therapies, and medications.*

•*DG: If referrals are made, consultations requested or advice sought, the record should indicate to whom or where the referral or consultation is made or from whom the advice is requested.*

Amount and/or Complexity of Data to be Reviewed

The amount and complexity of data to be reviewed is based on the types of diagnostic testing ordered or reviewed. A decision to obtain and review old medical records and/or obtain history from sources other than the patient increases the amount and complexity of data to be reviewed.

Discussion of contradictory or unexpected test results with the physician who performed or interpreted the test is an indication of the complexity of data being reviewed. On occasion the physician who ordered a test may personally review the image, tracing or specimen to supplement information from the physician who prepared the test report or interpretation; this is another indication of the complexity of data being reviewed.

•*DG: If a diagnostic service (test or procedure) is ordered, planned, scheduled, or performed at the time of the E/M encounter, the type of service, eg, lab or x-ray, should be documented.*

•*DG: The review of lab, radiology and/or other diagnostic tests should be documented. An entry in a progress note such as "WBC elevated" or "chest x-ray unremarkable" is acceptable. Alternatively, the review may be documented by initialing and dating the report containing the test results.*

•*DG: A decision to obtain old records or decision to obtain additional history from the family, caretaker or other source to supplement that obtained from the patient should be documented.*

•*DG: Relevant finding from the review of old records, and/or the receipt of additional history from the family, caretaker or other source should be documented. If there is no relevant information beyond that already obtained, that fact should be documented. A notation of "Old records reviewed" or "additional history obtained from family" without elaboration is insufficient.*

•*DG: The results of discussion of laboratory, radiology or other diagnostic tests with the physician who performed or interpreted the study should be documented.*

•*DG: The direct visualization and independent interpretation of an image, tracing or specimen previously or subsequently interpreted by another physician should be documented.*

Risk of Significant Complications, Morbidity, and/or Mortality

The risk of significant complications, morbidity, and/or mortality is based on the risks associated with the presenting problem(s), the diagnostic procedure(s), and the possible management options.

•*DG: Comorbidities/underlying diseases or other factors that increase the complexity of medical decision making by increasing the risk of complications, morbidity, and/or mortality should be documented.*

•*DG: If a surgical or invasive diagnostic procedure is ordered, planned or scheduled at the time of the E/M encounter, the type of procedure, eg, laparoscopy, should be documented.*

•*DG: If a surgical or invasive diagnostic procedure is performed at the time of the E/M encounter, the specific procedure should be documented.*

•*DG: The referral for or decision to perform a surgical or invasive diagnostic procedure on an urgent basis should be documented or implied.*

The following table may be used to help determine whether the risk of significant complications, morbidity, and/or mortality is **minimal, low, moderate,** or **high.** Because the determination of risk is complex and not readily quantifiable, the table includes common clinical examples rather than absolute measures of risk. The assessment of risk of the presenting problem(s) is based on the risk related to the disease process anticipated between the present encounter and the next one. The assessment of risk of selecting diagnostic procedures and management options is based on the risk during and immediately following any procedures or treatment. The highest level of risk in any one category (presenting problem(s), diagnostic procedure(s), or management options) determines the overall risk.

TABLE OF RISK

Level of Risk	Presenting Problem(s)	Diagnostic Procedure(s) Ordered	Management Options Selected
Minimal	• One self-limited or minor problem, eg, cold, insect bite, tinea corporis	• Laboratory tests requiring venipuncture • Chest x-rays • EKG/EEG • Urinalysis • Ultrasound, eg, echocardiography • KOH prep	• Rest • Gargles • Elastic bandages • Superficial dressings
Low	• Two or more self-limited or minor problems • One stable chronic illness, eg, well controlled hypertension, non-insulin dependent diabetes, cataract, BPH • Acute uncomplicated illness or injury, eg, cystitis, allergic rhinitis, simple sprain	• Physiologic tests not under stress, eg, pulmonary function tests • Non-cardiovascular imaging studies with contrast, eg, barium enema • Superficial needle biopsies • Clinical laboratory tests requiring arterial puncture • Skin biopsies	• Over-the-counter drugs • Minor surgery with no identified risk factors • Physical therapy • Occupational therapy • IV fluids without additives
Moderate	• One or more chronic illnesses with mild exacerbation, progression, or side effects of treatment • Two or more stable chronic illnesses • Undiagnosed new problem with uncertain prognosis, eg, lump in breast • Acute illness with systemic symptoms, eg, pyelonephritis, pneumonitis, colitis • Acute complicated injury, eg, head injury with brief loss of consciousness	• Physiologic tests under stress, eg, cardiac stress test, fetal contraction stress test • Diagnostic endoscopies with no identified risk factors • Deep needle or incisional biopsy • Cardiovascular imaging studies with contrast and no identified risk factors, eg, arteriogram, cardiac catheterization • Obtain fluid from body cavity, eg, lumbar puncture, thoracentesis, culdocentesis	• Minor surgery with identified risk factors • Elective major surgery (open, percutaneous or endoscopic) with no identified risk factors • Prescription drug management • Therapeutic nuclear medicine • IV fluids with additives • Closed treatment of fracture or dislocation without manipulation
High	• One or more chronic illnesses with severe exacerbation, progression, or side effects of treatment • Acute or chronic illnesses or injuries that pose a threat to life or bodily function, eg, multiple trauma, acute MI, pulmonary embolus, severe respiratory distress, progressive severe rheumatoid arthritis, psychiatric illness with potential threat to self or others, peritonitis, acute renal failure • An abrupt change in neurologic status, eg, seizure, TIA, weakness, sensory loss	• Cardiovascular imaging studies with contrast with identified risk factors • Cardiac electrophysiological tests • Diagnostic endoscopies with identified risk factors • Discography	• Elective major surgery (open, percutaneous or endoscopic) with identified risk factors • Emergency major surgery (open, percutaneous or endoscopic) • Parenteral controlled substances • Drug therapy requiring intensive monitoring for toxicity • Decision not to resuscitate or to de-escalate care because of poor prognosis

D. Documentation of an Encounter Dominated by Counseling or Coordination of Care

In the case where counseling and/or coordination of care dominates (more than 50%) of the physician/patient and/or family encounter (face-to-face time in the office or other outpatient setting or floor/unit time in the hospital or nursing facility), time is considered the key or controlling factor to qualify for a particular level of E/M services.

•*DG: If the physician elects to report the level of service based on counseling and/or coordination of care, the total length of time of the encounter (face-to-face or floor time, as appropriate) should be documented and the record should describe the counseling and/or activities to coordinate care.*

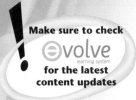

Make sure to check
evolve learning system
**for the latest
content updates**

1997 Documentation Guidelines for Evaluation and Management Services*

*Developed jointly by the American Medical Association (AMA) and the Health Care Financing Administration (HCFA) (now Centers for Medicare and Medicaid Services).

I. INTRODUCTION

What Is Documentation and Why Is It Important?

Medical record documentation is required to record pertinent facts, findings, and observations about an individual's health history including past and present illnesses, examinations, tests, treatments, and outcomes. The medical record chronologically documents the care of the patient and is an important element contributing to high quality care. The medical record facilitates:

- the ability of the physician and other health care professionals to evaluate and plan the patient's immediate treatment, and to monitor his/her health care over time.

- communication and continuity of care among physicians and other health care professionals involved in the patient's care;

- accurate and timely claims review and payment;

- appropriate utilization review and quality of care evaluations; and

- collection of data that may be useful for research and education.

An appropriately documented medical record can reduce many of the "hassles" associated with claims processing and may serve as a legal document to verify the care provided, if necessary.

What Do Payers Want and Why?

Because payers have a contractual obligation to enrollees, they may require reasonable documentation that services are consistent with the insurance coverage provided. They may request information to validate:

- the site of service;

- the medical necessity and appropriateness of the diagnostic and/or therapeutic services provided; and/or

- that services provided have been accurately reported.

II. GENERAL PRINCIPLES OF MEDICAL RECORD DOCUMENTATION

The principles of documentation listed below are applicable to all types of medical and surgical services in all settings. For Evaluation and Management (E/M) services, the nature and amount of physician work and documentation varies by type of service, place of service and the patient's status. The following list of general principles may be modified to account for these variable circumstances in providing E/M services.

1. The medical record should be complete and legible.

2. The documentation of each patient encounter should include:

   - reason for the encounter and relevant history, physical examination findings and prior diagnostic test results;

   - assessment, clinical impression or diagnosis;

   - plan for care; and

   - date and legible identity of the observer.

3. If not documented, the rationale for ordering diagnostic and other ancillary services should be easily inferred.

4. Past and present diagnoses should be accessible to the treating and/or consulting physician.

5. Appropriate health risk factors should be identified.

6. The patient's progress, response to and changes in treatment, and revision of diagnosis should be documented.

7. The CPT and ICD-9-CM codes reported on the health insurance claim form or billing statement should be supported by the documentation in the medical record.

III. DOCUMENTATION OF E/M SERVICES

This publication provides definitions and documentation guidelines for the three key components of E/M services and for visits which consist predominantly of counseling or coordination of care. The three *key* components—history, examination, and medical decision making—appear in the descriptors for office and other outpatient services, hospital observation services, hospital inpatient services, consultations, emergency department services, nursing facility services, domiciliary care services, and home services. While some of the text of CPT has been repeated in this publication, the reader should refer to CPT for the complete descriptors for E/M services and instructions for selecting a level of service. Documentation guidelines are identified by the symbol ■ *DG.*

The descriptors for the levels of E/M services recognize seven components which are used in defining the levels of E/M services. These components are:

- history;

- examination;

- medical decision making;

- counseling;

- coordination of care;

- nature of presenting problem; and

- time.

The first three of these components (i.e., history, examination and medical decision making) are the key components in selecting the level of E/M services. In the case of visits which consist *predominantly* of counseling or coordination of care, time is the key or controlling factor to qualify for a particular level of E/M service.

Because the level of E/M service is dependent on two or three key components, performance and documentation of one component (e.g., examination) at the highest level does not necessarily mean that the encounter in its entirety qualifies for the highest level of E/M service.

These Documentation Guidelines for E/M services reflect the needs of the typical adult population. For certain groups of patients, the recorded information may vary slightly from that described here. Specifically, the medical records of infants, children, adolescents and pregnant women may have additional or modified information recorded in each history and examination area.

As an example, newborn records may include under history of the present illness (HPI) the details of mother's pregnancy and the infant's status at birth; social history will focus on family structure; family history will focus on congenital anomalies and hereditary disorders in the family. In addition, the content of a pediatric examination will vary with the age and development of the child. Although not specifically defined in these documentation guidelines, these patient group variations on history and examination are appropriate.

A. Documentation of History

The levels of E/M services are based on four types of history (Problem Focused, Expanded Problem Focused, Detailed, and Comprehensive). Each type of history includes some or all of the following elements:

- Chief complaint (CC);

- History of present illness (HPI);

- Review of systems (ROS); and

- Past, family and/or social history (PFSH).

The extent of history of present illness, review of systems and past, family and/or social history that is obtained and documented is dependent upon clinical judgment and the nature of the presenting problem(s).

The chart below shows the progression of the elements required for each type of history. To qualify for a given type of history all three elements in the table must be met. (A chief complaint is indicated at all levels.)

History of Present Illness	Review of Systems (ROS)	Past, Family, and/ or Social History	Type of History
Brief	N/A	N/A	Problem Focused
Brief	Problem pertinent	N/A	Expanded Problem Focused
Extended	Extended	Pertinent	Detailed
Extended	Complete	Complete	Comprehensive

- DG: The CC, ROS, and PFSH may be listed as separate elements of history, or they may be included in the description of the history of the present illness.

- DG: A ROS and/or a PFSH obtained during an earlier encounter does not need to be re-recorded if there is evidence that the physician reviewed and updated the previous information. This may occur when a physician updates his or her own record or in an institutional setting or group practice where many physicians use a common record. The review and update may be documented by:

    - describing any new ROS and/or PFSH information or noting there has been no change in the information; and

    - noting the date and location of the earlier ROS and/or PFSH.

- DG: The ROS and/or PFSH may be recorded by ancillary staff or on a form completed by the patient. To document that the physician reviewed the information, there must be a notation supplementing or confirming the information recorded by others.

- DG: If the physician is unable to obtain a history from the patient or other source, the record should describe the patient's condition or other circumstance which precludes obtaining a history.

Definitions and specific documentation guidelines for each of the elements of history are in the following list.

Chief Complaint (CC)

The CC is a concise statement describing the symptom, problem, condition, diagnosis, physician recommended return, or other factor that is the reason for the encounter, usually stated in the patient's words.

- DG: The medical record should clearly reflect the chief complaint.

History of Present Illness (HPI)

The HPI is a chronological description of the development of the patient's present illness from the first sign and/or symptom or from the previous encounter to the present. It includes the following elements:

- location,
- quality,
- severity,
- duration,
- timing,
- context,
- modifying factors, and
- associated signs and symptoms.

Brief and *extended* HPIs are distinguished by the amount of detail needed to accurately characterize the clinical problem(s).
A *brief* HPI consists of one to three elements of the HPI.

- DG: The medical record should describe one to three elements of the present illness (HPI).

An *extended* HPI consists of at least four elements of the HPI or the status of at least three chronic or inactive conditions.

■ DG: The medical record should describe at least four elements of the present illness (HPI), or the status of at least three chronic or inactive conditions.

Review of Systems (ROS)

A ROS is an inventory of body systems obtained through a series of questions seeking to identify signs and/or symptoms which the patient may be experiencing or has experienced.

For purposes of ROS, the following systems are recognized:

■ Constitutional symptoms (e.g., fever, weight loss)

■ Eyes

■ Ears, Nose, Mouth, Throat

■ Cardiovascular

■ Respiratory

■ Gastrointestinal

■ Genitourinary

■ Musculoskeletal

■ Integumentary (skin and/or breast)

■ Neurological

■ Psychiatric

■ Endocrine

■ Hematologic/Lymphatic

■ Allergic/Immunologic

A *problem pertinent* ROS inquires about the system directly related to the problem(s) identified in the HPI.

■ DG: The patient's positive responses and pertinent negatives for the system related to the problem should be documented.

An *extended* ROS inquires about the system directly related to the problem(s) identified in the HPI and a limited number of additional systems.

■ DG: The patient's positive responses and pertinent negatives for two to nine systems should be documented.

A *complete* ROS inquires about the system(s) directly related to the problem(s) identified in the HPI *plus* all additional body systems.

■ DG: At least ten organ systems must be reviewed. Those systems with positive or pertinent negative responses must be individually documented. For the remaining systems, a notation indicating all other systems are negative is permissible. In the absence of such a notation, at least ten systems must be individually documented.

Past, Family and/or Social History (PFSH)

The PFSH consists of a review of three areas:

- past history (the patient's past experiences with illnesses, operations, injuries and treatments);

- family history (a review of medical events in the patient's family, including diseases which may be hereditary or place the patient at risk); and

- social history (an age appropriate review of past and current activities).

For certain categories of E/M services that include only an interval history, it is not necessary to record information about the PFSH. Those categories are subsequent hospital care, follow-up inpatient consultations and subsequent nursing facility care.

A *pertinent* PFSH is a review of the history area(s) directly related to the problem(s) identified in the HPI.

- DG: At least one specific item from any of the three history areas must be documented for a pertinent PFSH.

A *complete* PFSH is a review of two or all three of the PFSH history areas, depending on the category of the E/M service. A review of all three history areas is required for services that by their nature include a comprehensive assessment or reassessment of the patient. A review of two of the three history areas is sufficient for other services.

- DG: At least one specific item from two of the three history areas must be documented for a complete PFSH for the following categories of E/M services: office or other outpatient services, established patient; emergency department; domiciliary care, established patient; and home care, established patient.

- DG: At least one specific item from each of the three history areas must be documented for a complete PFSH for the following categories of E/M services: office or other outpatient services, new patient; hospital observation services; hospital inpatient services, initial care; consultations; comprehensive nursing facility assessments; domiciliary care, new patient; and home care, new patient.

B. Documentation of Examination

The levels of E/M services are based on four types of examination:

- *Problem Focused*—a limited examination of the affected body area or organ system.

- *Expanded Problem Focused*—a limited examination of the affected body area or organ system and any other symptomatic or related body area(s) or organ system(s).

- *Detailed*—an extended examination of the affected body area(s) or organ system(s) and any other symptomatic or related body area(s) or organ system(s).

- *Comprehensive*—a general multi-system examination, or complete examination of a single organ system and other symptomatic or related body area(s) or organ system(s).

These types of examinations have been defined for general multi-system and the following single organ systems:

- Cardiovascular

- Ears, Nose, Mouth and Throat

- Eyes

- Genitourinary (Female)

- Genitourinary (Male)

- Hematologic/Lymphatic/Immunologic

- Musculoskeletal

- Neurological

- Psychiatric

- Respiratory

- Skin

A general multi-system examination or a single organ system examination may be performed by any physician regardless of specialty. The type (general multi-system or single organ system) and content of examination are selected by the examining physician and are based upon clinical judgment, the patient's history, and the nature of the presenting problem(s).

The content and documentation requirements for each type and level of examination are summarized following and described in detail in tables beginning on page 113. In the tables, organ systems and body areas recognized by CPT for purposes of describing examinations are shown in the left column. The content, or individual elements, of the examination pertaining to that body area or organ system are identified by bullets (•) in the right column.

Parenthetical examples, "(e.g., . . .)," have been used for clarification and to provide guidance regarding documentation. Documentation for each element must satisfy any numeric requirements (such as "Measurement of *any three of the following seven . . .*") included in the description of the element. Elements with multiple components but with no specific numeric requirement (such as "Examination of *liver* and *spleen*") require documentation of at least one component. It is possible for a given examination to be expanded beyond what is defined here. When that occurs, findings related to the additional systems and/or areas should be documented.

- DG: Specific abnormal and relevant negative findings of the examination of the affected or symptomatic body area(s) or organ system(s) should be documented. A notation of "abnormal" without elaboration is insufficient.

- DG: Abnormal or unexpected findings of the examination of any asymptomatic body area(s) or organ system(s) should be described.

- DG: A brief statement or notation indicating "negative" or "normal" is sufficient to document normal findings related to unaffected area(s) or asymptomatic organ system(s).

General Multi-System Examinations

General multi-system examinations are described in detail beginning on page 113. To qualify for a given level of multi-system examination, the following content and documentation requirements should be met:

- *Problem Focused Examination*—should include performance and documentation of one to five elements identified by a bullet (•) in one or more organ system(s) or body area(s).

- *Expanded Problem Focused Examination*—should include performance and documentation of at least six elements identified by a bullet (•) in one or more organ system(s) or body area(s).

- *Detailed Examination*—should include at least six organ systems or body areas. For each system/area selected, performance and documentation of at least two elements identified by a bullet (•) is expected. Alternatively, a detailed examination may include performance and documentation of at least twelve elements identified by a bullet (•) in two or more organ systems or body areas.

- *Comprehensive Examination*—should include at least nine organ systems or body areas. For each system/area selected, all elements of the examination identified by a bullet (•) should be performed, unless specific directions limit the content of the examination. For each area/system, documentation of at least two elements identified by a bullet is expected.

Single Organ System Examinations

The single organ system examinations recognized by CPT are described in detail beginning on page 115. Variations among these examinations in the organ systems and body areas identified in the left columns and in the elements of the examinations described in the right columns reflect differing emphases among specialties. To qualify for a given level of single organ system examination, the following content and documentation requirements should be met:

- *Problem Focused Examination*—should include performance and documentation of one to five elements identified by a bullet (•), whether in a box with a shaded or unshaded border.

- *Expanded Problem Focused Examination*—should include performance and documentation of at least six elements identified by a bullet (•), whether in a box with a shaded or unshaded border.

- *Detailed Examination*—examinations other than the eye and psychiatric examinations should include performance and documentation of at least twelve elements identified by a bullet (•), whether in box with a shaded or unshaded border.

- Eye and psychiatric examinations should include the performance and documentation of at least nine elements identified by a bullet (•), whether in a box with a shaded or unshaded border.

- *Comprehensive Examination*—should include performance of all elements identified by a bullet (•), whether in a shaded or unshaded box. Documentation of every element in each box with a shaded border and at least one element in each box with an unshaded border is expected.

Content and Documentation Requirements

GENERAL MULTI-SYSTEM EXAMINATION

System/Body Area	Elements of Examination
Constitutional	• Measurement of any three of the following seven vital signs: 1) sitting or standing blood pressure, 2) supine blood pressure, 3) pulse rate and regularity, 4) respiration, 5) temperature, 6) height, 7) weight (may be measured and recorded by ancillary staff) • General appearance of patient (e.g., development, nutrition, body habitus, deformities, attention to grooming)
Eyes	• Inspection of conjunctivae and lids • Examination of pupils and irises (e.g., reaction to light and accommodation, size and symmetry) • Ophthalmoscopic examination of optic discs (e.g., size, C/D ratio, appearance) and posterior segments (e.g., vessel changes, exudates, hemorrhages)
Ears, Nose, Mouth and Throat	• External inspection of ears and nose (e.g., overall appearance, scars, lesions, masses) • Otoscopic examination of external auditory canals and tympanic membranes • Assessment of hearing (e.g., whispered voice, finger rub, tuning fork) • Inspection of nasal mucosa, septum and turbinates • Inspection of lips, teeth and gums • Examination of oropharynx: oral mucosa, salivary glands, hard and soft palates, tongue, tonsils and posterior pharynx
Neck	• Examination of neck (e.g., masses, overall appearance, symmetry, tracheal position, crepitus) • Examination of thyroid (e.g., enlargement, tenderness, mass)
Respiratory	• Assessment of respiratory effort (e.g., intercostal retractions, use of accessory muscles, diaphragmatic movement) • Percussion of chest (e.g., dullness, flatness, hyperresonance) • Palpation of chest (e.g., tactile fremitus) • Auscultation of lungs (e.g., breath sounds, adventitious sounds, rubs)
Cardiovascular	• Palpation of heart (e.g., location, size, thrills) • Auscultation of heart with notation of abnormal sounds and murmurs Examination of: • carotid arteries (e.g., pulse amplitude, bruits) • abdominal aorta (e.g., size, bruits) • femoral arteries (e.g., pulse amplitude, bruits) • pedal pulses (e.g., pulse amplitude) • extremities for edema and/or varicosities
Chest (Breasts)	• Inspection of breasts (e.g., symmetry, nipple discharge) • Palpation of breasts and axillae (e.g., masses or lumps, tenderness)

System/Body Area	Elements of Examination
Gastrointestinal (Abdomen)	• Examination of abdomen with notation of presence of masses or tenderness • Examination of liver and spleen
	• Examination for presence or absence of hernia • Examination (when indicated) of anus, perineum and rectum, including sphincter tone, presence of hemorrhoids, rectal masses • Obtain stool sample for occult blood test when indicated
Genitourinary	**Male:**
	• Examination of the scrotal contents (e.g., hydrocele, spermatocele, tenderness of cord, testicular mass) • Examination of the penis • Digital rectal examination of prostate gland (e.g., size, symmetry, nodularity, tenderness)
	Female:
	Pelvic examination (with or without specimen collection for smears and cultures), including • Examination of external genitalia (e.g., general appearance, hair distribution, lesions) and vagina (e.g., general appearance, estrogen effect, discharge, lesions, pelvic support, cystocele, rectocele) • Examination of urethra (e.g., masses, tenderness, scarring) • Examination of bladder (e.g., fullness, masses, tenderness) • Cervix (e.g., general appearance, lesions, discharge) • Uterus (e.g., size, contour, position, mobility, tenderness, consistency, descent or support) • Adnexa/parametria (e.g., masses, tenderness, organomegaly, nodularity)
Lymphatic	Palpation of lymph nodes in **two or more areas:** • Neck • Axillae • Groin • Other
Musculoskeletal	• Examination of gait and station • Inspection and/or palpation of digits and nails (e.g., clubbing, cyanosis,) inflammatory conditions, petechiae, ischemia, infections, nodes Examination of joints, bones and muscles of **one or more of the following six areas:** 1) head and neck; 2) spine, ribs and pelvis; 3) right upper extremity; 4) left upper extremity; 5) right lower extremity; and left lower extremity. The examination of a given area includes: • Inspection and/or palpation with notation of presence of any misalignment, asymmetry, crepitation, defects, tenderness, masses, effusions • Assessment of range of motion with notation of any pain, crepitation or contracture • Assessment of stability with notation of any dislocation (luxation), subluxation or laxity • Assessment of muscle strength and tone (e.g., flaccid, cog wheel, spastic) with notation of any atrophy or abnormal movements

System/Body Area	Elements of Examination
Skin	• Inspection of skin and subcutaneous tissue (e.g., rashes, lesions, ulcers) • Palpation of skin and subcutaneous tissue (e.g., induration, subcutaneous nodules, tightening)
Neurologic	• Test cranial nerves with notation of any deficits • Examination of deep tendon reflexes with notation of pathological reflexes (e.g., Babinski) • Examination of sensation (e.g., by touch, pin, vibration, proprioception)
Psychiatric	• Description of patient's judgment and insight Brief assessment of mental status including: • orientation to time, place and person • recent and remote memory • mood and affect (e.g., depression, anxiety, agitation)

Content and Documentation Requirements

LEVEL OF EXAM	PERFORM AND DOCUMENT
Problem Focused	**One to five** elements identified by a bullet.
Expanded Problem Focused	**At least six** elements identified by a bullet.
Detailed	**At least two** elements identified by a bullet **from each of six areas/systems** OR **at least twelve** elements identified by a bullet **in two or more areas/systems.**
Comprehensive	Perform **all elements** identified by a bullet in **at least nine** organ systems or body areas and document **at least two** elements identified by a bullet **from each of nine areas/systems.**

CARDIOVASCULAR EXAMINATION

System/Body Area	Elements of Examination
Constitutional	• Measurement of **any three of the following seven** vital signs: 1) sitting or standing blood pressure, 2) supine blood pressure, 3) pulse rate and regularity, 4) respiration, 5) temperature, 6) height, 7) weight (may be measured and recorded by ancillary staff) • General appearance of patient (e.g., development, nutrition, body habitus, deformities, attention to grooming)
Head and Face	
Eyes	• Inspection of conjunctivae and lids (e.g., xanthelasma)
Ears, Nose, Mouth and Throat	• Inspection of teeth, gums and palate • Inspection of oral mucosa with notation of presence of pallor or cyanosis
Neck	Examination of jugular veins (e.g., distension; a, v or cannon a waves)
	• Examination of thyroid (e.g., enlargement, tenderness, mass)

System/Body Area	Elements of Examination
Respiratory	• Assessment of respiratory effort (e.g., intercostal retractions, use of accessory muscles, diaphragmatic movement) • Auscultation of lungs (e.g., breath sounds, adventitious sounds, rubs)
Cardiovascular	• Palpation of heart (e.g., location, size and forcefulness of the point of maximal impact; thrills; lifts; palpable S3 or S4) • Auscultation of heart including sounds, abnormal sounds and murmurs • Measurement of blood pressure in two or more extremities when indicated (e.g., aortic dissection, coarctation) Examination of: • Carotid arteries (e.g., waveform, pulse amplitude, bruits, apical-carotid delay) • Abdominal aorta (e.g., size, bruits) • Femoral arteries (e.g., pulse amplitude, bruits) • Pedal pulses (e.g., pulse amplitude) • Extremities for peripheral edema and/or varicosities
Chest (Breasts)	
Gastrointestinal (Abdomen)	• Examination of abdomen with notation of presence of masses or tenderness • Examination of liver and spleen • Obtain stool sample for occult blood from patients who are being considered for thrombolytic or anticoagulant therapy
Genitourinary (Abdomen)	
Lymphatic	
Musculoskeletal	• Examination of the back with notation of kyphosis or scoliosis • Examination of gait with notation of ability to undergo exercise testing and/or participation in exercise programs • Assessment of muscle strength and tone (e.g., flaccid, cog wheel, spastic) with notation of any atrophy and abnormal movements
Extremities	• Inspection and palpation of digits and nails (e.g., clubbing, cyanosis, inflammation, petechiae, ischemia, infections, Osler's nodes)
Skin	• Inspection and/or palpation of skin and subcutaneous tissue (e.g., stasis dermatitis, ulcers, scars, xanthomas)
Neurologic/ Psychiatric	Brief assessment of mental status including • Orientation to time, place and person • Mood and affect (e.g., depression, anxiety, agitation)

Content and Documentation Requirements

LEVEL OF EXAM	PERFORM AND DOCUMENT
Problem Focused	**One to five** elements identified by a bullet.
Expanded Problem Focused	**At least six** elements identified by a bullet.
Detailed	**At least twelve** elements identified by a bullet.
Comprehensive	Perform **all** elements identified by a bullet; document every element in each box with a shaded border and at least one element in each box with an unshaded border.

EARS, NOSE AND THROAT EXAMINATION

System/Body Area	Elements of Examination
Constitutional	• Measurement of **any three of the following seven** vital signs: 1) sitting or standing blood pressure, 2) supine blood pressure, 3) pulse rate and regularity, 4) respiration, 5) temperature, 6) height, 7) weight (may be measured and recorded by ancillary staff) • General appearance of patient (e.g., development, nutrition, body habitus, deformities, attention to grooming) • Assessment of ability to communicate (e.g., use of sign language or other communication aids) and quality of voice
Head and Face	• Inspection of head and face (e.g., overall appearance, scars, lesions and masses) • Palpation and/or percussion of face with notation of presence or absence of sinus tenderness • Examination of salivary glands • Assessment of facial strength
Eyes	• Test ocular motility including primary gaze alignment
Ears, Nose, Mouth and Throat	• Otoscopic examination of external auditory canals and tympanic membranes including pneumo-otoscopy with notation of mobility of membranes • Assessment of hearing with tuning forks and clinical speech reception thresholds (e.g., whispered voice, finger rub) • External inspection of ears and nose (e.g., overall appearance, scars, lesions and masses) • Inspection of nasal mucosa, septum and turbinates • Inspection of lips, teeth and gums • Examination of oropharynx: oral mucosa, hard and soft palates, tongue, tonsils and posterior pharynx (e.g., asymmetry, lesions, hydration of mucosal surfaces) • Inspection of pharyngeal walls and pyriform sinuses (e.g., pooling of saliva, asymmetry, lesions) • Examination by mirror of larynx including the condition of the epiglottis, false vocal cords, true vocal cords and mobility of larynx (use of mirror not required in children) • Examination by mirror of nasopharynx including appearance of the mucosa, adenoids, posterior choanae and eustachian tubes (use of mirror not required in children)

System/Body Area	Elements of Examination
Neck	• Examination of neck (e.g., masses, overall appearance, symmetry, tracheal position, crepitus) • Examination of thyroid (e.g., enlargement, tenderness, mass)
Respiratory	• Inspection of chest including symmetry, expansion and/or assessment of respiratory effort (e.g., intercostal retractions, use of accessory muscles, diaphragmatic movement) • Auscultation of lungs (e.g., breath sounds, adventitious sounds, rubs)
Cardiovascular	• Auscultation of heart with notation of abnormal sounds and murmurs • Examination of peripheral vascular system by observation (e.g., swelling, varicosities) and palpation (e.g., pulses, temperature, edema, tenderness)
Chest (Breasts)	
Gastrointestinal (Abdomen)	
Genitourinary	
Lymphatic	• Palpation of lymph nodes in neck, axillae, groin and/or other location
Musculoskeletal	
Extremities	
Skin	
Neurological/ Psychiatric	• Test cranial nerves with notation of any deficits Brief assessment of mental status including • Orientation to time, place and person • Mood and affect (e.g., depression, anxiety, agitation)

Content and Documentation Requirements

LEVEL OF EXAM	PERFORM AND DOCUMENT
Problem Focused	**One to five** elements identified by a bullet.
Expanded Problem Focused	**At least six** elements identified by a bullet.
Detailed	**At least twelve** elements identified by a bullet.
Comprehensive	Perform **all** elements identified by a bullet; document every element in each box with a shaded border and at least one element in each box with an unshaded border.

EYE EXAMINATION

System/Body Area	Elements of Examination
Constitutional	
Head and Face	
Eyes	• Test visual acuity (does not include determination of refractive error) • Gross visual field testing by confrontation • Test ocular motility including primary gaze alignment • Inspection of bulbar and palpebral conjunctivae • Examination of ocular adnexae including lids (e.g., ptosis or lagophthalmos), lacrimal glands, lacrimal drainage, orbits and preauricular lymph nodes • Examination of pupils and irises including shape, direct and consensual reaction (afferent pupil), size (e.g., anisocoria) and morphology • Slit lamp examination of the corneas including epithelium, stroma, endothelium, and tear film • Slit lamp examination of the anterior chambers including depth, cells, and flare • Slit lamp examination of the lenses including clarity, anterior and posterior capsule, cortex, and nucleus • Measurement of intraocular pressures (except in children and patients with trauma or infectious disease) Ophthalmoscopic examination through dilated pupils (unless contraindicated) of • Optic discs including size, C/D ratio, appearance (e.g., atrophy, cupping, tumor elevation) and nerve fiber layer • Posterior segments including retina and vessels (e.g., exudates and hemorrhages)
Ears, Nose, Mouth and Throat	
Neck	
Respiratory	
Cardiovascular	
Chest (Breasts)	
Gastrointestinal (Abdomen)	
Genitourinary	
Lymphatic	
Musculoskeletal	
Extremities	
Skin	
Neurological/Psychiatric	Brief assessment of mental status including • Orientation to time, place and person • Mood and affect (e.g., depression, anxiety, agitation)

Content and Documentation Requirements

LEVEL OF EXAM	PERFORM AND DOCUMENT
Problem Focused	**One to five** elements identified by a bullet.
Expanded Problem Focused	**At least six** elements identified by a bullet.
Detailed	**At least twelve** elements identified by a bullet.
Comprehensive	Perform **all** elements identified by a bullet; document every element in each box with a shaded border and at least one element in each box with an unshaded border.

GENITOURINARY EXAMINATION

System/Body Area	Elements of Examination
Constitutional	• Measurement of **any three of the following seven** vital signs: 1) sitting or standing blood pressure, 2) supine blood pressure, 3) pulse rate and regularity, 4) respiration, 5) temperature, 6) height, 7) weight (may be measured and recorded by ancillary staff) • General appearance of patient (e.g., development, nutrition, body habitus, deformities, attention to grooming)
Head and Face	
Eyes	
Ears, Nose, Mouth and Throat	
Neck	• Examination of neck (e.g., masses, overall appearance, symmetry, tracheal position, crepitus) • Examination of thyroid (e.g., enlargement, tenderness, mass)
Respiratory	• Assessment of respiratory effort (e.g., intercostal retractions, use of accessory muscles, diaphragmatic movement) • Auscultation of lungs (e.g., breath sounds, adventitious sounds, rubs)
Cardiovascular	• Auscultation of heart with notation of abnormal sounds and murmurs • Examination of peripheral vascular system by observation (e.g., swelling, varicosities) and palpation (e.g., pulses, temperature, edema, tenderness)
Chest (Breasts)	[See genitourinary (female).]
Gastrointestinal (Abdomen)	• Examination of abdomen with notation of presence of masses or tenderness • Examination for presence or absence of hernia • Examination of liver and spleen • Obtain stool sample for occult blood test when indicated

System/Body Area	Elements of Examination
Genitourinary	**Male:**
	• Inspection of anus and perineum Examination (with or without specimen collection for smears and cultures) of genitalia including: • Scrotum (e.g., lesions, cysts, rashes) • Epididymides (e.g., size, symmetry, masses) • Testes (e.g., size, symmetry, masses) • Urethral meatus (e.g., size, location, lesions, discharge) • Penis (e.g., lesions, presence or absence of foreskin, foreskin retractability, plaque, masses, scarring, deformities) Digital rectal examination including: • Prostate gland (e.g., size, symmetry, nodularity, tenderness) • Seminal vesicles (e.g., symmetry, tenderness, masses, enlargement) • Sphincter tone, presence of hemorrhoids, rectal masses **Female:** Includes **at least seven of the following** eleven elements identified by bullets: • Inspection and palpation of breasts (e.g., masses or lumps, tenderness, symmetry, nipple discharge) • Digital rectal examination including sphincter tone, presence of hemorrhoids, rectal masses Pelvic examination (with or without specimen collection for smears and cultures) including: • External genitalia (e.g., general appearance, hair distribution, lesions) • Urethral meatus (e.g., size, location, lesions, prolapse) • Urethra (e.g., masses, tenderness, scarring) • Bladder (e.g., fullness, masses, tenderness) • Vagina (e.g., general appearance, estrogen effect, discharge, lesions, pelvic support, cystocele, rectocele) • Cervix (e.g., general appearance, lesions, discharge) • Uterus (e.g., size, contour, position, mobility, tenderness, consistency, descent or support) • Adnexa/parametria (e.g., masses, tenderness, organomegaly, nodularity) • Anus and perineum
Lymphatic	• Palpation of lymph nodes in neck, axillae, groin and/or other location
Musculoskeletal	
Extremities	
Skin	• Inspection and/or palpation of skin and subcutaneous tissue (e.g., rashes, lesions, ulcers)
Neurological/ Psychiatric	Brief assessment of mental status including • Orientation (e.g., time, place and person) and • Mood and affect (e.g., depression, anxiety, agitation)

Content and Documentation Requirements

LEVEL OF EXAM	PERFORM AND DOCUMENT
Problem Focused	**One to five** elements identified by a bullet.
Expanded Problem Focused	**At least six** elements identified by a bullet.
Detailed	**At least twelve** elements identified by a bullet.
Comprehensive	Perform **all** elements identified by a bullet; document every element in each box with a shaded border and at least one element in each box with an unshaded border.

HEMATOLOGIC/LYMPHATIC/IMMUNOLOGIC EXAMINATION

System/Body Area	Elements of Examination
Constitutional	• Measurement of **any three of the following seven** vital signs: 1) sitting or standing blood pressure, 2) supine blood pressure, 3) pulse rate and regularity, 4) respiration, 5) temperature, 6) height, 7) weight (may be measured and recorded by ancillary staff) • General appearance of patient (e.g., development, nutrition, body habitus, deformities, attention to grooming)
Head and Face	• Palpation and/or percussion of face with notation of presence or absence of sinus tenderness
Eyes	• Inspection of conjunctivae and lids
Ears, Nose, Mouth and Throat	• Otoscopic examination of external auditory canals and tympanic membranes • Inspection of nasal mucosa, septum and turbinates • Inspection of teeth and gums • Examination of oropharynx (e.g., oral mucosa, hard and soft palates, tongue, tonsils, posterior pharynx)
Neck	• Examination of neck (e.g., masses, overall appearance, symmetry, tracheal position, crepitus) • Examination of thyroid (e.g., enlargement, tenderness, mass)
Respiratory	• Assessment of respiratory effort (e.g., intercostal retractions, use of accessory muscles, diaphragmatic movement) • Auscultation of lungs (e.g., breath sounds, adventitious sounds, rubs)
Cardiovascular	• Auscultation of heart with notation of abnormal sounds and murmurs • Examination of peripheral vascular system by observation (e.g., swelling, varicosities) and palpation (e.g., pulses, temperature, edema, tenderness)
Chest (Breasts)	
Gastrointestinal (Abdomen)	• Examination of abdomen with notation of presence of masses or tenderness • Examination of liver and spleen
Genitourinary	
Lymphatic	• Palpation of lymph nodes in neck, axillae, groin, and/or other location
Musculoskeletal	

System/Body Area	Elements of Examination
Extremities	• Inspection and palpation of digits and nails (e.g., clubbing, cyanosis, inflammation, petechiae, ischemia, infections, nodes)
Skin	• Inspection and/or palpation of skin and subcutaneous tissue (e.g., rashes, lesions, ulcers, ecchymoses, bruises)
Neurological/ Psychiatric	Brief assessment of mental status including • Orientation to time, place and person • Mood and affect (e.g., depression, anxiety, agitation)

Content and Documentation Requirements

LEVEL OF EXAM	PERFORM AND DOCUMENT
Problem Focused	**One to five** elements identified by a bullet.
Expanded Problem Focused	**At least six** elements identified by a bullet.
Detailed	**At least twelve** elements identified by a bullet.
Comprehensive	Perform **all** elements identified by a bullet; document every element in each box with a shaded border and at least one element in each box with an unshaded border.

MUSCULOSKELETAL EXAMINATION

System/Body Area	Elements of Examination
Constitutional	• Measurement of **any three of the following seven** vital signs: 1) sitting or standing blood pressure, 2) supine blood pressure, 3) pulse rate and regularity, 4) respiration, 5) temperature, 6) height, 7) weight (may be measured and recorded by ancillary staff) • General appearance of patient (e.g., development, nutrition, body habitus, deformities, attention to grooming)
Head and Face	
Eyes	
Ears, Nose, Mouth and Throat	
Neck	
Respiratory	
Cardiovascular	• Examination of peripheral vascular system by observation (e.g., swelling, varicosities) and palpation (e.g., pulses, temperature, edema, tenderness)
Chest (Breasts)	
Gastrointestinal (Abdomen)	
Genitourinary	
Lymphatic	• Palpation of lymph nodes in neck, axillae, groin and/or other location

System/Body Area	Elements of Examination
Musculoskeletal	• Examination of gait and station Examination of joint(s), bone(s) and muscle(s)/tendon(s) **of four of the following six** areas: 1) head and neck; 2) spine, ribs and pelvis; 3) right upper extremity; 4) left upper extremity; 5) right lower extremity; and 6) left lower extremity. The examination of a given area includes: • Inspection, percussion and/or palpation with notation of any misalignment, asymmetry, crepitation, defects, tenderness, masses or effusions • Assessment of range of motion with notation of any pain (e.g., straight leg raising), crepitation or contracture • Assessment of stability with notation of any dislocation (luxation), subluxation or laxity • Assessment of muscle strength and tone (e.g., flaccid, cog wheel, spastic) with notation of any atrophy or abnormal movements *Note:* For the comprehensive level of examination, all four of the elements identified by a bullet must be performed and documented for each of four anatomic areas. For the three lower levels of examination, each element is counted separately for each body area. For example, assessing range of motion in two extremities constitutes two elements.
Extremities	[See musculoskeletal and skin.]
Skin	• Inspection and/or palpation of skin and subcutaneous tissue (e.g., scars, rashes, lesions, cafe-au-lait spots, ulcers) **in four of the following six** areas: 1) head and neck; 2) trunk; 3) right upper extremity; 4) left upper extremity; 5) right lower extremity; and 6) left lower extremity. *Note:* For the comprehensive level, the examination of all four anatomic areas must be performed and documented. For the three lower levels of examination, each body area is counted separately. For example, inspection and/or palpation of the skin and subcutaneous tissue of two extremities constitutes two elements.
Neurological/ Psychiatric	• Test coordination (e.g., finger/nose, heel/ knee/shin, rapid alternating movements in the upper and lower extremities, evaluation of fine motor coordination in young children) • Examination of deep tendon reflexes and/or nerve stretch test with notation of pathological reflexes (e.g., Babinski) • Examination of sensation (e.g., by touch, pin, vibration, proprioception) Brief assessment of mental status including • Orientation to time, place and person • Mood and affect (e.g., depression, anxiety, agitation)

Content and Documentation Requirements

LEVEL OF EXAM	PERFORM AND DOCUMENT
Problem Focused	**One to five** elements identified by a bullet.
Expanded Problem Focused	**At least six** elements identified by a bullet.
Detailed	**At least twelve** elements identified by a bullet.
Comprehensive	Perform **all** elements identified by a bullet; document every element in each box with a shaded border and at least one element in each box with an unshaded border.

NEUROLOGICAL EXAMINATION

System/Body Area	Elements of Examination
Constitutional	• Measurement of **any three of the following seven** vital signs: 1) sitting or standing blood pressure, 2) supine blood pressure, 3) pulse rate and regularity, 4) respiration, 5) temperature, 6) height, 7) weight (may be measured and recorded by ancillary staff) • General appearance of patient (e.g., development, nutrition, body habitus, deformities, attention to grooming)
Head and Face	
Eyes	• Ophthalmoscopic examination of optic discs (e.g., size, C/D ratio, appearance) and posterior segments (e.g., vessel changes, exudates, hemorrhages)
Ears, Nose, Mouth and Throat	
Neck	
Respiratory	
Cardiovascular	• Examination of carotid arteries (e.g., pulse amplitude, bruits) • Auscultation of heart with notation of abnormal sounds and murmurs • Examination of peripheral vascular system by observation (e.g., swelling, varicosities) and palpation (e.g., pulses, temperature, edema, tenderness)
Chest (Breasts)	
Gastrointestinal (Abdomen)	
Genitourinary	
Lymphatic	
Musculoskeletal	• Examination of gait and station Assessment of motor function including: • Muscle strength in upper and lower extremities • Muscle tone in upper and lower extremities (e.g., flaccid, cog wheel, spastic) with notation of any atrophy or abnormal movements (e.g., fasciculation, tardive dyskinesia)
Extremities	[See musculoskeletal.]
Skin	

System/Body Area	Elements of Examination
Neurological	Evaluation of higher integrative functions including: • Orientation to time, place and person • Recent and remote memory • Attention span and concentration • Language (e.g., naming objects, repeating phrases, spontaneous speech) • Fund of knowledge (e.g., awareness of current events, past history, vocabulary) Test the following cranial nerves: • 2nd cranial nerve (e.g., visual acuity, visual fields, fundi) • 3rd, 4th and 6th cranial nerves (e.g., pupils, eye movements) • 5th cranial nerve (e.g., facial sensation, corneal reflexes) • 7th cranial nerve (e.g., facial symmetry, strength) • 8th cranial nerve (e.g., hearing with tuning fork, whispered voice and/or finger rub) • 9th cranial nerve (e.g., spontaneous or reflex palate movement) • 11th cranial nerve (e.g., shoulder shrug strength) • 12th cranial nerve (e.g., tongue protrusion) • Examination of sensation (e.g., by touch, pin, vibration, proprioception) • Examination of deep tendon reflexes in upper and lower extremities with notation of pathological reflexes (e.g., Babinski) • Test coordination (e.g., finger/nose, heel/knee/shin, rapid alternating movements in the upper and lower extremities, evaluation of fine motor coordination in young children)
Psychiatric	

Content and Documentation Requirements

LEVEL OF EXAM	PERFORM AND DOCUMENT
Problem Focused	**One to five** elements identified by a bullet.
Expanded Problem Focused	**At least six** elements identified by a bullet.
Detailed	**At least twelve** elements identified by a bullet.
Comprehensive	Perform **all** elements identified by a bullet; document every element in each box with a shaded border and at least one element in each box with an unshaded border.

PSYCHIATRIC EXAMINATION

System/Body Area	Elements of Examination
Constitutional	• Measurement of **any three of the following seven** vital signs: 1) sitting or standing blood pressure, 2) supine blood pressure, 3) pulse rate and regularity, 4) respiration, 5) temperature, 6) height, 7) weight (may be measured and recorded by ancillary staff) • General appearance of patient (e.g., development, nutrition, body habitus, deformities, attention to grooming)

System/Body Area	Elements of Examination
Head and Face	
Eyes	
Ears, Nose, Mouth and Throat	
Neck	
Respiratory	
Cardiovascular	
Chest (Breasts)	
Gastrointestinal (Abdomen)	
Genitourinary	
Lymphatic	
Musculoskeletal	• Assessment of muscle strength and tone (e.g., flaccid, cog wheel, spastic) with notation of any atrophy and abnormal movements • Examination of gait and station
Extremities	
Skin	
Neurological	
Psychiatric	• Description of speech including: rate; volume; articulation; coherence; and spontaneity with notation of abnormalities (e.g., perseveration, paucity of language) • Description of thought processes including: rate of thoughts; content of thoughts (e.g., logical vs. illogical, tangential); abstract reasoning; and computation • Description of associations (e.g., loose, tangential, circumstantial, intact) • Description of abnormal or psychotic thoughts including: hallucinations; delusions; preoccupation with violence; homicidal or suicidal ideation; and obsessions • Description of the patient's judgment (e.g., concerning everyday activities and social situations) and insight (e.g., concerning psychiatric condition) Complete mental status examination including • Orientation to time, place and person • Recent and remote memory • Attention span and concentration • Language (e.g., naming objects, repeating phrases) • Fund of knowledge (e.g., awareness of current events, past history, vocabulary) • Mood and affect (e.g., depression, anxiety, agitation, hypomania, lability)

Content and Documentation Requirements

LEVEL OF EXAM	PERFORM AND DOCUMENT
Problem Focused	**One to five** elements identified by a bullet.
Expanded Problem Focused	**At least six** elements identified by a bullet.
Detailed	**At least twelve** elements identified by a bullet.
Comprehensive	Perform **all** elements identified by a bullet; document every element in each box with a shaded border and at least one element in each box with an unshaded border.

RESPIRATORY EXAMINATION

System/Body Area	Elements of Examination
Constitutional	• Measurement of **any three of the following seven** vital signs: 1) sitting or standing blood pressure, 2) supine blood pressure, 3) pulse rate and regularity, 4) respiration, 5) temperature, 6) height, 7) weight (may be measured and recorded by ancillary staff) • General appearance of patient (e.g., development, nutrition, body habitus, deformities, attention to grooming)
Head and Face	
Eyes	
Ears, Nose, Mouth and Throat	• Inspection of nasal mucosa, septum and turbinates • Inspection of teeth and gums • Examination of oropharynx (e.g., oral mucosa, hard and soft palates, tongue, tonsils and posterior pharynx)
Neck	• Examination of neck (e.g., masses, overall appearance, symmetry, tracheal position, crepitus) • Examination of thyroid (e.g., enlargement, tenderness, mass) • Examination of jugular veins (e.g., distension; a, v or cannon a waves)
Respiratory	• Inspection of chest with notation of symmetry and expansion • Assessment of respiratory effort (e.g., intercostal retractions, use of accessory muscles, diaphragmatic movement) • Percussion of chest (e.g., dullness, flatness, hyperresonance) • Palpation of chest (e.g., tactile fremitus) • Auscultation of lungs (e.g., breath sounds, adventitious sounds, rubs)
Cardiovascular	• Auscultation of heart including sounds, abnormal sounds and murmurs • Examination of peripheral vascular system by observation (e.g., swelling, varicosities) and palpation (e.g., pulses, temperature, edema, tenderness)
Chest (Breasts)	
Gastrointestinal (Abdomen)	• Examination of abdomen with notation of presence of masses or tenderness • Examination of liver and spleen
Genitourinary	

System/Body Area	Elements of Examination
Lymphatic	• Palpation of lymph nodes in neck, axillae, groin and/or other location
Musculoskeletal	• Assessment of muscle strength and tone (e.g., flaccid, cog wheel, spastic) with notation of any atrophy and abnormal movements • Examination of gait and station
Extremities	• Inspection and palpation of digits and nails (e.g., clubbing, cyanosis, inflammation, petechiae, ischemia, infections, nodes)
Skin	• Inspection and/or palpation of skin and subcutaneous tissue (e.g., rashes, lesions, ulcers)
Neurological/ Psychiatric	Brief assessment of mental status including • Orientation to time, place and person • Mood and affect (e.g., depression, anxiety, agitation)

Content and Documentation Requirements

LEVEL OF EXAM	PERFORM AND DOCUMENT
Problem Focused	**One to five** elements identified by a bullet.
Expanded Problem Focused	**At least six** elements identified by a bullet.
Detailed	**At least twelve** elements identified by a bullet.
Comprehensive	Perform **all** elements identified by a bullet; document every element in each box with a shaded border and at least one element in each box with an unshaded border.

SKIN EXAMINATION

System/Body Area	Elements of Examination
Constitutional	• Measurement of any **three of the following seven** vital signs: 1) sitting or standing blood pressure, 2) supine blood pressure, 3) pulse rate and regularity, 4) respiration, 5) temperature, 6) height, 7) weight (may be measured and recorded by ancillary staff) • General appearance of patient (e.g., development, nutrition, body habitus, deformities, attention to grooming)
Head and Face	
Eyes	• Inspection of conjunctivae and lids
Ears, Nose, Mouth and Throat	• Inspection of lips, teeth and gums • Examination of oropharynx (e.g., oral mucosa, hard and soft palates, tongue, tonsils, posterior pharynx)
Neck	• Examination of thyroid (e.g., enlargement, tenderness, mass)
Respiratory	
Cardiovascular	• Examination of peripheral vascular system by observation (e.g., swelling, varicosities) and palpation (e.g., pulses, temperature, edema, tenderness)
Chest (Breasts)	

System/Body Area	Elements of Examination
Gastrointestinal (Abdomen)	• Examination of liver and spleen • Examination of anus for condyloma and other lesions
Genitourinary	
Lymphatic	• Palpation of lymph nodes in neck, axillae, groin and/or other location
Musculoskeletal	
Extremities	• Inspection and palpation of digits and nails (e.g., clubbing, cyanosis, inflammation, petechiae, ischemia, infections, nodes)
Skin	• Palpation of scalp and inspection of hair of scalp, eyebrows, face, chest, pubic area (when indicated) and extremities • Inspection and/or palpation of skin and subcutaneous tissue (e.g., rashes, lesions, ulcers, susceptibility to and presence of photo damage) in **eight of the following ten** areas • Head, including the face and neck • Chest, including breasts and axillae • Abdomen • Genitalia, groin, buttocks • Back • Right upper extremity • Left upper extremity • Right lower extremity • Left lower extremity *Note:* For the comprehensive level, the examination of at least eight anatomic areas must be performed and documented. For the three lower levels of examination, each body area is counted separately. For example, inspection and/or palpation of the skin and subcutaneous tissue of the right upper extremity and the left upper extremity constitutes two elements. • Inspection of eccrine and apocrine glands of skin and subcutaneous tissue with identification and location of any hyperhidrosis, chromhidroses or bromhidrosis
Neurological/ Psychiatric	Brief assessment of mental status including • Orientation to time, place and person • Mood and affect (e.g., depression, anxiety, agitation)

Content and Documentation Requirements

LEVEL OF EXAM	PERFORM AND DOCUMENT
Problem Focused	**One to five** elements identified by a bullet.
Expanded Problem Focused	**At least six** elements identified by a bullet.
Detailed	**At least twelve** elements identified by a bullet.
Comprehensive	Perform **all** elements identified by a bullet; document every element in each box with a shaded border and at least one element in each box with an unshaded border.

C. Documentation of the Complexity of Medical Decision-Making

The levels of E/M services recognize four types of medical decision-making (straightforward, low complexity, moderate complexity and high complexity). Medical decision-making refers to the complexity of establishing a diagnosis and/or selecting a management option as measured by:

- the number of possible diagnoses and/or the number of management options that must be considered;

- the amount and/or complexity of medical records, diagnostic tests, and/or other information that must be obtained, reviewed and analyzed; and

- the risk of significant complications, morbidity and/or mortality, as well as comorbidities, associated with the patient's presenting problem(s), the diagnostic procedure(s) and/or the possible management options.

The following chart shows the progression of the elements required for each level of medical decision-making. To qualify for a given type of decision-making, **two of the three elements in the table must be either met or exceeded.**

Number of Diagnoses or Management Options	Amount and/or Complexity of Data to Be Reviewed	Risk of Complications and/or Morbidity or Mortality	Type of Decision Making
Minimal	Minimal or None	Minimal	*Straightforward*
Limited	Limited	Low	*Low Complexity*
Multiple	Moderate	Moderate	*Moderate Complexity*
Extensive	Extensive	High	*High Complexity*

Each of the elements of medical decision-making is described following.

Number of Diagnoses or Management Options

The number of possible diagnoses and/or the number of management options that must be considered is based on the number and types of problems addressed during the encounter, the complexity of establishing a diagnosis and the management decisions that are made by the physician.

Generally, decision-making with respect to a diagnosed problem is easier than that for an identified but undiagnosed problem. The number and type of diagnostic tests employed may be an indicator of the number of possible diagnoses. Problems which are improving or resolving are less complex than those which are worsening or failing to change as expected. The need to seek advice from others is another indicator of complexity of diagnostic or management problems.

- DG: For each encounter, an assessment, clinical impression, or diagnosis should be documented. It may be explicitly stated or implied in documented decisions regarding management plans and/or further evaluation.

  - For a presenting problem with an established diagnosis the record should reflect whether the problem is: a) improved, well controlled, resolving or resolved; or, b) inadequately controlled, worsening, or failing to change as expected.

■ For a presenting problem without an established diagnosis, the assessment or clinical impression may be stated in the form of differential diagnoses or as a "possible," "probable," or "rule out" (R/O) diagnosis.

■ DG: The initiation of, or changes in, treatment should be documented. Treatment includes a wide range of management options including patient instructions, nursing instructions, therapies, and medications.

■ DG: If referrals are made, consultations requested or advice sought, the record should indicate to whom or where the referral or consultation is made or from whom the advice is requested.

Amount and/or Complexity of Data to Be Reviewed

The amount and complexity of data to be reviewed is based on the types of diagnostic testing ordered or reviewed. A decision to obtain and review old medical records and/or obtain history from sources other than the patient increases the amount and complexity of data to be reviewed.

Discussion of contradictory or unexpected test results with the physician who performed or interpreted the test is an indication of the complexity of data being reviewed. On occasion the physician who ordered a test may personally review the image, tracing or specimen to supplement information from the physician who prepared the test report or interpretation; this is another indication of the complexity of data being reviewed.

■ DG: If a diagnostic service (test or procedure) is ordered, planned, scheduled, or performed at the time of the E/M encounter, the type of service, eg, lab or x-ray, should be documented.

■ DG: The review of lab, radiology and/or other diagnostic tests should be documented. A simple notation such as "WBC elevated" or "chest x-ray unremarkable" is acceptable. Alternatively, the review may be documented by initialing and dating the report containing the test results.

■ DG: A decision to obtain old records or decision to obtain additional history from the family, caretaker or other source to supplement that obtained from the patient should be documented.

■ DG: Relevant findings from the review of old records, and/or the receipt of additional history from the family, caretaker or other source to supplement that obtained from the patient should be documented. If there is no relevant information beyond that already obtained, that fact should be documented. A notation of "Old records reviewed" or "additional history obtained from family" without elaboration is insufficient.

■ DG: The results of discussion of laboratory, radiology or other diagnostic tests with the physician who performed or interpreted the study should be documented.

■ DG: The direct visualization and independent interpretation of an image, tracing or specimen previously or subsequently interpreted by another physician should be documented.

132

Risk of Significant Complications, Morbidity, and/or Mortality

The risk of significant complications, morbidity, and/or mortality is based on the risks associated with the presenting problem(s), the diagnostic procedure(s), and the possible management options.

- DG: Comorbidities/underlying diseases or other factors that increase the complexity of medical decision making by increasing the risk of complications, morbidity, and/or mortality should be documented.

- DG: If a surgical or invasive diagnostic procedure is ordered, planned or scheduled at the time of the E/M encounter, the type of procedure, e.g., laparoscopy, should be documented.

- DG: If a surgical or invasive diagnostic procedure is performed at the time of the E/M encounter, the specific procedure should be documented.

- DG: The referral for or decision to perform a surgical or invasive diagnostic procedure on an urgent basis should be documented or implied.

The following table may be used to help determine whether the risk of significant complications, morbidity, and/or mortality is *minimal, low, moderate,* or *high.* Because the determination of risk is complex and not readily quantifiable, the table includes common clinical examples rather than absolute measures of risk. The assessment of risk of the presenting problem(s) is based on the risk related to the disease process anticipated between the present encounter and the next one. The assessment of risk of selecting diagnostic procedures and management options is based on the risk during and immediately following any procedures or treatment. **The highest level of risk in any one category (presenting problem(s), diagnostic procedure(s), or management options) determines the overall risk.**

TABLE OF RISK

Level of Risk	Presenting Problem(s)	Diagnostic Procedure(s) Ordered	Management Options Selected
Minimal	• One self-limited or minor problem, eg, cold, insect bite, tinea corporis	• Laboratory tests requiring venipuncture • Chest x-rays • EKG/EEG • Urinalysis • Ultrasound, eg, echocardiography • KOH prep	• Rest • Gargles • Elastic bandages • Superficial dressings
Low	• Two or more self-limited or minor problems • One stable chronic illness, eg, well controlled hypertension, non-insulin dependent diabetes, cataract, BPH • Acute uncomplicated illness or injury, eg, cystitis, allergic rhinitis, simple sprain	• Physiologic tests not under stress, eg, pulmonary function tests • Non-cardiovascular imaging studies with contrast, eg, barium enema • Superficial needle biopsies • Clinical laboratory tests requiring arterial puncture • Skin biopsies	• Over-the-counter drugs • Minor surgery with no identified risk factors • Physical therapy • Occupational therapy • IV fluids without additives

Level of Risk	Presenting Problem(s)	Diagnostic Procedure(s) Ordered	Management Options Selected
Moderate	• One or more chronic illnesses with mild exacerbation, progression, or side effects of treatment • Two or more stable chronic illnesses • Undiagnosed new problem with uncertain prognosis, eg, lump in breast • Acute illness with systemic symptoms, eg, pyelonephritis, pneumonitis, colitis • Acute complicated injury, eg, head injury with brief loss of consciousness	• Physiologic tests under stress, eg, cardiac stress test, fetal contraction stress test • Diagnostic endoscopies with no identified risk factors • Deep needle or incisional biopsy • Cardiovascular imaging studies with contrast and no identified risk factors, eg, arteriogram, cardiac catheterization • Obtain fluid from body cavity, eg, lumbar puncture, thoracentesis, culdocentesis	• Minor surgery with identified risk factors • Elective major surgery (open, percutaneous or endoscopic) with no identified risk factors • Prescription drug management • Therapeutic nuclear medicine • IV fluids with additives • Closed treatment of fracture or dislocation without manipulation
High	• One or more chronic illnesses with severe exacerbation, progression, or side effects of treatment • Acute or chronic illnesses or injuries that pose a threat to life or bodily function, eg, multiple trauma, acute MI, pulmonary embolus, severe respiratory distress, progressive severe rheumatoid arthritis, psychiatric illness with potential threat to self or others, peritonitis, acute renal failure • An abrupt change in neurologic status, eg, seizure, TIA, weakness, sensory loss	• Cardiovascular imaging studies with contrast with identified risk factors • Cardiac electrophysiological tests • Diagnostic endoscopies with identified risk factors • Discography	• Elective major surgery (open, percutaneous or endoscopic) with identified risk factors • Emergency major surgery (open, percutaneous or endoscopic) • Parenteral controlled substances • Drug therapy requiring intensive monitoring for toxicity • Decision not to resuscitate or to de-escalate care because of poor prognosis

D. Documentation of an Encounter Dominated by Counseling or Coordination of Care

In the case where counseling and/or coordination of care dominates (more than 50%) of the physician/patient and/or family encounter (face-to-face time in the office or other or outpatient setting, floor/unit time in the hospital or nursing facility), time is considered the key or controlling factor to qualify for a particular level of E/M services.

■ DG: If the physician elects to report the level of service based on counseling and/or coordination of care, the total length of time of the encounter (face-to-face or floor time, as appropriate) should be documented and the record should describe the counseling and/or activities to coordinate care.

Internet Only Manual (IOM) 104, 30.6

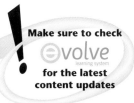

Make sure to check evolve *learning system* **for the latest content updates**

Reference: **https://www.cms.gov/regulations-and-guidance/guidance/manuals/downloads//clm104c12.pdf** (accessed 10/13/12)

Changes to the IOM 104, 30.6, will also be posted to the Evolve website.

30.6 - Evaluation and Management Service Codes - General (Codes 99201 - 99499)

30.6.1 - Selection of Level of Evaluation and Management Service

30.6.1.1 - Initial Preventive Physical Examination (IPPE) and Annual Wellness Visit (AWV)

30.6.2 - Billing for Medically Necessary Visit on Same Occasion as Preventive Medicine Service

30.6.3 - Payment for Immunosuppressive Therapy Management—Not Required Reading

30.6.4 - Evaluation and Management (E/M) Services Furnished Incident to Physician's Service by Nonphysician Practitioners

30.6.5 - Physicians in Group Practice

30.6.6 - Payment for Evaluation and Management Services Provided During Global Period of Surgery

30.6.7 - Payment for Office or Other Outpatient Evaluation and Management (E/M) Visits (Codes 99201 - 99215)

30.6.8 - Payment for Hospital Observation Services and Observation or Inpatient Care Services (Including Admission and Discharge Services)

30.6.9 - Payment for Inpatient Hospital Visits - General

30.6.9.1 - Payment for Initial Hospital Care Services and Observation or Inpatient Care Services (Including Admission and Discharge Services)

30.6.9.2 - Subsequent Hospital Visits and Hospital Discharge Day Management Services (Codes 99231 - 99239)

30.6.10 - Consultation Services

30.6.11 - Emergency Department Visits (Codes 99281 - 99288)

30.6.12 - Critical Care Visits and Neonatal Intensive Care (Codes 99291 - 99292)

30.6 - EVALUATION AND MANAGEMENT SERVICE CODES - GENERAL (CODES 99201 - 99499)

(Rev. 178, 05-14-04)

B3-15501-15501.1

30.6.1 - SELECTION OF LEVEL OF EVALUATION AND MANAGEMENT SERVICE

(Rev. 1875, Issued: 12-14-09, Effective: 01-01-10, Implementation: 01-04-10)

A. Use of CPT Codes

Advise physicians to use CPT codes (level 1 of HCPCS) to code physician services, including evaluation and management services. Medicare will pay for E/M services for specific non-physician practitioners (i.e., nurse practitioner (NP), clinical nurse specialist (CNS) and certified nurse midwife (CNM)) whose Medicare benefit permits them to bill these services. A physician assistant (PA) may also provide a physician service, however, the physician collaboration and general supervision rules as well as all billing rules apply to all the above non-physician practitioners. The service provided must be medically necessary and the service must be within the scope of practice for a non-physician practitioner in the State in which he/she practices. Do not pay for CPT evaluation and management codes billed by physical therapists in independent practice or by occupational therapists in independent practice.

Medical necessity of a service is the overarching criterion for payment in addition to the individual requirements of a CPT code. It would not be medically necessary or appropriate to bill a higher level of evaluation and management service when a lower level of service is warranted. The volume of documentation should not be the primary influence upon which a specific level of service is billed. Documentation should support the level of service reported. The service should be documented during, or as soon as practicable after it is provided in order to maintain an accurate medical record.

B. Selection of Level of Evaluation and Management Service

Instruct physicians to select the code for the service based upon the content of the service. The duration of the visit is an ancillary factor and does not control the level of the service to be billed unless more than 50 percent of the face-to-face time (for non-inpatient services) or more than 50 percent of the floor time (for inpatient services) is spent providing counseling or coordination of care as described in subsection C.

Any physician or non-physician practitioner (NPP) authorized to bill Medicare services will be paid by the carrier at the appropriate physician fee schedule amount based on the rendering UPIN/PIN.

"Incident to" Medicare Part B payment policy is applicable for office visits when the requirements for "incident to" are met (refer to sections 60.1, 60.2, and 60.3, chapter 15 in IOM 100-02).

SPLIT/SHARED E/M SERVICE

OFFICE/CLINIC SETTING

In the office/clinic setting when the physician performs the E/M service the service must be reported using the physician's UPIN/PIN. When an E/M service is a shared/split encounter between a physician and a non-physician practitioner (NP, PA, CNS or CNM), the service is considered to have been performed "incident to" if the requirements for "incident to" are met and the patient is an established patient. If "incident to" requirements are not met for the shared/split E/M service, the service must be billed under the NPP's UPIN/PIN, and payment will be made at the appropriate physician fee schedule payment.

HOSPITAL INPATIENT/OUTPATIENT/EMERGENCY DEPARTMENT SETTING

When a hospital inpatient/hospital outpatient or emergency department E/M is shared between a physician and an NPP from the same group practice and the physician provides any face-to-face portion of the E/M encounter with the patient, the service may be billed under either the physician's or the NPP's UPIN/PIN number. However, if there was no face-to-face encounter between the patient and the physician (e.g., even if the physician participated in the service by only reviewing the patient's medical record) then the service may only be billed under the NPP's UPIN/PIN. Payment will be made at the appropriate physician fee schedule rate based on the UPIN/PIN entered on the claim.

EXAMPLES OF SHARED VISITS

1. If the NPP sees a hospital inpatient in the morning and the physician follows with a later face-to-face visit with the patient on the same day, the physician or the NPP may report the service.

2. In an office setting the NPP performs a portion of an E/M encounter and the physician completes the E/M service. If the "incident to" requirements are met, the physician reports the service. If the "incident to" requirements are not met, the service must be reported using the NPP's UPIN/PIN.

In the rare circumstance when a physician (or NPP) provides a service that does not reflect a CPT code description, the service must be reported as an unlisted service with CPT code 99499. A description of the service provided must accompany the claim. The carrier has the discretion to value the service when the service does not meet the full terms of a CPT code description (e.g., only a history is performed). The carrier also determines the payment based on the applicable percentage of the physician fee schedule depending on whether the claim is paid at the physician rate or the non-physician practitioner rate. CPT modifier -52 (reduced services) must not be used with an evaluation and management service. Medicare does not recognize modifier -52 for this purpose.

C. Selection Of Level Of Evaluation and Management Service Based On Duration Of Coordination of Care and/or Counseling

Advise physicians that when counseling and/or coordination of care dominates (more than 50 percent) the face-to-face physician/patient encounter or the floor time (in the case of inpatient services), time is the key or controlling factor in selecting the level of service. In general, to bill an E/M code, the physician must complete at least 2 out of 3 criteria applicable to the type/level of service provided. However, the physician may document time spent with the patient in conjunction with the medical decision-making involved and a description of the coordination of care or counseling provided. Documentation must be in sufficient detail to support the claim.

EXAMPLE: A cancer patient has had all preliminary studies completed and a medical decision to implement chemotherapy. At an office visit the physician discusses the treatment options and subsequent lifestyle effects of treatment the patient may encounter or is experiencing. The physician need not complete a history and physical examination in order to select the level of service. The time spent in counseling/coordination of care and medical decision-making will determine the level of service billed.

The code selection is based on the total time of the face-to-face encounter or floor time, not just the counseling time. The medical record must be documented in sufficient detail to justify the selection of the specific code if time is the basis for selection of the code.

In the office and other outpatient setting, counseling and/or coordination of care must be provided in the presence of the patient if the time spent providing those services is used to determine the level of service reported. Face-to-face time refers to the time with the physician only. Counseling by other staff is not considered to be part of the face-to-face physician/patient encounter time. Therefore, the time spent by the other staff is not considered in selecting the appropriate level of service. The code used depends upon the physician service provided.

In an inpatient setting, the counseling and/or coordination of care must be provided at the bedside or on the patient's hospital floor or unit that is associated with an individual patient. Time spent counseling the patient or coordinating the patient's care after the patient has left the office or the physician has left the patient's floor or begun to care for another patient on the floor is not considered when selecting the level of service to be reported.

The duration of counseling or coordination of care that is provided face-to-face or on the floor may be estimated but that estimate, along with the total duration of the visit, must be recorded when time is used for the selection of the level of a service that involves predominantly coordination of care or counseling.

D. Use of Highest Levels of Evaluation and Management Codes

Contractors must advise physicians that to bill the highest levels of visit codes, the services furnished must meet the definition of the code (e.g., to bill a Level 5 new patient visit, the history must meet CPT's definition of a comprehensive history).

The comprehensive history must include a review of all the systems and a complete past (medical and surgical) family and social history obtained at that visit. In the case of an established patient, it is acceptable for a physician to review the existing record and update it to reflect only changes in the patient's medical, family, and social history from the last encounter, but the physician must review the entire history for it to be considered a comprehensive history.

The comprehensive examination may be a complete single system exam such as cardiac, respiratory, psychiatric, or a complete multi-system examination.

30.6.1.1 – Initial Preventive Physical Examination (IPPE) and Annual Wellness Visit (AWV)

(Rev. 2159, Issued: 02-15-11, Effective: 01-01-11, Implementation: 04-04-11)

A. Definitions

1. Initial Preventive Physical Examination (IPPE)

The initial preventive physical examination (IPPE), or "Welcome to Medicare Visit" (WMV) is a preventive evaluation and management service (E/M), allowed by Section 611 of the Medicare Prescription Drug Improvement and Modernization Act (MMA) of 2003, that includes:

(1) review of the individual's medical and social history with attention to modifiable risk factors for disease detection,

(2) review of the individual's potential (risk factors) for depression or other mood disorders,

(3) review of the individual's functional ability and level of safety,

(4) a physical examination to include measurement of the individual's height, weight, blood pressure, a visual acuity screen, and other factors as deemed appropriate by the examining physician or qualified nonphysician practitioner (NPP),

(5) performance and interpretation of an electrocardiogram (EKG),

(6) education, counseling, and referral, as deemed appropriate, based on the results of the review and evaluation services described in the previous 5 elements, and,

(7) education, counseling, and referral including a brief written plan (e.g., a checklist or alternative) provided to the individual for obtaining the appropriate screening and other preventive services.

Effective January 1, 2007, Section 5112 of the Deficit Reduction Act of 2005 allows for one ultrasound screening for Abdominal Aortic Aneurysm (AAA), HCPCS code G0389, as a result of a referral from an IPPE. This service is not subject to the Part B annual deductible. For AAA physician/practitioner billing, correct coding, and payment policy, refer to chapter 18, §110, of this manual.

Effective January 1, 2009, Section 101 (b) of the Medicare Improvement for Patients and Providers Act (MIPPA) of 2008 requires the addition of the measurement of an individual's body mass index and, upon an individual's consent, end-of-life planning, to the IPPE. Also, effective January 1, 2009, MIPPA removes the screening electrocardiogram (EKG) as a mandatory service of the IPPE. MIPPA requires that there be education, counseling, and referral for an EKG, as appropriate. This is a once-in-a-lifetime screening EKG as a result of a referral from an IPPE.

The MIPPA of 2008 allows for possible future payment for additional preventive services not otherwise described in Title XVIII of the Social Security Act (the Act) that identify medical conditions or risk factors for eligible individuals if the Secretary determines through the national coverage determination (NCD) process (as defined in Section 1869(f)(1)(B) of the Act) that they are: (1) reasonable and necessary for the prevention or early detection of illness or disability, (2) recommended with a grade of A or B by the United States Preventive Services Task Force (USPSTF), and, (3) appropriate for individuals entitled to benefits under Part A or enrolled under Part B, or both. MIPPA requires that there be education, counseling, and referral for additional preventive services, as appropriate, under the IPPE, if the Secretary determines in the future that such services are covered.

2. Annual Wellness Visit (AWV)

Effective January 1, 2011, Section 4103 of the Affordable Care Act (ACA), allows for a preventive physical examination, called the annual wellness visit (AWV), and includes personal prevention plan services (PPPS). The AWV is a new annual Medicare preventive physical examination, available for eligible beneficiaries, and identified by new HCPCS codes G0438 (Annual wellness visit, including PPPS, first visit) and G0439 (Annual wellness visit, including PPPS, subsequent visit). Definitions relative to the AWV are included at Pub. 100-02, Medicare Benefit Policy Manual, chapter 15, section 280.5.

First AWV services providing PPPS (HCPCS G0438) are a 'one time' allowed Medicare benefit and include the following key elements furnished to an eligible beneficiary by a health professional:

- Establishment of the individual's medical/family history,

- Measurement of the individual's height, weight, body mass index (or waist circumference, if appropriate), blood pressure (BP), and other routine measurements as deemed appropriate, based on the individual's medical and family history,

- Establishment of a list of current providers and suppliers that are regularly involved in providing medical care to the individual,

- Detection of any cognitive impairment that the individual may have,

- Review of an individual's potential risk factors for depression , including current or past experiences with depression or other mood disorders, based on the use of an appropriate screening instrument for persons without a current diagnosis of depression, which the health professional may select from various available standardized screening tests designed for this purpose and recognized by national professional medical organizations,

- Review of the individual's functional ability and level of safety, based on direct observation of the individual, or the use of appropriate screening questions or a screening questionnaire, which the health professional may select from various available screening questions or standardized questionnaires designed for this purpose and recognized by national professional medical organizations,

- Establishment of a written screening schedule for the individual, such as a checklist for the next 5 to 10 years, as appropriate, based on recommendations of the USPSTF and Advisory Committee of Immunizations Practices (ACIP), the individual's health status, screening history, and age-appropriate preventive services covered by Medicare,

- Establishment of a list of risk factors and conditions of which primary, secondary, or tertiary interventions are recommended or underway for the individual, including any mental health conditions or any such risk factors or conditions that have been identified through an IPPE, and a list of treatment options and their associated risks and benefits,

- Provision of personalized health advice to the individual and a referral, as appropriate, to health education or preventive counseling services or programs aimed at reducing identified risk factors and improving self-management or community-based lifestyle interventions to reduce health risks and promote self-management and wellness, including weight loss, physical activity, smoking cessation, fall prevention, and nutrition, and,

- Any other element(s) determined appropriate by the Secretary through the NCD process.

Subsequent AWV services providing PPPS (HCPCS G0439) include the following key elements furnished to an eligible beneficiary by a health professional:

- Update to the individual's medical /family history,

- Measurements of an individual's weight (or waist circumference), BP, and other routine measurements as deemed appropriate, based on the individual's medical and family history,

- Update to the list of the individual's current medical providers and suppliers that are regularly involved in providing medical care to the individual as that list was developed for the first AWV providing PPPS,

- Detection of any cognitive impairment that the individual may have,

- Update to the individual's written screening schedule as developed at the first AWV providing PPPS,

- Update to the individual's list of risk factors and conditions for which primary, secondary, or tertiary interventions are recommended or are underway for the individual, as that list was developed at the first AWV providing PPPS,

- Furnish appropriate personalized health advice to the individual and a referral, as appropriate, to health education or preventive counseling services or programs, and,

- Any other element determined appropriate by the Secretary through the NCD process.

Preventive services are separately covered under Medicare Part B. See chapter 18 of this manual.

B. Who May Perform

The IPPE and the AWV may be performed by a doctor of medicine or osteopathy as defined in Section 1861(r) (1) of the Act, by a qualified NPP (nurse practitioner, physician assistant or clinical nurse specialist), or for the AWV, by a health professional (a medical professional including a health educator, registered dietitian, nutrition professional, or other licensed practitioner) or a team of such medical professionals who are working under the direct supervision of a physician. The contractor pays the appropriate physician fee schedule amount based on the rendering National Provider Identification (NPI) number.

C. Eligibility

1. IPPE

As a result of the MMA 2003, Medicare will pay for one IPPE per beneficiary per lifetime. A beneficiary is eligible when he/she first enrolls in Medicare Part B. For beneficiaries enrolled on or after January 1, 2005, beneficiaries must have received their IPPE within the first 6 months of Medicare coverage. The MIPPA extends the eligibility period for an IPPE to 12 months effective January 1, 2009.

Beneficiaries in their first 12 months of Part B coverage will continue to be eligible for only the IPPE. Medicare continues to pay for only one IPPE per beneficiary per lifetime.

2. AWV

As a result of the ACA, effective January 1, 2011, Medicare will pay for an AWV for a beneficiary who is no longer within 12 months after the effective date of his/her first Medicare Part B coverage period, and he/she has not received either an IPPE or an AWV providing PPPS within the past 12 months. Medicare pays for only one first AWV (HCPCS G0438), per beneficiary per lifetime, and all subsequent wellness visits must be billed as a subsequent AWV (HCPCS G0439).

Beneficiaries in their first 12 months of Part B coverage will continue to be eligible for only the IPPE (see 30.6.1.1.A.1).

D. Deductible and Coinsurance

1. IPPE

The Medicare deductible and coinsurance apply for the IPPE provided before January 1, 2009.

The Medicare deductible is waived effective for the IPPE provided on or after January 1, 2009. However, the applicable coinsurance continues to apply for the IPPE provided on or after January 1, 2009.

As a result of the ACA, effective for the IPPE provided on or after January 1, 2011, the Medicare deductible and coinsurance (for HCPCS code G0402 only) are waived.

2. AWV

As a result of the ACA, effective January 1, 2011, the Medicare deductible and coinsurance for the AWV (HCPCS G0438 and G0439) are waived.

E. The EKG Component of the IPPE

Under the MMA of 2003, if the physician or qualified NPP is not able to perform both the examination and the screening EKG, an arrangement may be made to ensure that another physician or entity performs the screening EKG and reports the EKG separately using the appropriate HCPCS G code(s) identified in F.1. of this section. When the screening EKG is performed, the primary physician or qualified NPP shall document the results of the screening EKG into the beneficiary's medical record to complete and bill for the IPPE benefit.

NOTE: Both components of the IPPE (the examination and the screening EKG) must be performed before the claims can be submitted by the physician, qualified NPP, and/or entity.

MIPPA 2008 changes the once-in-a-lifetime screening EKG from a mandated service to a service that may be performed, as appropriate, with a referral from an IPPE. When an EKG is furnished with the IPPE, the deductible and coinsurance will continue to apply for EKG services only.

F. HCPCS Codes Used to Bill the IPPE or AWV

1. HCPCS Codes Used to Bill the IPPE

For IPPE and EKG services provided prior to January 1, 2009, the physician or qualified NPP shall bill HCPCS code G0344 for the physical examination performed face-to-face, and HCPCS code G0366 for performing a screening EKG that includes both the interpretation and report. If the primary physician or qualified NPP performs only the examination, he/she shall bill HCPCS code G0344 only. The physician or entity that performs the screening EKG that includes both the interpretation and report shall bill HCPCS code G0366. The physician or entity that performs the screening EKG tracing only (without interpretation and report) shall bill HCPCS code G0367. The physician or entity that performs the interpretation and report only (without the EKG tracing) shall bill HCPCS code G0368. Medicare will pay for a screening EKG only as part of the IPPE. HCPCS codes G0344, G0366, G0367 and G0368 will not be billable codes effective on or after January 1, 2009.

Effective for a beneficiary who has the IPPE on or after January 1, 2009, and within his/her 12-month enrollment period of Medicare Part B, the IPPE and screening EKG services are billable with the appropriate HCPCS G code(s).

The physician or qualified NPP shall bill HCPCS code G0402 for the physical examination performed face-to-face with the patient.

The physician or entity shall bill HCPCS code G0403 for performing the complete screening EKG that includes the tracing, interpretation and report.

The physician or entity that performs the screening EKG tracing only (without interpretation and report) shall bill HCPCS code G0404.

The physician or entity that performs the screening EKG interpretation and report only, (without the EKG tracing) shall bill HCPCS code G0405.

2. HCPCS Codes Used to Bill the AWV

For the first AWV provided on or after January 1, 2011, the health professional shall bill HCPCS G0438 (Annual wellness visit, including PPPS, first visit). This is a once per beneficiary per lifetime allowable Medicare benefit.

All subsequent AWVs shall be billed with HCPCS G0439 (Annual Wellness Visit, including PPPS, subsequent visit). In the event that a beneficiary selects a new health professional to complete a subsequent AWV, the new health professional will continue to bill the subsequent AWV with HCPCS G0439.

NOTE: For an IPPE or AWV performed during the global period of surgery refer to chapter 12, §30.6.6 of this manual for reporting instructions.

G. Documentation for the IPPE or AWV

The physician and qualified NPP, or for AWV the health professional, shall use the appropriate screening tools typically used in routine physician practice. Physicians, qualified NPPs, and medical professionals are required to use the 1995 and 1997 E/M documentation guidelines to document the medical record with the appropriate clinical information. (http://www.cms.hhs.gov/

MLNEdWebGuide/25_EMDOC.asp). All referrals and a written medical plan must be included in this documentation.

H. Reporting a Medically Necessary E/M Service Furnished During the Same Encounter as an IPPE or AWV

When the physician or qualified NPP, or for AWV the health professional, provides a significant, separately identifiable medically necessary E/M service in addition to the IPPE or an AWV, CPT codes 99201 - 99215 may be reported depending on the clinical appropriateness of the circumstances. CPT Modifier –25 shall be appended to the medically necessary E/M service identifying this service as a significant, separately identifiable service from the IPPE or AWV code reported (HCPCS code G0344 or G0402, whichever applies based on the date the IPPE is performed, or HCPCS code G0438 or G0439 whichever AWV code applies).

NOTE: Some of the components of a medically necessary E/M service (e.g., a portion of history or physical exam portion) may have been part of the IPPE or AWV and should not be included when determining the most appropriate level of E/M service to be billed for the medically necessary, separately identifiable, E/M service.

30.6.2 - BILLING FOR MEDICALLY NECESSARY VISIT ON SAME OCCASION AS PREVENTIVE MEDICINE SERVICE

(Rev. 1, 10-01-03)

See Chapter 18 for payment for covered preventive services.

When a physician furnishes a Medicare beneficiary a covered visit at the same place and on the same occasion as a noncovered preventive medicine service (CPT codes 99381 - 99397), consider the covered visit to be provided in lieu of a part of the preventive medicine service of equal value to the visit. A preventive medicine service (CPT codes 99381 - 99397) is a noncovered service. The physician may charge the beneficiary, as a charge for the noncovered remainder of the service, the amount by which the physician's current established charge for the preventive medicine service exceeds his/her current established charge for the covered visit. Pay for the covered visit based on the lesser of the fee schedule amount or the physician's actual charge for the visit. The physician is not required to give the beneficiary written advance notice of noncoverage of the part of the visit that constitutes a routine preventive visit. However, the physician is responsible for notifying the patient in advance of his/her liability for the charges for services that are not medically necessary to treat the illness or injury.

There could be covered and noncovered procedures performed during this encounter (e.g., screening x-ray, EKG, lab tests.). These are considered individually. Those procedures which are for screening for asymptomatic conditions are considered noncovered and, therefore, no payment is made. Those procedures ordered to diagnose or monitor a symptom, medical condition, or treatment are evaluated for medical necessity and, if covered, are paid.

30.6.3 - PAYMENT FOR IMMUNOSUPPRESSIVE THERAPY MANAGEMENT

(Rev. 1, 10-01-03)
B3-4820-4824

Physicians bill for management of immunosuppressive therapy using the office or subsequent hospital visit codes that describe the services furnished. If the physician who is managing the immunotherapy is also the transplant surgeon, he or she bills these visits with modifier "-24" indicating that the visit during the global period is not related to the original procedure if the physician also performed the transplant surgery and submits documentation that shows that the visit is for immunosuppressive therapy.

30.6.4 - EVALUATION AND MANAGEMENT (E/M) SERVICES FURNISHED INCIDENT TO PHYSICIAN'S SERVICE BY NONPHYSICIAN PRACTITIONERS

(Rev. 1, 10-01-03)

When evaluation and management services are furnished incident to a physician's service by a nonphysician practitioner, the physician may bill the CPT code that describes the evaluation and management service furnished.

When evaluation and management services are furnished incident to a physician's service by a nonphysician employee of the physician, not as part of a physician service, the physician bills code 99211 for the service.

A physician is not precluded from billing under the "incident to" provision for services provided by employees whose services cannot be paid for directly under the Medicare program. Employees of the physician may provide services incident to the physician's service, but the physician alone is permitted to bill Medicare.

Services provided by employees as "incident to" are covered when they meet all the requirements for incident to and are medically necessary for the individual needs of the patient.

30.6.5 - PHYSICIANS IN GROUP PRACTICE

(Rev. 1, 10-01-03)

Physicians in the same group practice who are in the same specialty must bill and be paid as though they were a single physician. If more than one evaluation and management (face-to-face) service is provided on the same day to the same patient by the same physician or more than one physician in the same specialty in the same group, only one evaluation and management service may be reported unless the evaluation and management services are for unrelated problems. Instead of billing separately, the physicians should select a level of service representative of the combined visits and submit the appropriate code for that level.

Physicians in the same group practice but who are in different specialties may bill and be paid without regard to their membership in the same group.

30.6.6 - PAYMENT FOR EVALUATION AND MANAGEMENT SERVICES PROVIDED DURING GLOBAL PERIOD OF SURGERY

(Rev. 954, Issued: 05-19-06, Effective: 06-01-06, Implementation: 08-20-06)

A. CPT Modifier "-24" - Unrelated Evaluation and Management Service by Same Physician During Postoperative Period

Carriers pay for an evaluation and management service other than inpatient hospital care before discharge from the hospital following surgery (CPT codes 99221 - 99238) if it was provided during the postoperative period of a surgical procedure, furnished by the same physician who performed the procedure, billed with CPT modifier "-24," and accompanied by documentation that supports that the service is not related to the postoperative care of the procedure. They do not pay for inpatient hospital care that is furnished during the hospital stay in which the surgery occurred unless the doctor is also treating another medical condition that is unrelated to the surgery. All care provided during the inpatient stay in which the surgery occurred is compensated through the global surgical payment.

B. CPT Modifier "-25" - Significant Evaluation and Management Service by Same Physician on Date of Global Procedure

Medicare requires that Current Procedural Terminology (CPT) modifier -25 should only be used on claims for evaluation and management (E/M) services, and only when these services are provided by the same physician (or same qualified nonphysician practitioner) to the same patient on the same day as another procedure or other service. Carriers pay for an E/M service provided on the day of a procedure with a global fee period if the physician indicates that the service is for a significant, separately identifiable E/M service that is above and beyond the usual pre- and post-operative work of the procedure. Different diagnoses are not required for reporting the E/M service on the same date as the procedure or other service. Modifier -25 is added to the E/M code on the claim.

Both the medically necessary E/M service and the procedure must be appropriately and sufficiently documented by the physician or qualified nonphysician practitioner in the patient's medical record to support the claim for these services, even though the documentation is not required to be submitted with the claim.

If the physician bills the service with the CPT modifier "-25," carriers pay for the service in addition to the global fee without any other requirement for documentation unless one of the following conditions is met:

• When inpatient dialysis services are billed (CPT codes 90935, 90945, 90947, and 93937), the physician must document that the service was unrelated to the dialysis and could not be performed during the dialysis procedure;

• When preoperative critical care codes are being billed on the date of the procedure, the diagnosis must support that the service is unrelated to the performance of the procedure; or

• When a carrier has conducted a specific medical review process and determined, after reviewing the data, that an individual or a group has high use of modifier "-25" compared to other physicians, has done a case-by-case review of the records to verify that the use of modifier was inappropriate, and has educated the individual or group, the carrier may impose prepayment screens or documentation requirements for that provider or group.
When a carrier has completed a review and determined that a high usage rate of modifier "-57," the carrier must complete a case-by-case review of the records. Based upon this review, the carrier will educate providers regarding the appropriate use of modifier "-57." If high usage rates continue, the carrier may impose prepayment screens or documentation requirements for that provider or group.

Carriers may not permit the use of CPT modifier "-25" to generate payment for multiple evaluation and management services on the same day by the same physician, notwithstanding the CPT definition of the modifier.

C. CPT Modifier "-57" - Decision for Surgery Made Within Global Surgical Period

Carriers pay for an evaluation and management service on the day of or on the day before a procedure with a 90-day global surgical period if the physician uses CPT modifier "-57" to indicate that the service resulted in the decision to perform the procedure. Carriers may no pay for an evaluation and management service billed with the CPT modifier "-57" if it was provided on the day of or the day before a procedure with a 0 or 10-day global surgical period.

30.6.7 - PAYMENT FOR OFFICE OR OTHER OUTPATIENT EVALUATION AND MANAGEMENT (E/M) VISITS (CODES 99201 - 99215)

(Rev. 731, Issued: 10-28-05, Effective: 01-01-04 Chemotherapy and Non-Chemotherapy drug infusion codes/01-01-05 Therapeutic and Diagnostic injection codes, Implementation: 01-03-06)

A Definition of New Patient for Selection of E/M Visit Code

Interpret the phrase "new patient" to mean a patient who has not received any professional services, i.e., E/M service or other face-to-face service (e.g., surgical procedure) from the physician or physician group practice (same physician specialty) within the previous 3 years. For example, if a professional component of a previous procedure is billed in a 3 year time period, e.g., a lab interpretation is billed and no E/M service or other face-to-face service with the patient is performed, then this patient remains a new patient for the initial visit. An interpretation of a diagnostic test, reading an x-ray or EKG etc., in the absence of an E/M service or other face-to-face service with the patient does not affect the designation of a new patient.

B Office/Outpatient E/M Visits Provided on Same Day for Unrelated Problems

As for all other E/M services except where specifically noted, carriers may not pay two E/M office visits billed by a physician (or physician of the same specialty from the same group practice) for the same beneficiary on the same day unless the physician documents that the visits were for unrelated problems in the office or outpatient setting which could not be provided during the same encounter (e.g., office visit for blood pressure medication evaluation, followed five hours later by a visit for evaluation of leg pain following an accident).

C Office/Outpatient or Emergency Department E/M Visit on Day of Admission to Nursing Facility

Carriers may not pay a physician for an emergency department visit or an office visit **and** a comprehensive nursing facility assessment on the same day. Bundle E/M visits on the same date provided in sites other than the nursing facility into the initial nursing facility care code when performed on the same date as the nursing facility admission by the same physician.

D Drug Administration Services and E/M Visits Billed on Same Day of Service

Carriers must advise physicians that CPT code 99211 cannot be paid if it is billed with a drug administration service such as a chemotherapy or nonchemotherapy drug infusion code (effective January 1, 2004). This drug administration policy was expanded in the Physician Fee Schedule Final Rule,

November 15, 2004, to also include a therapeutic or diagnostic injection code (effective January 1, 2005). Therefore, when a medically necessary, significant and separately identifiable E/M service (which meets a higher complexity level than CPT code 99211) is performed, in addition to one of these drug administration services, the appropriate E/M CPT code should be reported with modifier -25. Documentation should support the level of E/M service billed. For an E/M service provided on the same day, a different diagnosis is not required.

30.6.8 - PAYMENT FOR HOSPITAL OBSERVATION SERVICES AND OBSERVATION OR INPATIENT CARE SERVICES (INCLUDING ADMISSION AND DISCHARGE SERVICES)

(Rev. 2282, Issued: 08-26-11, Effective: 01-01-11, Implementation: 11-28-11)

A. Who May Bill Observation Care Codes

Observation care is a well-defined set of specific, clinically appropriate services, which include ongoing short term treatment, assessment, and reassessment, that are furnished while a decision is being made regarding whether patients will require further treatment as hospital inpatients or if they are able to be discharged from the hospital. Observation services are commonly ordered for patients who present to the emergency department and who then require a significant period of treatment or monitoring in order to make a decision concerning their admission or discharge.

In only rare and exceptional cases do reasonable and necessary outpatient observation services span more than 48 hours. In the majority of cases, the decision whether to discharge a patient from the hospital following resolution of the reason for the observation care or to admit the patient as an inpatient can be made in less than 48 hours, usually in less than 24 hours.

Contractors pay for initial observation care billed by only the physician who ordered hospital outpatient observation services and was responsible for the patient during his/her observation care. A physician who does not have inpatient admitting privileges but who is authorized to furnish hospital outpatient observation services may bill these codes.

For a physician to bill observation care codes, there must be a medical observation record for the patient which contains dated and timed physician's orders regarding the observation services the patient is to receive, nursing notes, and progress notes prepared by the physician while the patient received observation services. This record must be in addition to any record prepared as a result of an emergency department or outpatient clinic encounter.

Payment for an initial observation care code is for all the care rendered by the ordering physician on the date the patient's observation services began. All other physicians who furnish consultations or additional evaluations or services while the patient is receiving hospital outpatient observation services must bill the appropriate outpatient service codes.

For example, if an internist orders observation services and asks another physician to additionally evaluate the patient, only the internist may bill the initial and subsequent observation care codes. The other physician who evaluates the patient must bill the new or established office or other outpatient visit codes as appropriate.

For information regarding hospital billing of observation services, see Chapter 4, §290.

B. Physician Billing for Observation Care Following Initiation of Observation Services

Similar to initial observation codes, payment for a subsequent observation care code is for all the care rendered by the treating physician on the day(s) other than the initial or discharge date. All other physicians who furnish consultations or additional evaluations or services while the patient is receiving hospital outpatient observation services must bill the appropriate outpatient service codes.

When a patient receives observation care for less than 8 hours on the same calendar date, the Initial Observation Care, from CPT code range 99218 - 99220, shall be reported by the physician. The Observation Care Discharge Service, CPT code 99217, shall not be reported for this scenario.

When a patient is admitted for observation care and then is discharged on a different calendar date, the physician shall report Initial Observation Care, from CPT code range 99218 - 99220, and CPT observation care discharge CPT code 99217. On the rare occasion when a patient remains in observation care for 3 days, the physician shall report an initial observation care code (99218 - 99220) for the first day of observation care, a subsequent observation care code (99224 - 99226) for the second day of observation care, and an observation care discharge CPT code 99217 for the observation care on the discharge date. When observation care continues beyond 3 days, the physician shall report a subsequent observation care code (99224 - 99226) for each day between the first day of observation care and the discharge date.

When a patient receives observation care for a minimum of 8 hours, but less than 24 hours, and is discharged on the same calendar date, Observation or Inpatient Care Services (Including Admission and Discharge Services) from CPT code range 99234 - 99236 shall be reported. The observation discharge, CPT code 99217, cannot also be reported for this scenario.

C. Documentation Requirements for Billing Observation or Inpatient Care Services (Including Admission and Discharge Services)

The physician shall satisfy the E/M documentation guidelines for furnishing observation care or inpatient hospital care. In addition to meeting the documentation requirements for history, examination, and medical decision making, documentation in the medical record shall include:

- Documentation stating the stay for observation care or inpatient hospital care involves 8 hours, but less than 24 hours;

- Documentation identifying the billing physician was present and personally performed the services; and

- Documentation identifying the order for observation services, progress notes, and discharge notes were written by the billing physician.

In the rare circumstance when a patient receives observation services for more than 2 calendar dates, the physician shall bill observation services furnished on day(s) other than the initial or discharge date using subsequent observation care codes. The physician may not use the subsequent hospital care codes since the patient is not an inpatient of the hospital.

D. Admission to Inpatient Status Following Observation Care

If the same physician who ordered hospital outpatient observation services also admits the patient to inpatient status before the end of the date on which the patient began receiving hospital outpatient observation services, pay only an initial hospital visit for the evaluation and management services provided on that date. Medicare payment for the initial hospital visit includes all services provided to the patient on the date of admission by that physician, regardless of the site of service. The physician may not bill an initial or subsequent observation care code for services on the date that he or she admits the patient to inpatient status. If the patient is admitted to inpatient status from hospital outpatient observation care subsequent to the date of initiation of observation services, the physician must bill an initial hospital visit for the services provided on that date. The physician may not bill the hospital observation discharge management code (code 99217) or an outpatient/office visit for the care provided while the patient received hospital outpatient observation services on the date of admission to inpatient status.

E. Hospital Observation Services During Global Surgical Period

The global surgical fee includes payment for hospital observation (codes 99217, 99218, 99219, 99220, 99224, 99225, 99226, 99234, 99235, and 99236) services unless the criteria for use of CPT modifiers "-24," "-25," or "-57" are met. Contractors must pay for these services in addition to the global surgical fee only if both of the following requirements are met:

- The hospital observation service meets the criteria needed to justify billing it with CPT modifiers "-24," "-25," or "-57" (decision for major surgery); and

- The hospital observation service furnished by the surgeon meets all of the criteria for the hospital observation code billed.

Examples of the decision for surgery during a hospital observation period are:

- An emergency department physician orders hospital outpatient observation services for a patient with a head injury. A neurosurgeon is called in to evaluate the need for surgery while the patient is receiving observation services and decides that the patient requires surgery. The surgeon would bill a new or established office or other outpatient visit code as appropriate with the "-57" modifier to indicate that the decision for surgery was made during the evaluation. The surgeon must bill the office or other outpatient visit code because the patient receiving hospital outpatient observation services is not an inpatient of the hospital. Only the physician who ordered hospital outpatient observation services may bill for observation care.

- A neurosurgeon orders hospital outpatient observation services for a patient with a head injury. During the observation period, the surgeon makes the decision for surgery. The surgeon would bill the appropriate level of hospital observation code with the "-57" modifier to indicate that the decision for surgery was made while the surgeon was providing hospital observation care.

Examples of hospital observation services during the postoperative period of a surgery are:

- A surgeon orders hospital outpatient observation services for a patient with abdominal pain from a kidney stone on the 80th day following a TURP (performed by that surgeon). The surgeon decides that the patient does not require surgery. The surgeon would bill the observation code with CPT modifier "-24" and documentation to support that the observation services are unrelated to the surgery.

- A surgeon orders hospital outpatient observation services for a patient with abdominal pain on the 80th day following a TURP (performed by that surgeon). While the patient is receiving hospital outpatient observation services, the surgeon decides that the patient requires kidney surgery. The surgeon would bill the observation code with HCPCS modifier "-57" to indicate that the decision for surgery was made while the patient was receiving hospital outpatient observation services. The subsequent surgical procedure would be reported with modifier "-79."

- A surgeon orders hospital outpatient observation services for a patient with abdominal pain on the 20th day following a resection of the colon (performed by that surgeon). The surgeon determines that the patient requires no further colon surgery and discharges the patient. The surgeon may not bill for the observation services furnished during the global period because they were related to the previous surgery.

An example of a billable hospital observation service on the same day as a procedure is when a physician repairs a laceration of the scalp in the emergency department for a patient with a head injury and then subsequently orders hospital outpatient observation services for that patient. The physician would bill the observation code with a CPT modifier 25 and the procedure code.

30.6.9 - PAYMENT FOR INPATIENT HOSPITAL VISITS - GENERAL

(Rev. 2282, Issued: 08-26-11, Effective: 01-01-11, Implementation: 11-28-11)

A. Hospital Visit and Critical Care on Same Day

When a hospital inpatient or office/outpatient evaluation and management service (E/M) are furnished on a calendar date at which time the patient does not require critical care and the patient subsequently requires critical care both the critical Care Services (CPT codes 99291 and 99292) and the previous E/M service may be paid on the same date of service. Hospital emergency department services are not paid for the same date as critical care services when provided by the same physician to the same patient.

During critical care management of a patient those services that do not meet the level of critical care shall be reported using an inpatient hospital care service with CPT Subsequent Hospital Care using a code from CPT code range 99231 - 99233.

Both Initial Hospital Care (CPT codes 99221 - 99223) and Subsequent Hospital Care codes are "per diem" services and may be reported only once per day by the same physician or physicians of the same specialty from the same group practice.

Physicians and qualified nonphysician practitioners (NPPs) are advised to retain documentation for discretionary contractor review should claims be questioned for both hospital care and critical care claims. The retained documentation shall support claims for critical care when the same physician or physicians of the same specialty in a group practice report critical care services for the same patient on the same calendar date as other E/M services.

B. Two Hospital Visits Same Day

Contractors pay a physician for only one hospital visit per day for the same patient, whether the problems seen during the encounters are related or not. The inpatient hospital visit descriptors contain the phrase "per day" which means that the code and the payment established for the code represent all services provided on that date. The physician should select a code that reflects all services provided during the date of the service.

C. Hospital Visits Same Day But by Different Physicians

In a hospital inpatient situation involving one physician covering for another, if physician A sees the patient in the morning and physician B, who is covering for A, sees the same patient in the evening, contractors do not pay physician B for the second visit. The hospital visit descriptors include the phrase "per day" meaning care for the day.

If the physicians are each responsible for a different aspect of the patient's care, pay both visits if the physicians are in different specialties and the visits are billed with different diagnoses. There are circumstances where concurrent care may be billed by physicians of the same specialty.

D. Visits to Patients in Swing Beds

If the inpatient care is being billed by the hospital as inpatient hospital care, the hospital care codes apply. If the inpatient care is being billed by the hospital as nursing facility care, then the nursing facility codes apply.

30.6.9.1 - Payment for Initial Hospital Care Services and Observation or Inpatient Care Services (Including Admission and Discharge Services)

(Rev. 2282, Issued: 08-26-11, Effective: 01-01-11, Implementation: 11-28-11)

A. Initial Hospital Care From Emergency Room

Contractors pay for an initial hospital care service if a physician sees a patient in the emergency room and decides to admit the person to the hospital. They do not pay for both E/M services. Also, they do not pay for an emergency department visit by the same physician on the same date of service. When the patient is admitted to the hospital via another site of service (e.g., hospital emergency department, physician's office, nursing facility), all services provided by the physician in conjunction with that admission are considered part of the initial hospital care when performed on the same date as the admission.

B. Initial Hospital Care on Day Following Visit

Contractors pay both visits if a patient is seen in the office on one date and admitted to the hospital on the next date, even if fewer than 24 hours has elapsed between the visit and the admission.

C. Initial Hospital Care and Discharge on Same Day

When the patient is admitted to inpatient hospital care for less than 8 hours on the same date, then Initial Hospital Care, from CPT code range 99221 - 99223, shall be reported by the physician. The Hospital Discharge Day Management service, CPT codes 99238 or 99239, shall not be reported for this scenario.

When a patient is admitted to inpatient initial hospital care and then discharged on a different calendar date, the physician shall report an Initial Hospital Care from CPT code range 99221 - 99223 and a Hospital Discharge Day Management service, CPT code 99238 or 99239.

When a patient has been admitted to inpatient hospital care for a minimum of 8 hours but less than 24 hours and discharged on the same calendar date, Observation or Inpatient Hospital Care Services (Including Admission and Discharge Services), from CPT code range 99234 - 99236, shall be reported.

D. Documentation Requirements for Billing Observation or Inpatient Care Services (Including Admission and Discharge Services)

The physician shall satisfy the E/M documentation guidelines for admission to and discharge from inpatient observation or hospital care. In addition to meeting the documentation requirements for history, examination and medical decision making documentation in the medical record shall include:

- Documentation stating the stay for hospital treatment or observation care status involves 8 hours but less than 24 hours;

- Documentation identifying the billing physician was present and personally performed the services; and

- Documentation identifying the admission and discharge notes were written by the billing physician.

E. Physician Services Involving Transfer From One Hospital to Another; Transfer Within Facility to Prospective Payment System (PPS) Exempt Unit of Hospital; Transfer From One Facility to Another Separate Entity Under Same Ownership and/or Part of Same Complex; or Transfer From One Department to Another Within Single Facility

Physicians may bill both the hospital discharge management code and an initial hospital care code when the discharge and admission do not occur on the same day if the transfer is between:

- Different hospitals;

- Different facilities under common ownership which do not have merged records; or

- Between the acute care hospital and a PPS exempt unit within the same hospital when there are no merged records.

In all other transfer circumstances, the physician should bill only the appropriate level of subsequent hospital care for the date of transfer.

F. Initial Hospital Care Service History and Physical That Is Less Than Comprehensive

When a physician performs a visit that meets the definition of a Level 5 office visit several days prior to an admission and on the day of admission performs less than a comprehensive history and physical, he or she should report the office visit that reflects the services furnished and also report the lowest level initial hospital care code (i.e., code 99221) for the initial hospital admission. Contractors pay the office visit as billed and the Level 1 initial hospital care code.

Physicians who provide an initial visit to a patient during inpatient hospital care that meets the minimum key component work and/or medical necessity requirements shall report an initial hospital care code (99221 - 99223). The principal physician of record shall append modifier "-AI" (Principal Physician of Record) to the claim for the initial hospital care code. This modifier will identify the physician who oversees the patient's care from all other physicians who may be furnishing specialty care.

Physicians may bill initial hospital care service codes (99221 - 99223), for services that were reported with CPT consultation codes (99241 - 99255) prior to January 1, 2010, when the furnished service and documentation meet the minimum key component work and/or medical necessity requirements. Physicians must meet all the requirements of the initial hospital care codes, including "a detailed or comprehensive history" and "a detailed or comprehensive examination" to report CPT code 99221, which are greater than the requirements for consultation codes 99251 and 99252.

Subsequent hospital care CPT codes 99231 and 99232, respectively, require "a problem focused interval history" and "an expanded problem focused interval history." An E/M service that could be described by CPT consultation code 99251 or 99252 could potentially meet the component work and medical necessity requirements to report 99231 or 99232. Physicians may report a subsequent hospital care CPT code for services that were reported as CPT consultation codes (99241 - 99255) prior to January 1, 2010, where the medical record appropriately demonstrates that the work and medical necessity requirements are met for reporting a subsequent hospital care code (under the level selected), even though the reported code is for the provider's first E/M service to the inpatient during the hospital stay.

Reporting CPT code 99499 (Unlisted evaluation and management service) should be limited to cases where there is no other specific E/M code payable by Medicare that describes that service. Reporting CPT code 99499 requires submission of medical records and contractor manual medical review of the service prior to payment. Contractors shall expect reporting under these circumstances to be unusual.

G. Initial Hospital Care Visits by Two Different M.D.s or D.O.s When They Are Involved in Same Admission

In the inpatient hospital setting all physicians (and qualified nonphysician practitioners where permitted) who perform an initial evaluation may bill the initial hospital care codes (99221 - 99223) or nursing facility care codes (99304 - 99306). Contractors consider only one M.D. or D.O. to be the principal physician of record (sometimes referred to as the admitting physician.) The principal physician of record is identified in Medicare as the physician who oversees the patient's care from other physicians who may be furnishing specialty care. Only the principal physician of record shall append modifier "-AI" (Principal Physician of Record) in addition to the E/M code. Follow-up visits in the facility setting shall be billed as subsequent hospital care visits and subsequent nursing facility care visits.

30.6.9.2 - Subsequent Hospital Visit and Hospital Discharge Day Management (Codes 99231 - 99239)

(Rev. 1460, Issued: 02-22-08, Effective: 04-01-08, Implementation: 04-07-08)

A. Subsequent Hospital Visits During the Global Surgery Period

(Refer to §§40-40.4 on global surgery)

The Medicare physician fee schedule payment amount for surgical procedures includes all services (e.g., evaluation and management visits) that are part of the global surgery payment; therefore, contractors shall not pay more than that amount when a bill is fragmented for staged procedures.

B. Hospital Discharge Day Management Service

Hospital Discharge Day Management Services, CPT code 99238 or 99239 is a face-to-face evaluation and management (E/M) service between the attending physician and the patient. The E/M discharge day management visit shall be reported for the date of the actual visit by the physician or qualified nonphysician practitioner even if the patient is discharged from the facility on a different calendar date. Only one hospital discharge day management service is payable per patient per hospital stay.

Only the attending physician of record reports the discharge day management service. Physicians or qualified nonphysician practitioners, other than the attending physician, who have been managing concurrent health care problems not primarily managed by the attending physician, and who are not acting on behalf of the attending physician, shall use Subsequent Hospital Care (CPT code range 99231 - 99233) for a final visit.

Medicare pays for the paperwork of patient discharge day management through the pre- and post- service work of an E/M service.

C. Subsequent Hospital Visit and Discharge Management on Same Day

Pay only the hospital discharge management code on the day of discharge (unless it is also the day of admission, in which case, refer to §30.6.9.1 C for the policy on Observation or Inpatient Care Services (Including Admission and Discharge Services CPT Codes 99234 - 99236). Contractors do not pay both a subsequent hospital visit in addition to hospital discharge day management service on the same day by the same physician. Instruct physicians that they may not bill for both a hospital visit and hospital discharge management for the same date of service.

D. Hospital Discharge Management (CPT Codes 99238 and 99239) and Nursing Facility Admission Code When Patient Is Discharged From Hospital and Admitted to Nursing Facility on Same Day

Contractors pay the hospital discharge code (codes 99238 or 99239) in addition to a nursing facility admission code when they are billed by the same physician with the same date of service.

If a surgeon is admitting the patient to the nursing facility due to a condition that is not as a result of the surgery during the postoperative period of a service with the global surgical period, he/she bills for the nursing facility admission and care with a modifier "-24" and provides documentation that the service is unrelated to the surgery (e.g., return of an elderly patient to the nursing facility in which he/she has resided for five years following discharge from the hospital for cholecystectomy).

Contractors do not pay for a nursing facility admission by a surgeon in the postoperative period of a procedure with a global surgical period if the patient's admission to the nursing facility is to receive post operative care related to the surgery (e.g., admission to a nursing facility to receive physical therapy following a hip replacement). Payment for the nursing facility admission and subsequent nursing facility services are included in the global fee and cannot be paid separately.

E. Hospital Discharge Management and Death Pronouncement

Only the physician who personally performs the pronouncement of death shall bill for the face-to-face Hospital Discharge Day Management Service, CPT code 99238 or 99239. The date of the pronouncement shall reflect the calendar date of service on the day it was performed even if the paperwork is delayed to a subsequent date.

30.6.10 - CONSULTATION SERVICES

(Rev. 2282, Issued: 08-26-11, Effective: 01-01-11, Implementation: 11-28-11)
Consultation Services versus Other Evaluation and Management (E/M) Visits
Effective January 1, 2010, the consultation codes are no longer recognized for Medicare Part B payment. Physicians shall code patient evaluation and management visits with E/M codes that represent where the visit occurs and that identify the complexity of the visit performed.

In the inpatient hospital setting and the nursing facility setting, physicians (and qualified nonphysician practitioners where permitted) may bill the most appropriate initial hospital care code (99221 - 99223), subsequent hospital care code (99231 and 99232), initial nursing facility care code (99304 - 99306), or subsequent nursing facility care code (99307 - 99310) that reflects the services the physician or practitioner furnished. Subsequent hospital care codes could potentially meet the component work and medical necessity requirements to be reported for an E/M service that could be described by CPT consultation code 99251 or 99252. Contractors shall not find fault in cases where the medical record appropriately demonstrates that the work and medical necessity requirements are met for reporting a subsequent hospital care code (under the level selected), even though the reported code is for the provider's first E/M service to the inpatient during the hospital stay. Unlisted evaluation and management service (code 99499) shall only be reported for consultation services when an E/M service that could be described by codes 99251 or 99252 is furnished, and there is no other specific E/M code payable by Medicare that describes that service. Reporting code 99499 requires submission of medical records and contractor manual medical review of the service prior to payment. CMS expects reporting under these circumstances to be unusual. The principal physician of record is identified in Medicare as the physician who oversees the patient's care from other physicians who may be furnishing specialty care. The principal physician of record shall append modifier "-AI" (Principal Physician of Record), in addition to the E/M code. Follow-up visits in the facility setting shall be billed as subsequent hospital care visits and subsequent nursing facility care visits.

In the CAH setting, those CAHs that use method II shall bill the appropriate new or established visit code for those physician and non-physician practitioners who have reassigned their billing rights, depending on the relationship status between the physician and patient.

In the office or other outpatient setting where an evaluation is performed, physicians and qualified nonphysician practitioners shall use the CPT codes (99201 - 99215) depending on the complexity of the visit and whether the patient is a new or established patient to that physician. All physicians and qualified nonphysician practitioners shall follow the E/M documentation guidelines for all E/M services. These rules are applicable for Medicare secondary payer claims as well as for claims in which Medicare is the primary payer.

30.6.11 - EMERGENCY DEPARTMENT VISITS (CODES 99281 - 99288)

(Rev. 1875, Issued: 12-14-09, Effective: 01-01-10, Implementation: 01-04-10)

A. Use of Emergency Department Codes by Physicians Not Assigned to Emergency Department

Any physician seeing a patient registered in the emergency department may use emergency department visit codes (for services matching the code description). It is not required that the physician be assigned to the emergency department.

B. Use of Emergency Department Codes In Office

Emergency department coding is not appropriate if the site of service is an office or outpatient setting or any sight of service other than an emergency department. The emergency department codes should only be used if the patient is seen in the emergency department and the services described by the HCPCS code definition are provided. The emergency department is defined as an organized hospital-based facility for the provision of unscheduled or episodic services to patients who present for immediate medical attention.

C. Use of Emergency Department Codes to Bill Nonemergency Services

Services in the emergency department may not be emergencies. However the codes (99281 - 99288) are payable if the described services are provided.

However, if the physician asks the patient to meet him or her in the emergency department as an alternative to the physician's office and the patient is not registered as a patient in the emergency department, the physician should bill the appropriate office/outpatient visit codes. Normally a lower level emergency department code would be reported for a nonemergency condition.

D. Emergency Department or Office/Outpatient Visits on Same Day As Nursing Facility Admission

Emergency department visit provided on the same day as a comprehensive nursing facility assessment are not paid. Payment for evaluation and management services on the same date provided in sites other than the nursing facility are included in the payment for initial nursing facility care when performed on the same date as the nursing facility admission.

E. Physician Billing for Emergency Department Services Provided to Patient by Both Patient's Personal Physician and Emergency Department Physician

If a physician advises his/her own patient to go to an emergency department (ED) of a hospital for care and the physician subsequently is asked by the ED physician to come to the hospital to evaluate the patient and to advise the ED physician as to whether the patient should be admitted to the hospital or be sent home, the physicians should bill as follows:

- If the patient is admitted to the hospital by the patient's personal physician, then the patient's regular physician should bill only the appropriate level of the initial hospital care (codes 99221 - 99223) because all evaluation and management services provided by that physician in conjunction with that admission are considered part of the initial hospital care when performed on the same date as the admission. The ED physician who saw the patient in the emergency department should bill the appropriate level of the ED codes.

- If the ED physician, based on the advice of the patient's personal physician who came to the emergency department to see the patient, sends the patient home, then the ED physician should bill the appropriate level of emergency department service. The patient's personal physician should also bill the level of emergency department code that describes the service he or she provided in the emergency department. If the patient's personal physician does not come to the hospital to see the patient, but only advises the emergency department physician by telephone, then the patient's personal physician may not bill.

F. Emergency Department Physician Requests Another Physician to See the Patient in Emergency Department or Office/Outpatient Setting

If the emergency department physician requests that another physician evaluate a given patient, the other physician should bill an emergency department visit code. If the patient is admitted to the hospital by the second physician performing the evaluation, he or she should bill an initial hospital care code and not an emergency department visit code.

30.6.12 - CRITICAL CARE VISITS AND NEONATAL INTENSIVE CARE (CODES 99291 - 99292)

(Rev. 1548, Issued: 07-089-08; Effective Date: 07-01-08; Implementation Date: 07-07-08)
CRITICAL CARE SERVICES (CODES 99291 - 99292)

A. Use of Critical Care Codes

Pay for services reported with CPT codes 99291 and 99292 when all the criteria for critical care and critical care services are met. Critical care is defined as the direct delivery by a physician(s) medical care for a critically ill or critically injured patient. A critical illness or injury acutely impairs one or more vital organ systems such that there is a high probability of imminent or life threatening deterioration in the patient's condition.

Critical care involves high complexity decision making to assess, manipulate, and support vital system functions(s) to treat single or multiple vital organ system failure and/or to prevent further life threatening deterioration of the patient's condition.

Examples of vital organ system failure include, but are not limited to: central nervous system failure, circulatory failure, shock, renal, hepatic, metabolic, and/or respiratory failure. Although critical care typically requires interpretation of multiple physiologic parameters and/or application of advanced technology(s), critical care may be provided in life threatening situations when these elements are not present.

Providing medical care to a critically ill, injured, or post-operative patient qualifies as a critical care service only if both the illness or injury and the treatment being provided meet the above requirements.

Critical care is usually, but not always, given in a critical care area such as a coronary care unit, intensive care unit, respiratory care unit, or the emergency department. However, payment may be made for critical care services provided in any location as long as the care provided meets the definition of critical care.

Consult the American Medical Association (AMA) CPT Manual for the applicable codes and guidance for critical care services provided to neonates, infants and children.

B. Critical Care Services and Medical Necessity

Critical care services must be medically necessary and reasonable. Services provided that do not meet critical care services or services provided for a patient who is not critically ill or injured in accordance with the above definitions and criteria but who happens to be in a critical care, intensive care, or other specialized care unit should be reported using another appropriate E/M code (e.g., subsequent hospital care, CPT codes 99231 - 99233).

As described in Section A, critical care services encompass both treatment of "vital organ failure" and "prevention of further life threatening deterioration of the patient's condition." Therefore, although critical care may be delivered in a moment of crisis or upon being called to the patient's bedside emergently, this is not a requirement for providing critical care service. The treatment and management of the patient's condition, while not necessarily emergent, shall be required, based on the threat of imminent deterioration (i.e., the patient shall be critically ill or injured at the time of the physician's visit).

Chronic Illness and Critical Care:

Examples of patients whose medical condition may not warrant critical care services:

1. Daily management of a patient on chronic ventilator therapy does not meet the criteria for critical care unless the critical care is separately identifiable from the chronic long term management of the ventilator dependence.

2. Management of dialysis or care related to dialysis for a patient receiving ESRD hemodialysis does not meet the criteria for critical care unless the critical care is separately identifiable from the chronic long term management of the dialysis dependence (refer to Chapter 8, §160.4). When a separately identifiable condition (e.g., management of seizures or pericardial tamponade related to renal failure) is being managed, it may be billed as critical care if critical care requirements are met. Modifier –25 should be appended to the critical care code when applicable in this situation.

Examples of patients whose medical condition may warrant critical care services:

1. An 81 year old male patient is admitted to the intensive care unit following abdominal aortic aneurysm resection. Two days after surgery he requires fluids and pressors to maintain adequate perfusion and arterial pressures. He remains ventilator dependent.

2. A 67 year old female patient is 3 days status post mitral valve repair. She develops petechiae, hypotension and hypoxia requiring respiratory and circulatory support.

3. A 70 year old admitted for right lower lobe pneumococcal pneumonia with a history of COPD becomes hypoxic and hypotensive 2 days after admission.

4. A 68 year old admitted for an acute anterior wall myocardial infarction continues to have symptomatic ventricular tachycardia that is marginally responsive to antiarrhythmic therapy.

Examples of patients who may not satisfy Medicare medical necessity criteria, or do not meet critical care criteria or who do not have a critical care illness or injury and therefore not eligible for critical care payment:

1. Patients admitted to a critical care unit because no other hospital beds were available;

2. Patients admitted to a critical care unit for close nursing observation and/or frequent monitoring of vital signs (e.g., drug toxicity or overdose); and

3. Patients admitted to a critical care unit because hospital rules require certain treatments (e.g., insulin infusions) to be administered in the critical care unit.

Providing medical care to a critically ill patient should not be automatically deemed to be a critical care service for the sole reason that the patient is critically ill or injured. While more than one physician may provide critical care services to a patient during the critical care episode of an illness or injury each physician must be managing one or more critical illness(es) or injury(ies) in whole or in part.

EXAMPLE: A dermatologist evaluates and treats a rash on an ICU patient who is maintained on a ventilator and nitroglycerine infusion that are being managed by an intensivist. The dermatologist should not report a service for critical care.

C. Critical Care Services and Full Attention of the Physician

The duration of critical care services to be reported is the time the physician spent evaluating, providing care and managing the critically ill or injured patient's care. That time must be spent at the immediate bedside or elsewhere on the floor or unit so long as the physician is immediately available to the patient.

For example, time spent reviewing laboratory test results or discussing the critically ill patient's care with other medical staff in the unit or at the nursing station on the floor may be reported as critical care, even when it does not occur at the bedside, if this time represents the physician's full attention to the management of the critically ill/injured patient.

For any given period of time spent providing critical care services, the physician must devote his or her full attention to the patient and, therefore, cannot provide services to any other patient during the same period of time.

D. Critical Care Services and Qualified Non-Physician Practitioners (NPP)

Critical care services may be provided by qualified NPPs and reported for payment under the NPP's National Provider Identifier (NPI) when the services meet the definition and requirements of critical care services in Sections A and B. The provision of critical care services must be within the scope of practice and licensure requirements for the State in which the qualified NPP practices and provides the service(s). Collaboration, physician supervision and billing requirements must also be met. A physician assistant shall meet the general physician supervision requirements.

E. Critical Care Services and Physician Time

Critical care is a time- based service, and for each date and encounter entry, the physician's progress note(s) shall document the total time that critical care services were provided. More than one physician can provide critical care at another time and be paid if the service meets critical care, is medically necessary and is not duplicative care. Concurrent care by more than one physician (generally representing different physician specialties) is payable if these requirements are met (refer to the Medicare Benefit Policy Manual, Pub. 100-02, Chapter 15, §30 for concurrent care policy discussion).

The CPT critical care codes 99291 and 99292 are used to report the total duration of time spent by a physician providing critical care services to a critically ill or critically injured patient, even if the time spent by the physician on that date is not continuous. Non-continuous time for medically necessary critical care services may be aggregated. Reporting CPT code 99291 is a prerequisite to reporting CPT code 99292. Physicians of the same specialty within the same group practice bill and are paid as though they were a single physician (§30.6.5).

1. Off the Unit/Floor

   Time spent in activities (excluding those identified previously in Section C) that occur outside of the unit or off the floor (i.e., telephone calls, whether taken at home, in the office, or elsewhere in the hospital) may not be reported as critical care because the physician is not immediately available to the patient. This time is regarded as pre- and post service work bundled in evaluation and management services.

2. Split/Shared Service

   A split/shared E/M service performed by a physician and a qualified NPP of the same group practice (or employed by the same employer) cannot be reported as a critical care service. Critical care services are reflective of the care and management of a critically ill or critically injured patient by an individual physician or qualified non-physician practitioner for the specified reportable period of time.

   Unlike other E/M services where a split/shared service is allowed the critical care service reported shall reflect the evaluation, treatment and management of a patient by an individual physician or qualified non-physician practitioner and shall not be representative of a combined service between a physician and a qualified NPP.

   When CPT code time requirements for both 99291 and 99292 and critical care criteria are met for a medically necessary visit by a qualified NPP the service shall be billed using the appropriate individual NPI number. Medically necessary visit(s) that do not meet these requirements shall be reported as subsequent hospital care services.

3. Unbundled Procedures

   Time involved performing procedures that are not bundled into critical care (i.e., billed and paid separately) may not be included and counted toward critical care time. The physician's progress note(s) in the medical record should document that time involved in the performance of separately billable procedures was not counted toward critical care time.

4. Family Counseling/Discussions

Critical care CPT codes 99291 and 99292 include pre and post service work. Routine daily updates or reports to family members and or surrogates are considered part of this service. However, time involved with family members or other surrogate decision makers, whether to obtain a history or to discuss treatment options (as described in CPT), may be counted toward critical care time when these specific criteria are met:

a) The patient is unable or incompetent to participate in giving a history and/ or making treatment decisions, and

b) The discussion is necessary for determining treatment decisions.

For family discussions, the physician should document:

a. The patient is unable or incompetent to participate in giving history and/ or making treatment decisions

b. The necessity to have the discussion (e.g., "no other source was available to obtain a history" or "because the patient was deteriorating so rapidly I needed to immediately discuss treatment options with the family",

c. Medically necessary treatment decisions for which the discussion was needed, and

d. A summary in the medical record that supports the medical necessity of the discussion

All other family discussions, no matter how lengthy, may not be additionally counted towards critical care. Telephone calls to family members and or surrogate decision-makers may be counted towards critical care time, but only if they meet the same criteria as described in the aforementioned paragraph.

5. Inappropriate Use of Time for Payment of Critical Care Services.

Time involved in activities that do not directly contribute to the treatment of the critically ill or injured patient may not be counted towards the critical care time, even when they are performed in the critical care unit at a patient's bedside (e.g., review of literature, and teaching sessions with physician residents whether conducted on hospital rounds or in other venues).

F. Hours and Days of Critical Care that May Be Billed

Critical care service is a time-based service provided on an hourly or fraction of an hour basis. Payment should not be restricted to a fixed number of hours, a fixed number of physicians, or a fixed number of days, on a per patient basis, for medically necessary critical care services. Time counted towards critical care services may be continuous or intermittent and aggregated in time increments (e.g., 50 minutes of continuous clock time or (5) 10 minute blocks of time spread over a given calendar date). Only one physician may bill for critical care services during any one single period of time even if more than one physician is providing care to a critically ill patient.

For Medicare Part B physician services paid under the physician fee schedule, critical care is not a service that is paid on a "shift" basis or a "per day" basis. Documentation may be requested for any claim to determine medical necessity. Examples of critical care billing that may require further review could include: claims from several physicians submitting multiple units of critical care for a single patient, and submitting claims for more than 12 hours of critical care time by a physician for one or more patients on the same given calendar date.

Physicians assigned to a critical care unit (e.g., hospitalist, intensivist, etc.) may not report critical care for patients based on a 'per shift" basis.

The CPT code 99291 is used to report the first 30 - 74 minutes of critical care on a given calendar date of service. It should only be used once per calendar date per patient by the same physician or physician group of the same specialty. CPT code 99292 is used to report additional block(s) of time, of up to 30 minutes each beyond the first 74 minutes of critical care (See table below). Critical care of <u>less than 30 minutes total duration on a given calendar date</u> is not reported separately using the critical care codes. This service should be reported using another appropriate E/M code such as subsequent hospital care.

<u>Clinical Example of Correct Billing of Time</u>:

A patient arrives in the emergency department in cardiac arrest. The emergency department physician provides 40 minutes of critical care services. A cardiologist is called to the ED and assumes responsibility for the patient, providing 35 minutes of critical care services. The patient stabilizes and is transferred to the CCU. In this instance, the ED physician provided 40 minutes of critical care services and reports only the critical care code (CPT code 99291) and not also emergency department services. The cardiologist may report the 35 minutes of critical care services (also CPT code 99291) provided in the ED. Additional critical care services by the cardiologist in the CCU may be reported on the same calendar date using 99292 or another appropriate E/M code depending on the clock time involved.

G. Counting of Units of Critical Care Services

The CPT code 99291 (critical care, first hour) is used to report the services of a physician providing full attention to a critically ill or critically injured patient from 30-74 minutes on a given date. Only one unit of CPT code 99291 may be billed by a physician for a patient on a given date. Physicians of the same specialty within the same group practice bill and are paid as though they were a single physician and would not each report CPT 99291on the same date of service.

The following illustrates the correct reporting of critical care services:

Total Duration of Critical Care	Codes
Less than 30 minutes	99232 or 99233 or other appropriate E/M code
30 - 74 minutes	99291 × 1
75 - 104 minutes	99291 × 1 and 99292 × 1
105 - 134 minutes	99291 × 1 and 99292 × 2
135 - 164 minutes	99291 × 1 and 99292 × 3
165 - 194 minutes	99291 × 1 and 99292 × 4
194 minutes or longer	99291 - 99292 as appropriate (per the above illustrations)

H. Critical Care Services and Other Evaluation and Management Services Provided on Same Day

When critical care services are required upon the patient's presentation to the hospital emergency department, only critical care codes 99291 - 99292 may be reported. An emergency department visit code may not also be reported.

When critical care services are provided on a date where an inpatient hospital or office/outpatient evaluation and management service was furnished earlier on the same date at which time the patient did not require critical care, both the critical care and the previous evaluation and management service may be paid. Hospital emergency department services are not payable for the same calendar date as critical care services when provided by the same physician to the same patient.

Physicians are advised to submit documentation to support a claim when critical care is additionally reported on the same calendar date as when other evaluation and management services are provided to a patient by the same physician or physicians of the same specialty in a group practice.

I. Critical Care Services Provided by Physicians in Group Practice(s)

Medically necessary critical care services provided on the same calendar date to the same patient by physicians representing different medical specialties that are not duplicative services are payable. The medical specialists may be from the same group practice or from different group practices.

Critically ill or critically injured patients may require the care of more than one physician medical specialty. Concurrent critical care services provided by each physician must be medically necessary and not provided during the same instance of time. Medical record documentation must support the medical necessity of critical care services provided by each physician (or qualified NPP). Each physician must accurately report the service(s) he/she provided to the patient in accordance with any applicable global surgery rules or concurrent care rules. (Refer to Medicare Claims Processing Manual, Pub. 100-04, Chapter 12, §40, and the Medicare Benefit Policy Manual, Pub. 100-02, Chapter 15, §30.)

CPT Code 99291

The initial critical care time, billed as CPT code 99291, must be met by a single physician or qualified NPP. This may be performed in a single period of time or be cumulative by the same physician on the same calendar date. A history or physical exam performed by one group partner for another group partner in order for the second group partner to make a medical decision would not represent critical care services.

CPT Code 99292

Subsequent critical care visits performed on the same calendar date are reported using CPT code 99292. The service may represent aggregate time met by a single physician or physicians in the same group practice with the same medical specialty in order to meet the duration of minutes required for CPT code 99292. The aggregated critical care visits must be medically necessary and each aggregated visit must meet the definition of critical care in order to combine the times.

Physicians in the same group practice who have the same specialty may not each report CPT initial critical care code 99291 for critical care services to the same patient on the same calendar date. Medicare payment policy states that physicians in the same group practice who are in the same specialty must bill and be paid as though each were the single physician. (Refer to the Medicare Claims Processing Manual, Pub. 100-04, Chapter 12, §30.6.)

Physician specialty means the self-designated primary specialty by which the physician bills Medicare and is known to the contractor that adjudicates the claims. Physicians in the same group practice who have different medical specialties may bill and be paid without regard to their membership in the same group. For example, if a cardiologist and an endocrinologist are group partners and the critical care services of each are medically necessary and not duplicative, the critical care services may be reported by each regardless of their group practice relationship.

Two or more physicians in the same group practice who have different specialties and who provide critical care to a critically ill or critically injured patient may not in all cases each report the initial critical care code (CPT 99291) on the same date. When the group physicians are providing care that is unique to his/her individual medical specialty and managing at least one of the patient's critical illness(es) or critical injury(ies) then the initial critical care service may be payable to each.

However, if a physician or qualified NPP within a group provides "staff coverage" or "follow-up" for each other after the first hour of critical care services was provided on the same calendar date by the previous group clinician (physician or qualified NPP), the subsequent visits by the "covering" physician or qualified NPP in the group shall be billed using CPT critical care add-on code 99292. The appropriate individual NPI number shall be reported on the claim. The services will be paid at the specific physician fee schedule rate for the individual clinician (physician or qualified NPP) billing the service.

Clinical Examples of Critical Care Services

1. Drs. Smith and Jones, pulmonary specialists, share a group practice. On Tuesday Dr. Smith provides critical care services to Mrs. Benson who is comatose and has been in the intensive care unit for 4 days following a motor vehicle accident. She has multiple organ dysfunction including cerebral hematoma, flail chest and pulmonary contusion. Later on the same calendar date Dr. Jones covers for Dr. Smith and provides critical care services. Medically necessary critical care services provided at the different time periods may be reported by both Drs. Smith and Jones. Dr. Smith would report CPT code 99291 for the initial visit and Dr. Jones, as part of the same group practice would report CPT code 99292 on the same calendar date if the appropriate time requirements are met.

2. Mr. Marks, a 79 year old comes to the emergency room with vague joint pains and lethargy. The ED physician evaluates Mr. Marks and phones his primary care physician to discuss his medical evaluation. His primary care physician visits the ER and admits Mr. Marks to the observation unit for monitoring, and diagnostic and laboratory tests. In observation Mr. Marks has a cardiac arrest. His primary care physician provides 50 minutes of critical care services. Mr. Marks' is admitted to the intensive care unit. On the same calendar day Mr. Marks' condition deteriorates and he requires intermittent critical care services. In this scenario the ED physician should report an emergency department visit and the primary care physician should report both an initial hospital visit and critical care services.

J. Critical Care Services and Other Procedures Provided on the Same Day by the Same Physician as Critical Care Codes 99291 - 99292

The following services when performed on the day a physician bills for critical care are included in the critical care service and should not be reported separately:

- The interpretation of cardiac output measurements (CPT 93561, 93562);
- Chest x-rays, professional component (CPT 71010, 71015, 71020);

- Blood draw for specimen (CPT 36415);

- Blood gases, and information data stored in computers (e.g., ECGs, blood pressures, hematologic data-CPT 99090);

- Gastric intubation (CPT 43752, 91105);

- Pulse oximetry (CPT 94760, 94761, 94762);

- Temporary transcutaneous pacing (CPT 92953);

- Ventilator management (CPT 94002 - 94004, 94660, 94662); and

- Vascular access procedures (CPT 36000, 36410, 36415, 36591, 36600).

No other procedure codes are bundled into the critical care services. Therefore, other medically necessary procedure codes may be billed separately.

K. Global Surgery

Critical care services shall not be paid on the same calendar date the physician also reports a procedure code with a global surgical period unless the critical care is billed with CPT modifier -25 to indicate that the critical care is a significant, separately identifiable evaluation and management service that is above and beyond the usual pre and post operative care associated with the procedure that is performed.

Services such as endotracheal intubation (CPT code 31500) and the insertion and placement of a flow directed catheter e.g., Swan-Ganz (CPT code 93503) are not bundled into the critical care codes. Therefore, separate payment may be made for critical care in addition to these services if the critical care was a significant, separately identifiable service and it was reported with modifier -25. The time spent performing the pre, intra, and post procedure work of these unbundled services, e.g., endotracheal intubation, shall be excluded from the determination of the time spent providing critical care.

This policy applies to any procedure with a 0, 10 or 90 day global period including cardiopulmonary resuscitation (CPT code 92950). CPR has a global period of 0 days and is not bundled into critical care codes. Therefore, critical care may be billed in addition to CPR if critical care was a significant, separately identifiable service and it was reported with modifier -25. The time spent performing CPR shall be excluded from the determination of the time spent providing critical care. In this instance it must be the physician who performs the resuscitation who bills for this service. Members of a code team must not each bill Medicare Part B for this service.

When postoperative critical care services (for procedures with a global surgical period) are provided by a physician other than the surgeon, no modifier is required unless all surgical postoperative care has been officially transferred from the surgeon to the physician performing the critical care services. In this situation, CPT modifiers "-54" (surgical care only) and "-55"(postoperative management only) must be used by the surgeon and intensivist who are submitting claims. Medical record documentation by the surgeon and the physician who assumes a transfer (e.g., intensivist) is required to support claims for services when CPT modifiers -54 and -55 are used indicating the transfer of care from the surgeon to the intensivist. Critical care services must meet all the conditions previously described in this manual section.

L. Critical Care Services Provided During Preoperative Portion and Postoperative Portion of Global Period of Procedure with 90 Day Global Period in Trauma and Burn Cases

Preoperative

Preoperative critical care may be paid in addition to a global fee if the patient is critically ill and requires the full attention of the physician, and the critical care is unrelated to the specific anatomic injury or general surgical procedure performed. Such patients may meet the definition of being critically ill and criteria for conditions where there is a high probability of imminent or life threatening deterioration in the patient's condition.

Preoperatively, in order for these services to be paid, two reporting requirements must be met. Codes 99291 - 99292 and modifier -25 (significant, separately identifiable evaluation and management services by the same physician on the day of the procedure) must be used, and documentation identifying that the critical care was unrelated to the specific anatomic injury or general surgical procedure performed shall be submitted. An ICD-9-CM code in the range 800.0 through 959.9 (except 930.0 - 939.9), which clearly indicates that the critical care was unrelated to the surgery, is acceptable documentation.

Postoperative

Postoperatively, in order for critical care services to be paid, two reporting requirements must be met. Codes 99291 - 99292 and modifier -24 (unrelated evaluation and management service by the same physician during a postoperative period) must be used, and documentation that the critical care was unrelated to the specific anatomic injury or general surgical procedure performed must be submitted. An ICD-9-CM code in the range 800.0 through 959.9 (except 930.0 - 939.9), which clearly indicates that the critical care was unrelated to the surgery, is acceptable documentation.

Medicare policy allows separate payment to the surgeon for postoperative critical care services during the surgical global period when the patient has suffered trauma or burns. When the surgeon provides critical care services during the global period, for reasons unrelated to the surgery, these are separately payable as well.

M. Teaching Physician Criteria

In order for the teaching physician to bill for critical care services the teaching physician must meet the requirements for critical care described in the preceding sections. For CPT codes determined on the basis of time, such as critical care, the teaching physician must be present for the entire period of time for which the claim is submitted. For example, payment will be made for 35 minutes of critical care services only if the teaching physician is present for the full 35 minutes. (See IOM, Pub 100-04, Chapter12, §100.1.4)

1. Teaching

Time spent teaching may not be counted towards critical care time. Time spent by the resident, in the absence of the teaching physician, cannot be billed by the teaching physician as critical care or other time-based services. Only time spent by the resident and teaching physician together with the patient or the teaching physician alone with the patient can be counted toward critical care time.

2. Documentation

A combination of the teaching physician's documentation and the resident's documentation may support critical care services. Provided that all requirements for critical care services are met, the teaching physician documentation may tie into the resident's documentation. The teaching physician may refer to the resident's documentation for specific patient history, physical findings and medical assessment. However, the teaching physician medical record documentation must provide substantive information including: (1) the time the teaching physician spent providing critical care, (2) that the patient was critically ill during the time the teaching physician saw the patient, (3) what made the patient critically ill, and (4) the nature of the treatment and management provided by the teaching physician. The medical review criteria are the same for the teaching physician as for all physicians. (See the Medicare Claims Processing, Pub. 100-04, Chapter 12, §100.1.1 for teaching physician documentation guidance.)

Unacceptable Example of Documentation:

"I came and saw (the patient) and agree with (the resident)".

Acceptable Example of Documentation:

"Patient developed hypotension and hypoxia; I spent 45 minutes while the patient was in this condition, providing fluids, pressor drugs, and oxygen. I reviewed the resident's documentation and I agree with the resident's assessment and plan of care."

N. Ventilator Management

Medicare recognizes the ventilator codes (CPT codes 94002 - 94004, 94660 and 94662) as physician services payable under the physician fee schedule. Medicare Part B under the physician fee schedule does not pay for ventilator management services in addition to an evaluation and management service (e.g., critical care services, CPT codes 99291 - 99292) on the same day for the patient even when the evaluation and management service is billed with CPT modifier -25.

30.6.13 - NURSING FACILITY SERVICES

(Rev. 2282, Issued: 08-26-11, Effective: 01-01-11, Implementation: 11-28-11)

A. Visits to Perform the Initial Comprehensive Assessment and Annual Assessments

The distinction made between the delegation of physician visits and tasks in a skilled nursing facility (SNF) and in a nursing facility (NF) is based on the Medicare Statute. Section 1819 (b) (6) (A) of the Social Security Act (the Act) governs SNFs while section 1919 (b) (6) (A) of the Act governs NFs. For further information refer to Medlearn Matters article number SE0418 at www.cms.hhs.gov/medlearn/matters.

The federally mandated visits in a SNF and NF must be performed by the physician except as otherwise permitted (42 CFR 483.40 (c) (4) and (f)). The principal physician of record must append the modifier "-AI", (Principal Physician of Record), to the initial nursing facility care code. This modifier will identify the physician who oversees the patient's care from other physicians who may be furnishing specialty care. All other physicians or qualified NPPs who perform an initial evaluation in the NF or SNF may bill the initial nursing facility care code. The initial federally mandated visit is defined in S&C-04-08

(see www.cms.hhs.gov/medlearn/matters) as the initial comprehensive visit during which the physician completes a thorough assessment, develops a plan of care, and writes or verifies admitting orders for the nursing facility resident. For Survey and Certification requirements, a visit must occur no later than 30 days after admission.

Further, per the Long Term Care regulations at 42 CFR 483.40 (c) (4) and (e) (2), in a SNF the physician may not delegate a task that the physician must personally perform. Therefore, as stated in S&C-04-08 the physician may not delegate the initial federally mandated comprehensive visit in a SNF.

The only exception, as to who performs the initial visit, relates to the NF setting. In the NF setting, a qualified NPP (i.e., a nurse practitioner (NP), physician assistant (PA), or a clinical nurse specialist (CNS)), who is not employed by the facility, may perform the initial visit when the State law permits. The evaluation and management (E/M) visit shall be within the State scope of practice and licensure requirements where the E/M visit is performed and the requirements for physician collaboration and physician supervision shall be met.

Under Medicare Part B payment policy, other medically necessary E/M visits may be performed and reported prior to and after the initial visit, if the medical needs of the patient require an E/M visit. A qualified NPP may perform medically necessary E/M visits prior to and after the initial visit if all the requirements for collaboration, general physician supervision, licensure, and billing are met.

The CPT Nursing Facility Services codes shall be used with place of service (POS) 31 (SNF) if the patient is in a Part A SNF stay. They shall be used with POS 32 (nursing facility) if the patient does not have Part A SNF benefits or if the patient is in a NF or in a non-covered SNF stay (e.g., there was no preceding 3-day hospital stay). The CPT Nursing Facility code definition also includes POS 54 (Intermediate Care Facility/Mentally Retarded) and POS 56 (Psychiatric Residential Treatment Center). For further guidance on POS codes and associated CPT codes refer to §30.6.14.

Effective January 1, 2006, the Initial Nursing Facility Care codes 99301 - 99303 are deleted.

Beginning January 1, 2006, the new CPT codes, Initial Nursing Facility Care, per day, (99304 - 99306) shall be used to report the initial federally mandated visit. Only a physician may report these codes for an initial federally mandated visit performed in a SNF or NF (with the exception of the qualified NPP in the NF setting who is not employed by the facility and when State law permits, as explained above).

A readmission to a SNF or NF shall have the same payment policy requirements as an initial admission in both the SNF and NF settings.

A physician who is employed by the SNF/NF may perform the E/M visits and bill independently to Medicare Part B for payment. An NPP who is employed by the SNF or NF may perform and bill Medicare Part B directly for those services where it is permitted as discussed above. The employer of the PA shall always report the visits performed by the PA. A physician, NP or CNS has the option to bill Medicare directly or to reassign payment for his/her professional service to the facility.

As with all E/M visits for Medicare Part B payment policy, the E/M documentation guidelines apply.

MEDICALLY NECESSARY VISITS

Qualified NPPs may perform medically necessary E/M visits prior to and after the physician's initial federally mandated visit in both the SNF and NF. Medically necessary E/M visits for the diagnosis or treatment of an illness or injury or to improve the functioning of a malformed body member are payable under the physician fee schedule under Medicare Part B. A physician or NPP may bill the most appropriate initial nursing facility care code (CPT codes 99304 - 99306) or subsequent nursing facility care code (CPT codes 99307 - 99310), even if the E/M service is provided prior to the initial federally mandated visit.

SNF SETTING–PLACE OF SERVICE CODE 31

Following the initial federally mandated visit by the physician, the physician may delegate alternate federally mandated physician visits to a qualified NPP who meets collaboration and physician supervision requirements and is licensed as such by the State and performing within the scope of practice in that State.

NF SETTING–PLACE OF SERVICE CODE 32

Per the regulations at 42 CFR 483.40 (f), a qualified NPP, who meets the collaboration and physician supervision requirements, the State scope of practice and licensure requirements, and who is not employed by the NF, may at the option of the State, perform the initial federally mandated visit in a NF, and may perform any other federally mandated physician visit in a NF in addition to performing other medically necessary E/M visits.

Questions pertaining to writing orders or certification and recertification issues in the SNF and NF settings shall be addressed to the appropriate State Survey and Certification Agency departments for clarification.

B. Visits to Comply With Federal Regulations (42 CFR 483.40 (c) (1)) in the SNF and NF

Payment is made under the physician fee schedule by Medicare Part B for federally mandated visits. Following the initial federally mandated visit by the physician or qualified NPP where permitted, payment shall be made for federally mandated visits that monitor and evaluate residents at least once every 30 days for the first 90 days after admission and at least once every 60 days thereafter.

Effective January 1, 2006, the Subsequent Nursing Facility Care, per day, codes 99311 - 99313 are deleted.

Beginning January 1, 2006, the new CPT codes, Subsequent Nursing Facility Care, per day, (99307 - 99310) shall be used to report federally mandated physician E/M visits and medically necessary E/M visits.

Carriers shall not pay for more than one E/M visit performed by the physician or qualified NPP for the same patient on the same date of service. The Nursing Facility Services codes represent a "per day" service.

The federally mandated E/M visit may serve also as a medically necessary E/M visit if the situation arises (i.e., the patient has health problems that need attention on the day the scheduled mandated physician E/M visit occurs). The physician/qualified NPP shall bill only one E/M visit.

Beginning January 1, 2006, the new CPT code, Other Nursing Facility Service (99318), may be used to report an annual nursing facility assessment visit on the required schedule of visits on an annual basis. For Medicare Part B payment policy, an annual nursing facility assessment visit code may substitute as meeting one of the federally mandated physician visits if the code requirements for CPT code 99318 are fully met and in lieu of reporting a Subsequent Nursing Facility Care, per day, service (codes 99307 - 99310). It shall not be performed in addition to the required number of federally mandated physician visits. The new CPT annual assessment code does not represent a new benefit service for Medicare Part B physician services.

Qualified NPPs, whether employed or not by the SNF, may perform alternating federally mandated physician visits, at the option of the physician, after the initial federally mandated visit by the physician in a SNF.

Qualified NPPs in the NF setting, who are not employed by the NF and who are working in collaboration with a physician, may perform federally mandated physician visits, at the option of the State.

Medicare Part B payment policy does not pay for additional E/M visits that may be required by State law for a facility admission or for other additional visits to satisfy facility or other administrative purposes. E/M visits, prior to and after the initial federally mandated physician visit, that are reasonable and medically necessary to meet the medical needs of the individual patient (unrelated to any State requirement or administrative purpose) are payable under Medicare Part B.

C. Visits by Qualified Nonphysician Practitioners

All E/M visits shall be within the State scope of practice and licensure requirements where the visit is performed and all the requirements for physician collaboration and physician supervision shall be met when performed and reported by qualified NPPs. General physician supervision and employer billing requirements shall be met for PA services in addition to the PA meeting the State scope of practice and licensure requirements where the E/M visit is performed.

MEDICALLY NECESSARY VISITS

Qualified NPPs may perform medically necessary E/M visits prior to and after the physician's initial visit in both the SNF and NF. Medically necessary E/M visits for the diagnosis or treatment of an illness or injury or to improve the functioning of a malformed body member are payable under the physician fee schedule under Medicare Part B. A physician or NPP may bill the most appropriate initial nursing facility care code (CPT codes 99304 - 99306) or subsequent nursing facility care code (CPT codes 99307 - 99310), even if the E/M service is provided prior to the initial federally mandated visit.

SNF SETTING–PLACE OF SERVICE CODE 31

Following the initial federally mandated visit by the physician, the physician may delegate alternate federally mandated physician visits to a qualified NPP who meets collaboration and physician supervision requirements and is licensed as such by the State and performing within the scope of practice in that State.

NF SETTING–PLACE OF SERVICE CODE 32

Per the regulations at 42 CFR 483.40 (f), a qualified NPP, who meets the collaboration and physician supervision requirements, the State scope of practice and licensure requirements, and who is not employed by the NF, may at the option of the State, perform the initial federally mandated visit in a NF, and may perform any other federally mandated physician visit in a NF in addition to performing other medically necessary E/M visits.

Questions pertaining to writing orders or certification and recertification issues in the SNF and NF settings shall be addressed to the appropriate State Survey and Certification Agency departments for clarification.

D. Medically Complex Care

Payment is made for E/M visits to patients in a SNF who are receiving services for medically complex care upon discharge from an acute care facility when the visits are reasonable and medically necessary and documented in the medical record. Physicians and qualified NPPs shall report initial nursing facility care codes for their first visit with the patient. The principal physician of record must append the modifier "-AI" (Principal Physician of Record), to the initial nursing facility care code when billed to identify the physician who oversees the patient's care from other physicians who may be furnishing specialty care. Follow-up visits shall be billed as subsequent nursing facility care visits.

E. Incident to Services

Where a physician establishes an office in a SNF/NF, the "incident to" services and requirements are confined to this discrete part of the facility designated as his/her office. "Incident to" E/M visits, provided in a facility setting, are not payable under the Physician Fee Schedule for Medicare Part B. Thus, visits performed outside the designated "office" area in the SNF/NF would be subject to the coverage and payment rules applicable to the SNF/NF setting and shall not be reported using the CPT codes for office or other outpatient visits or use place of service code 11.

F. Use of the Prolonged Services Codes and Other Time-Related Services

Beginning January 1, 2008, typical/average time units for E/M visits in the SNF/NF settings are reestablished. Medically necessary prolonged services for E/M visits (codes 99356 and 99357) in a SNF or NF may be billed with the Nursing Facility Services in the code ranges (99304 - 99306, 99307 - 99310 and 99318).

COUNSELING AND COORDINATION OF CARE VISITS

With the reestablishment of typical/average time units, medically necessary E/M visits for counseling and coordination of care, for Nursing Facility Services in the code ranges (99304 - 99306, 99307 - 99310 and 99318) that are time-based services, may be billed with the appropriate prolonged services codes (99356 and 99357).

G. Multiple Visits

The complexity level of an E/M visit and the CPT code billed must be a covered and medically necessary visit for each patient (refer to §§1862 (a)(1)(A) of the Act). Claims for an unreasonable number of daily E/M visits by the same physician to multiple patients at a facility within a 24-hour period may result in medical review to determine medical necessity for the visits. The E/M visit (Nursing Facility Services) represents a "per day" service per patient as defined by the CPT code. The medical record must be personally documented by the physician or qualified NPP who performed the E/M visit and the documentation shall support the specific level of E/M visit to each individual patient.

H. Split/Shared E/M Visit

A split/shared E/M visit cannot be reported in the SNF/NF setting. A split/shared E/M visit is defined by Medicare Part B payment policy as a medically necessary encounter with a patient where the physician and a qualified NPP each personally perform a substantive portion of an E/M visit face-to-face with the same patient on the same date of service. A substantive portion of an E/M visit involves all or some portion of the history, exam or medical decision making key components of an E/M service. The physician and the qualified NPP must be in the same group practice or be employed by the same employer. The split/shared E/M visit applies only to selected E/M visits and settings (i.e., hospital inpatient, hospital outpatient, hospital observation, emergency department, hospital discharge, office and non facility clinic visits, and prolonged visits associated with these E/M visit codes). The split/shared E/M policy does not apply to critical care services or procedures.

I. SNF/NF Discharge Day Management Service

Medicare Part B payment policy requires a face-to-face visit with the patient provided by the physician or the qualified NPP to meet the SNF/NF discharge day management service as defined by the CPT code. The E/M discharge day management visit shall be reported for the date of the actual visit by the physician or qualified NPP even if the patient is discharged from the facility on a different calendar date. The CPT codes 99315 - 99316 shall be reported for this visit. The Discharge Day Management Service may be reported using CPT code 99315 or 99316, depending on the code requirement, for a patient who has expired, but only if the physician or qualified NPP personally performed the death pronouncement.

30.6.14 - HOME CARE AND DOMICILIARY CARE VISITS (CODES 99324 - 99350)

(Rev. 775, Issued: 12-02-05, Effective: 01-01-06, Implementation: 01-03-06)
Physician Visits to Patients Residing in Various Places of Service
The American Medical Association's <u>Current Procedural Terminology</u> (CPT) 2006 new patient codes 99324 - 99328 and established patient codes 99334 - 99337(new codes beginning January 2006), for Domiciliary, Rest Home (e.g., Boarding Home), or Custodial Care Services, are used to report evaluation and management (E/M) services to residents residing in a facility which provides room, board, and other personal assistance services, generally on a long-term basis. These CPT codes are used to report E/M services in facilities assigned places of service (POS) codes 13 (Assisted Living Facility), 14 (Group Home), 33 (Custodial Care Facility) and 55 (Residential Substance Abuse Facility). Assisted living facilities may also be known as adult living facilities.

Physicians and qualified nonphysician practitioners (NPPs) furnishing E/M services to residents in a living arrangement described by one of the POS listed above must use the level of service code in the CPT code range 99324 - 99337 to report the service they provide. The CPT codes 99321 - 99333 for Domiciliary, Rest Home (e.g., Boarding Home), or Custodial Care Services are deleted beginning January, 2006.

Beginning in 2006, reasonable and medically necessary, face-to-face, prolonged services, represented by CPT codes 99354 - 99355, may be reported with the appropriate companion E/M codes when a physician or qualified NPP, provides a prolonged service involving direct (face-to-face) patient contact that is beyond the usual E/M visit service for a Domiciliary, Rest Home (e.g., Boarding Home) or Custodial Care Service. All the requirements for prolonged services at §30.6.15.1 must be met.

The CPT codes 99341 through 99350, <u>Home Services</u> codes, are used to report E/M services furnished to a patient residing in his or her own private residence (e.g., private home, apartment, town home) and not residing in any type of congregate/shared facility living arrangement including assisted living facilities and group homes. The Home Services codes apply only to the specific 2-digit POS 12 (Home). <u>Home Services</u> codes may not be used for billing E/M services provided in settings other than in the private residence of an individual as described above.

Beginning in 2006, E/M services provided to patients residing in a Skilled Nursing Facility (SNF) or a Nursing Facility (NF) must be reported using the appropriate CPT level of service code within the range identified for Initial Nursing Facility Care (new CPT codes 99304 - 99306) and Subsequent Nursing Facility Care (new CPT codes 99307 - 99310). Use the CPT code, Other Nursing Facility Services (new CPT code 99318), for an annual nursing facility assessment. Use CPT codes 99315 - 99316 for SNF/NF discharge services. The CPT codes 99301 - 99303 and 99311 - 99313 are deleted beginning January, 2006. The Home Services codes should not be used for these places of service.

The CPT SNF/NF code definition includes intermediate care facilities (ICFs) and long term care facilities (LTCFs). These codes are limited to the specific 2-digit POS 31 (SNF), 32 (Nursing Facility), 54 (Intermediate Care Facility/ Mentally Retarded) and 56 (Psychiatric Residential Treatment Center).

The CPT nursing facility codes should be used with POS 31 (SNF) if the patient is in a Part A SNF stay and POS 32 (nursing facility) if the patient does not have Part A SNF benefits. There is no longer a different payment amount for a Part A or Part B benefit period in these POS settings.

30.6.14.1 - Home Services (Codes 99341 - 99350)

(Rev. 1, 10-01-03)
B3-15515, B3-15066

A. Requirement for Physician Presence

Home services codes 99341 - 99350 are paid when they are billed to report evaluation and management services provided in a private residence. A home visit cannot be billed by a physician unless the physician was actually present in the beneficiary's home.

B. Homebound Status

Under the home health benefit the beneficiary must be confined to the home for services to be covered. For home services provided by a physician using these codes, the beneficiary does not need to be confined to the home. The medical record must document the medical necessity of the home visit made in lieu of an office or outpatient visit.

C. Fee Schedule Payment for Services to Homebound Patients under General Supervision

Payment may be made in some medically underserved areas where there is a lack of medical personnel and home health services for injections, EKGs, and venipunctures that are performed for homebound patients under general physician supervision by nurses and paramedical employees of physicians or physician-directed clinics. Section 10 provides additional information on the provision of services to homebound Medicare patients.

30.6.15 - PROLONGED SERVICES AND STANDBY SERVICES (CODES 99354 - 99360)

(Rev. 1, 10-01-03)
B3-15511-15511.3

30.6.15.1 - Prolonged Services With Direct Face-to-Face Patient Contact Service (ZZZ codes)

(Rev. 2282, Issued: 08-26-11, Effective: 01-01-11, Implementation: 11-28-11)

A. Definition

Prolonged physician services (CPT code 99354) in the office or other outpatient setting with direct face-to-face patient contact which require 1 hour beyond the usual service are payable when billed on the same day by the same physician or qualified nonphysician practitioner (NPP) as the companion evaluation and management codes. The time for usual service refers to the typical/average time units associated with the companion evaluation and management service as noted in the CPT code. Each additional 30 minutes of direct face-to-face patient contact following the first hour of prolonged services may be reported by CPT code 99355.

Prolonged physician services (code 99356) in the inpatient setting, with direct face-to-face patient contact which require 1 hour beyond the usual service are payable when they are billed on the same day by the same physician or qualified NPP as the companion evaluation and management codes. Each additional 30 minutes of direct face-to-face patient contact following the first hour of prolonged services may be reported by CPT code 99357.

Prolonged service of less than 30 minutes total duration on a given date is not separately reported because the work involved is included in the total work of the evaluation and management codes.

Code 99355 or 99357 may be used to report each additional 30 minutes beyond the first hour of prolonged services, based on the place of service. These codes may be used to report the final 15 - 30 minutes of prolonged service on a given date, if not otherwise billed. Prolonged service of less than 15 minutes beyond the first hour or less than 15 minutes beyond the final 30 minutes is not reported separately.

B. Required Companion Codes

The companion evaluation and management codes for 99354 are the Office or Other Outpatient visit codes (99201 - 99205, 99212 - 99215), the Domiciliary, Rest Home, or Custodial Care Services codes (99324 - 99328, 99334 - 99337), the Home Services codes (99341 - 99345, 99347 - 99350);

The companion codes for 99355 are 99354 and one of the evaluation and management codes required for 99354 to be used;

The companion evaluation and management codes for 99356 are the Initial Hospital Care codes and Subsequent Hospital Care codes (99221 - 99223, 99231 - 99233); Nursing Facility Services codes (99304 - 99318); or

The companion codes for 99357 are 99356 and one of the evaluation and management codes required for 99356 to be used.
Prolonged services codes 99354 - 99357 are not paid unless they are accompanied by the companion codes as indicated.

C. Requirement for Physician Presence

Physicians may count only the duration of direct face-to-face contact between the physician and the patient (whether the service was continuous or not) beyond the typical/average time of the visit code billed to determine whether prolonged services can be billed and to determine the prolonged services codes that are allowable. In the case of prolonged office services, time spent by office staff with the patient, or time the patient remains unaccompanied in the office cannot be billed. In the case of prolonged hospital services, time spent reviewing charts or discussion of a patient with house medical staff and not with direct face-to-face contact with the patient, or waiting for test results, for changes in the patient's condition, for end of a therapy, or for use of facilities cannot be billed as prolonged services.

D. Documentation

Documentation is not required to accompany the bill for prolonged services unless the physician has been selected for medical review. Documentation is required in the medical record about the duration and content of the medically necessary evaluation and management service and prolonged services billed. The medical record must be appropriately and sufficiently documented by the physician or qualified NPP to show that the physician or qualified NPP personally furnished the direct face-to-face time with the patient specified in the CPT code definitions. The start and end times of the visit shall be documented in the medical record along with the date of service.

E. Use of the Codes

Prolonged services codes can be billed only if the total duration of the physician or qualified NPP direct face-to-face service (including the visit) equals or exceeds the threshold time for the evaluation and management service the physician or qualified NPP provided (typical/average time associated with the CPT E/M code plus 30 minutes). If the total duration of direct face-to-face time does not equal or exceed the threshold time for the level of evaluation and management service the physician or qualified NPP provided, the physician or qualified NPP may not bill for prolonged services.

F. Threshold Times for Codes 99354 and 99355 (Office or Other Outpatient Setting)

If the total direct face-to-face time equals or exceeds the threshold time for code 99354, but is less than the threshold time for code 99355, the physician should bill the evaluation and management visit code and code 99354. No more than one unit of 99354 is acceptable. If the total direct face-to-face time equals or exceeds the threshold time for code 99355 by no more than 29 minutes, the physician should bill the visit code 99354 and one unit of code 99355. One additional unit of code 99355 is billed for each additional increment of 30 minutes extended duration. Contractors use the following threshold times to determine if the prolonged services codes 99354 and/or 99355 can be billed with the office or other outpatient settings including domiciliary, rest home, or custodial care services and home services codes.

Threshold Time for Prolonged Visit Codes 99354 and/or 99355 Billed with Office/Outpatient

Code	Typical Time for Code	Threshold Time to Bill Code 99354	Threshold Time to Bill Codes 99354 and 99355
99201	10	40	85
99202	20	50	95
99203	30	60	105
99204	45	75	120
99205	60	90	135
99212	10	40	85
99213	15	45	90
99214	25	55	100
99215	40	70	115
99324	20	50	95
99325	30	60	105
99326	45	75	120
99327	60	90	135
99328	75	105	150
99334	15	45	90
99335	25	55	100
99336	40	70	115
99337	60	90	135
99341	20	50	95
99342	30	60	105
99343	45	75	120
99344	60	90	135
99345	75	105	150
99347	15	45	90
99348	25	55	100
99349	40	70	115
99350	60	90	135

Add 30 minutes to the threshold time for billing codes 99354 and 99355 to get the threshold time for billing code 99354 and two units of code 99355. For example, to bill code 99354 and two units of code 99355 when billing a code 99205, the threshold time is 150 minutes.

G. Threshold Times for Codes 99356 and 99357

(Inpatient Setting) If the total direct face-to-face time equals or exceeds the threshold time for code 99356, but is less than the threshold time for code 99357, the physician should bill the visit and code 99356. Contractors do not accept more than one unit of code 99356. If the total direct face-to-face time equals or exceeds the threshold time for code 99356 by no more than 29 minutes, the physician bills the visit code 99356 and one unit of code 99357. One additional unit of code 99357 is billed for each additional increment of 30 minutes extended duration. Contractors use the following threshold times to determine if the prolonged services codes 99356 and/or 99357 can be billed with the inpatient setting codes.

Threshold Time for Prolonged Visit Codes 99356 and/or 99357 Billed with Inpatient Setting Codes

Code	Typical Time for Code	Threshold Time to Bill Code 99356	Threshold Time to Bill Codes 99356 and 99357
99221	30	60	105
99222	50	80	125
99223	70	100	145
99231	15	45	90
99232	25	55	100

Add 30 minutes to the threshold time for billing codes 99356 and 99357 to get the threshold time for billing code 99356 and two units of 99357.

H. Prolonged Services Associated With Evaluation and Management Services Based on Counseling and/or Coordination of Care (Time-Based)

When an evaluation and management service is dominated by counseling and/or coordination of care (the counseling and/or coordination of care represents more than 50% of the total time with the patient) in a face-to-face encounter between the physician or qualified NPP and the patient in the office/clinic or the floor time (in the scenario of an inpatient service), then the evaluation and management code is selected based on the typical/average time associated with the code levels. The time approximation must meet or exceed the specific CPT code billed (determined by the typical/average time associated with the evaluation and management code) and should not be "rounded" to the next higher level.

In those evaluation and management services in which the code level is selected based on time, prolonged services may only be reported with the highest code level in that family of codes as the companion code.

I.   Examples of Billable Prolonged Services

EXAMPLE 1

A physician performed a visit that met the definition of an office visit code 99213 and the total duration of the direct face-to-face services (including the visit) was 65 minutes. The physician bills code 99213 and one unit of code 99354.

EXAMPLE 2

A physician performed a visit that met the definition of a domiciliary, rest home care visit code 99327 and the total duration of the direct face-to-face contact (including the visit) was 140 minutes. The physician bills codes 99327, 99354, and one unit of code 99355.

EXAMPLE 3

A physician performed an office visit to an established patient that was predominantly counseling, spending 75 minutes (direct face-to-face) with the patient. The physician should report CPT code 99215 and one unit of code 99354.

J. Examples of Nonbillable Prolonged Services

EXAMPLE 1

A physician performed a visit that met the definition of visit code 99212 and the total duration of the direct face-to-face contact (including the visit) was 35 minutes. The physician cannot bill prolonged services because the total duration of direct face-to-face service did not meet the threshold time for billing prolonged services.

EXAMPLE 2

A physician performed a visit that met the definition of code 99213 and, while the patient was in the office receiving treatment for 4 hours, the total duration of the direct face-to-face service of the physician was 40 minutes. The physician cannot bill prolonged services because the total duration of direct face-to-face service did not meet the threshold time for billing prolonged services.

EXAMPLE 3

A physician provided a subsequent office visit that was predominantly counseling, spending 60 minutes (face-to-face) with the patient. The physician cannot code 99214, which has a typical time of 25 minutes, and one unit of code 99354. The physician must bill the highest level code in the code family (99215 which has 40 minutes typical/average time units associated with it). The additional time spent beyond this code is 20 minutes and does not meet the threshold time for billing prolonged services.

30.6.15.2 - Prolonged Services Without Direct Face-to-Face Patient Contact Service (Codes 99358 - 99359)

(Rev. 1490, Issued: 04-11-08, Effective: 07-01-08, Implementation: 07-07-08)
Contractors may not pay prolonged services codes 99358 and 99359, which do not require any direct patient face-to-face contact (e.g., telephone calls). Payment for these services is included in the payment for direct face-to-face services that physicians bill. The physician cannot bill the patient for these services since they are Medicare covered services and payment is included in the payment for other billable services.

30.6.15.3 - Physician Standby Service (Code 99360)

(Rev. 1, 10-01-03)

Standby services are not payable to physicians. Physicians may not bill Medicare or beneficiaries for standby services. Payment for standby services is included in the Part A payment to the facility. Such services are a part of hospital costs to provide quality care. If hospitals pay physicians for standby services, such services are part of hospital costs to provide quality care.

30.6.15.4 – Power Mobility Devices (PMDs) (Code G0372)

(Rev. 748, Issued: 11-04-05; Effective/Implementation Dates: 10-25-05)

Section 302(a)(2)(E)(iv) of the Medicare Prescription Drug, Improvement, and Modernization Act of 2003 (MMA) sets forth revised conditions for Medicare payment of Power Mobility Devices (PMDs). This section of the MMA states that payment for motorized or power wheelchairs may not be made unless a physician (as defined in §1861(r)(1) of the Act), a physician assistant, nurse practitioner, or a clinical nurse specialist (as those terms are defined in §1861(aa)(5)) has conducted a face-to-face examination of the beneficiary and written a prescription for the PMD.

Payment for the history and physical examination will be made through the appropriate evaluation and management (E&M) code corresponding to the history and physical examination of the patient. Due to the MMA requirement that the physician or treating practitioner create a written prescription and a regulatory requirement that the physician or treating practitioner prepare pertinent parts of the medical record for submission to the durable medical equipment supplier, code G0372 (physician service required to establish and document the need for a power mobility device) has been established to recognize additional physician services and resources required to establish and document the need for the PMD.

The G code indicates that all of the information necessary to document the PMD prescription is included in the medical record, and the prescription and supporting documentation is delivered to the PMD supplier within 30 days after the face-to-face examination.

Effective October 25, 2005, G0372 will be used to recognize additional physician services and resources required to establish and document the need for the PMD and will be added to the Medicare physician fee schedule.

30.6.16 - CASE MANAGEMENT SERVICES (CODES 99362 AND 99371 - 99373)

(Rev. 1, 10-01-03)
B3-15512

A. Team Conferences

Team conferences (codes 99361 - 99362) may not be paid separately. Payment for these services is included in the payment for the services to which they relate.

B. Telephone Calls

Telephone calls (codes 99371 - 99373) may not be paid separately. Payment for telephone calls is included in payment for billable services (e.g., visit, surgery, diagnostic procedure results).

Unit 1, Evaluation and Management Practice Answers

Practice 1, Report A

ICD-9-CM

Rationale:

A. Incorrect because the key components of this evaluation consist of an expanded problem focused (EPF) history, detailed expanded problem focused examination and low medical decision making (MDM). 99212 would be undercoding.

B. Incorrect because even though 99213 is the correct service code, the diagnosis of cough (786.2) would not be coded because it is a symptom of the acute bronchitis.

C. **Correct because the service code is for an established office service, which consists of an expanded problem focused history, expanded problem focused examination, and moderate MDM. Office and Other Outpatient Services codes require 2 of the 3 key components to qualify for assignment and the documentation supports assignment of this code. The diagnosis is correct with 466.0 (Bronchitis, acute) reported for the bronchitis since the documentation does specify the type (acute).**

D. Incorrect because 99202 is for a new patient, and this note states that the patient is established.

ICD-10-CM

Rationale:

A. Incorrect because the key components of this evaluation consist of an expanded problem focused (EPF) history, detailed expanded problem focused examination and low medical decision making (MDM). 99212 would be undercoding.

B. Incorrect because even though 99213 is the correct service code, the diagnosis of cough (R05) would not be coded because it is a symptom of the acute bronchitis.

C. **Correct because the service code is for an established office service, which consists of an expanded problem focused history, expanded problem focused examination, and moderate MDM. Office and Other Outpatient Services codes require 2 of the 3 key components to qualify for assignment and the documentation supports assignment of this code. The diagnosis is correct with J20.9 (Bronchitis, acute) reported for the bronchitis since the documentation does specify the type (acute).**

D. Incorrect because 99202 is for a new patient, and this note states that the patient is established.

Practice 1, Report B

Professional Services: 99213 (Evaluation and Management, Office and Other Outpatient)

ICD-9-CM: 577.0 (Pancreatitis, acute), 577.2 (Pseudocyst, pancreas)

ICD-10-CM: K85.9 (Pancreatitis, acute), K86.3 (Pseudocyst, pancreas)

Rationale: The patient is an established patient. The history of present illness (HPI) includes the location (abdomen), duration (4 months), and associated signs and symptoms (fever) for a total of 3, which is a level 2 or expanded problem focused HPI. One review of systems (ROS) (gastrointestinal) was performed for a level 2 or expanded problem focused ROS. Only the patient's past medical history (cholecystectomy) was discussed for a level 3 or detailed past, family, and social history (PFSH). All 3 elements of a patient's history have to be at the same level or higher when choosing the level of history. This documentation contained a level 2 or problem focused HPI, a level 2 or problem focused ROS and a level 3 or problem focused PFSH. The history level would therefore be a level 2 or expanded problem focused history because the lowest level is 2.

The examination included only 1 element of constitutional (general appearance) for 1 OS. The abdomen was soft for 1 BA. No organ systems were examined. There is a total of 2 BAs/OSs examined for an expanded problem focused or level 2 examination.

The MDM consisted of multiple diagnoses (acute pancreatitis, pseudocyst, past surgery to consider), limited data were reviewed, and the patient has a moderate risk of complication (established problem, not improving). To qualify for a given level of MDM complexity, 2 of 3 elements must be met or exceeded and this MDM is a level 3 or moderate.

The levels included level 2 or expanded problem focused history; level 2 or expanded problem focused examination, and a level 3 or moderate MDM. Because this is an established patient, only 2 of the 3 key components need to be met or exceeded to assign the code. The documentation qualifies for assignment of 99213.

ICD-9-CM: The primary reason for the office service is the persisting generalized abdominal pain (789.07); the report states she has acute pancreatitis (577.0) and since abdominal pain is a symptom of pancreatitis, it is not reported. A pseudocyst of the pancreas (577.2) was found on CT scan. The correct diagnoses are acute pancreatitis (577.0) and pseudocyst of the pancreas (577.2).

ICD-10-CM: The primary reason for the office service is the persisting generalized abdominal pain (R10.84); the report states she has acute pancreatitis (K85.9) and since abdominal pain is a symptom of pancreatitis, it is not reported. A pseudocyst of the pancreas (K86.3) was found on CT scan. The correct diagnoses are acute pancreatitis (K85.9) and pseudocyst of the pancreas (K86.3).

HISTORY ELEMENTS	Documented
HISTORY OF PRESENT ILLNESS (HPI)	
1. Location (site on body)	✗
2. Quality (characteristic: throbbing, sharp)	
3. Severity (1/10 or how intense)	
4. Duration* (how long for problem or episode)	✗
5. Timing (when it occurs)	
6. Context (under what circumstances does it occur)	
7. Modifying factors (what makes it better or worse)	
8. Associated signs and symptoms (what else is happening when it occurs)	✗

*Duration not in CPT as HPI Element	TOTAL	3
	LEVEL	2

REVIEW OF SYSTEMS (ROS)	Documented
1. Constitutional (e.g., weight loss, fever)	
2. Ophthalmologic (eyes)	
3. Otolaryngologic (ears, nose, mouth, throat)	
4. Cardiovascular	
5. Respiratory	
6. Gastrointestinal	✗
7. Genitourinary	
8. Musculoskeletal	
9. Integumentary (skin and/or breasts)	
10. Neurological	
11. Psychiatric	
12. Endocrine	
13. Hematologic/Lymphatic	
14. Allergic/Immunologic	

	TOTAL	1
	LEVEL	2

PAST, FAMILY, AND/OR SOCIAL HISTORY (PFSH)	Documented
1. Past illness, operations, injuries, treatments, and current medications	✗
2. Family medical history for heredity and risk	
3. Social activities, both past and present	

	TOTAL	1
	LEVEL	3

History Level	1	2	3	4
	Problem Focused	Expanded Problem Focused	Detailed	Comprehensive
HPI	Brief 1-3	Brief 1-3	Extended 4+	Extended 4+
ROS	None	Problem Pertinent 1	Extended 2-9	Complete 10+
PFSH	None	None	Pertinent 1	Complete 2-3
			HISTORY LEVEL	2

EXAMINATION ELEMENTS	Documented
CONSTITUTIONAL (OS)	
• Blood pressure, sitting	
• Blood pressure, lying	
• Pulse	
• Respirations	
• Temperature	
• Height	
• Weight	
• General appearance	✗

(Counts as only 1) NUMBER	1

BODY AREAS (BA)	Documented
1. Head (including face)	
2. Neck	
3. Chest (including breasts and axillae)	
4. Abdomen	✗
5. Genitalia, groin, buttocks	
6. Back (including spine)	
7. Each extremity	

	NUMBER	1

ORGAN SYSTEMS (OS)	Documented
1. Ophthalmologic (eyes)	
2. Otolaryngologic (ears, nose, mouth, throat)	
3. Cardiovascular	
4. Respiratory	
5. Gastrointestinal	
6. Genitourinary	
7. Musculoskeletal	
8. Integumentary (skin)	
9. Neurologic	
10. Psychiatric	
11. Hematologic/Lymphatic/Immunologic	

	NUMBER	0
	TOTAL BA/OS	2

Exam Level	1	2	3	4
	Problem Focused	Expanded Problem Focused	Detailed	Comprehensive
	Limited to affected BA/OS	Limited to affected BA/OS & other related OS(s)	Extended of affected BA(s) & other related OS(s)	General multi-system (OSs only)
# of OS or BA	1	2-7 limited	2-7 extended	8+
			EXAMINATION LEVEL	2

MDM ELEMENTS	Documented
# OF DIAGNOSIS/MANAGEMENT OPTIONS	
1. Minimal	
2. Limited	
3. Multiple	✗
4. Extensive	

	LEVEL	3

AMOUNT AND/OR COMPLEXITY OF DATA TO REVIEW	Documented
1. Minimal/None	
2. Limited	✗
3. Moderate	
4. Extensive	

	LEVEL	2

RISK OF COMPLICATION OR DEATH IF NOT TREATED	Documented
1. Minimal	
2. Low	
3. Moderate	✗
4. High	

	LEVEL	3

MDM*	1	2	3	4
	Straightforward	Low	Moderate	High
Number of DX or management options	Minimal	Limited	Multiple	Extensive
Amount and/or complexity of data	Minimal/None	Limited	Moderate	Extensive
Risks	Minimal	Low	Moderate	High
			MDM LEVEL	3

*To qualify for a given type of MDM complexity, 2 of 3 elements in the table must be met or exceeded.

History: Expanded Problem Focused

Examination: Expanded Problem Focused

MDM: Moderate

Number of Key Components: 2 of 3

Code: 99213

PRACTICE 2, HOSPITAL OBSERVATION SERVICES

Practice 2, Report A

ICD-9-CM:

Rationale:

A. Incorrect because the elements documented do not support a 99220 level of service. Diagnosis coding is incorrect.

B. Incorrect because prolonged service exclusions do not permit assignment of 99354 and 99355 with 99218. Diagnosis coding is also incorrect.

C. Incorrect because the cough 786.2 and abnormal findings on radiological examination (793.19) are missing and a CT scan was ordered for next week to assess these two conditions. The Index indicates that 583.81, which is missing, should be coded with 250.42. CPT coding is correct.

D. **Correct answer because the elements documents, detailed history, detailed exam and high MDM make the Observation level 99218. The patient presents with uncontrolled type 2 diabetes (250.42) and end stage renal disease (585.6) treated with peritoneal dialysis (V45.11). The Index shows 250.4 [583.81] indicating that diabetes with nephropathy, 250.42, must be followed by 583.81 to indicate nephrosis/nephritis in diseases classified elsewhere. End-stage renal disease 585.6 follows to indicate the severity of the diabetic nephropathy. The report states that the patient is going to be admitted for observation primarily to control his blood sugar levels, so the 5th digit 2 in 250.42 indicates uncontrolled diabetes. The patient has a cough (786.2) and bilateral lung infiltrates on chest x-ray (793.19), and a CT is to be scheduled the following week to assess both of these conditions. Also noted in the report is the elevated protein (790.99) and low albumin (790.99). The code is only reported once, 790.99. The leg edema (782.3) and depression (311) may be considered; however, these conditions were not addressed so are not reported. Noncompliance with medical treatment (V15.81) and long-term (current) use of insulin (V48.67) could also be reported for this case.**

ICD-10-CM

Rationale:

A. Incorrect because the elements documented do not support a 99220 level of service. Diagnosis coding is incorrect.

B. Incorrect because prolonged service exclusions do not permit assignment of 99354 and 99355 with 99218. Diagnosis coding is also incorrect.

C. Incorrect because the cough R05 and abnormal findings on radiological examinations (R91.8) are missing and a CT scan was ordered for next week to assess these two conditions. The diabetes type 2 with diabetic nephropathy (E11.21) and insulin use (Z79.4) should be reported. CPT coding is correct.

D. **Correct answer because the elements documents, detailed history, detailed exam and high MDM make the Observation level 99218. The patient presents with uncontrolled type 2 diabetes with diabetic nephropathy (E11.21 and E11.65 (Hyperglycemia)) and end stage renal disease (N18.6) treated with peritoneal dialysis (Z99.2). End-stage renal disease [N18.6] follows to indicate the severity of the diabetic nephropathy. The patient has a cough (R05) and bilateral lung infiltrates on chest x-ray (R91.8), and a**

CT is to be scheduled the following week to assess both of these conditions. Also noted in the report is the elevated protein (R78.9) and low albumin (R77.0). Report also the use of insulin (Z79.4). The leg edema (R60.9) and depression (F32.9) may be considered; however, these conditions were not addressed so are not reported. Noncompliance with medical treatment (Z91.19) could also be reported for this case.

Practice 2, Report B

Professional Services: 99217 (Evaluation and Management, Hospital Service, Observation Care)

ICD-9-CM: 440.1 (Stenosis, renal artery), 997.72 (Complications, surgical procedures, vascular, renal artery), 458.9 (Hypotension), 403.90 (Disease/diseased, renovascular), 585.9 (Disease/diseased, renal, chronic), 285.1 (Anemia, due to, blood loss, chronic)

ICD-10-CM: I70.1 (Stenosis, renal artery), T81.711A (Complications, surgical procedure, vascular, artery, renal), I95.9 (Hypotension), I12.9 (Hypertension, kidney, with, stage 1 through stage 4 chronic kidney disease), N18.9 (Disease/diseased, kidney, chronic), D50.0 (Anemia, due to, blood loss [chronic])

Rationale: There is no audit form with this case because the hospital observation discharge service is not based on the key components of history, exam, and MDM. There is only one CPT code for a hospital observation discharge—99217.

ICD-9-CM: This patient was admitted to Observation after an outpatient angioplasty for renal stenosis. The Guidelines, Section IV.A.2. Observation stay state that when a patient presents for outpatient surgery and develops complications requiring admission for observation, code the reason for the surgery as the first-reported diagnosis (reason for the encounter), followed by codes for the complications as secondary diagnoses. The first-listed diagnosis then is renal stenosis (440.1) followed by the complications of peri-procedural bleeding (997.72) that caused hypotension (458.9). This patient has chronic renal failure secondary to hypertensive renovascular disease.

According to the Official Guidelines for Coding and Reporting, Section I.C.7.a.3: "Assign codes from category 403, Hypertensive chronic kidney disease, when conditions classified to categories 585 are present. Unlike hypertension with heart disease, ICD-9-CM presumes a cause-and-effect relationship and classifies chronic kidney disease (CKD) with hypertension as hypertensive chronic kidney disease. Fifth digits for category 403 should be assigned as follows: 0 with CKD stage I through stage IV, or unspecified. 1 with CKD stage V or end stage renal disease. The appropriate code from category 585, Chronic kidney disease, should be used as a secondary code with a code from category 403 to identify the stage of chronic kidney disease." Therefore, the renovascular disease is reported with 403.90, with fifth digit 0 to indicate unspecified or chronic kidney disease stages I through IV. 585.9 is reported for the CRF (chronic renal failure). Code 285.1 (Anemia secondary to blood loss, acute) is also reported as it has been addressed.

ICD-10-CM: This patient was admitted to Observation after an outpatient angioplasty for renal stenosis. The Guidelines, Section IV.A.2. Observation stay state that when a patient presents for outpatient surgery and develops complications requiring admission for observation, code the reason for the surgery as the first reported diagnosis (reason for the encounter), followed by the codes for the complications as secondary diagnoses. The first-listed diagnosis then is renal artery stenosis (I70.1) followed by the complications of peri-procedural bleeding (T81.711A) that caused hypotension (I95.9). This patient has chronic renal failure secondary to hypertensive renovascular disease. According to the Official Guidelines for Coding and Reporting, Section I.C.9.2.a: "Assign codes from category I12, Hypertensive chronic kidney disease, when conditions, classified to categories N18 are present. Unlike hypertension with heart disease, ICD-10-CM presumes a cause-and-effect relationship and classifies chronic kidney disease (CKD) with hypertension as hypertensive chronic kidney disease. Fourth characters for category I12 should be assigned as follows: 0 hypertensive chronic kidney disease with stage 5 chronic kidney disease or end stage renal disease. 9 hypertensive chronic kidney disease with stage 1 through stage 4 chronic kidney disease, or unspecified chronic kidney disease. The appropriate code from category N18 should be used as a secondary code with a code from category I12 to identify the stage of chronic kidney disease." Therefore, the renovascular disease is reported with I12, with fourth character 9 to indicate unspecified or chronic kidney disease stages 1 through 4. N18.9 is reported for the CRF (chronic renal failure). Code D50.0 (Anemia secondary to blood loss, acute) is also reported as it has been addressed.

PRACTICE 3, HOSPITAL INPATIENT SERVICES

Practice 3, Report A

Rationale:
A. This choice is incorrect because 99205, initial office service, would not be reported, because only one E/M service is billable per provider per day, and the service provided by the physician in the office would be "bundled" into the documentation for the initial hospital service.

B. Is correct. 99223 is reported because the office visit and all services provided in that setting are considered when choosing the hospital admission code. To assign a code from this subcategory all three key components must meet or exceed the level in the code. The history and examination were comprehensive and the MDM was high.

C. This choice is incorrect. CPT 99215 is for an established patient office service and would not be reported because only one E/M service is billable per provider per day and the work done by the physician in the office would be "bundled" into the documentation for the initial hospital service.

D. This choice is incorrect. 99221 is for a level 1 initial hospital service. The history and exam are comprehensive, but the MDM documented is high, rather than straightforward or low, making this incorrect.

Practice 3, Report B

Professional Services: 99238 (Evaluation and Management, Hospital, Discharge)

ICD-9-CM: 578.9 (GI Bleed), 285.1 (Anemia, due to blood loss, acute); 414.00 (Arteriosclerosis/arteriosclerotic, coronary, artery), 443.9 (Disease/diseased, peripheral vascular); 496 (Disease/diseased, lung, obstructive [chronic], COPD); V45.82 (Status [post], angioplasty, percutaneous transluminal, coronary)

ICD-10-CM: K92.2 (Bleeding, gastrointestinal), D50.0 (Anemia, due to blood loss, acute). I25.10 (Stenosis, coronary, artery), I73.9 (Disease/diseased peripheral, vascular NOS), J44.9 (Disease/diseased, lung, obstructive [chronic], COPD), Z98.61 (Status [post], angioplasty [peripheral], coronary artery)

Rationale: Hospital discharges are based on time. If the documentation does not specify time spent discharging the patient, then the lowest level code must be assigned (99238). No audit form is needed with time based codes. The service may or may not include an examination of the patient.

ICD-9-CM: The diagnoses are stated in the final diagnosis area of the discharge summary. The acute GI bleed (458.9) and anemia due to blood loss (285.1) are reported even though they are listed as stable, which means that the condition is under control. When referencing the Index under "Disease, artery, coronary," you are directed to "see Arteriosclerosis, coronary" (414.00). The fifth digit of "0" is assigned because the documentation does not state if this disease is in the patient's native vessel or in a previously grafted vessel; however, *Coding Clinic* states to report "1" is unknown (414.01). The PVD (peripheral vascular disease) (443.9), COPD (496), and the post-procedural status of stent placement (V45.82) are reported.

ICD-10-CM: The diagnoses are stated in the final diagnosis area of the discharge summary. The acute GI bleed (K92.2) and anemia due to blood loss (D50.0) are reported even though they are listed as stable, which means that the condition is under control. The coronary arteriosclerosis is reported with (I25.10). The fifth character "0" is assigned because the documentation does not state if this disease is "with angina pectoris." The PVD (peripheral vascular disease) (I73.9), COPD (J44.9) and the post-procedural status of stent placement (Z98.61) are also reported. Code J44.9 describes COPD, and Z98.61 describes Coronary angioplasty status.

PRACTICE 4. CONSULTATIONS

Practice 4, Report A

Rationale:

A. Is the correct answer. The service is a consultation, based on the opening statement thanking for the referral and the reason for it. The consultation codes require 3 of 3 elements. This case had a detailed history and physical exam and moderate MDM, a level 3 consultation. To assign the level 4 requires a comprehensive history and physical exam components.

B. This choice is incorrect. CPT 99244 requires a comprehensive history and physical exam, and the documentation in this scenario did not meet those criteria. The decision making is moderate and meets this level, but 3 of 3 key components must be met or exceeded to select a level and only MDM meets this level.

C. This choice is incorrect. CPT 99203 is for a new patient office service, and this scenario is for a consultation.

D. This choice is incorrect. CPT 99215 is for an established patient office service, and this scenario is for a consultation.

Practice 4, Report B

Professional Services: 99253 (Evaluation and Management, Consultation)

ICD-9-CM: 787.01 (Nausea, with vomiting), 789.00 (Pain[s], abdominal, unspecified site), 790.4 (Elevation, transaminase), 250.60 (Diabetes with gastroparesis), 536.3 (Diabetic gastroparalysis), V58.69 (Long-term [current] drug use, methadone/opioids [for pain control]), V58.67 (Long-term [current] drug use, insulin), V44.2 (Status, gastrostomy)

ICD-10-CM: R11.2 (Nausea, with vomiting). R10.9 (Pain[s], abdominal), R74.0 (Elevation, transaminase level), E11.43 (Diabetes, with, gastroparesis), Z79.891 (Long-term [current] drug use, methadone for pain management), Z79.4 (Long-term [current] drug use, insulin), Z93.1 (Status gastrostomy)

Rationale: The physician has been asked to evaluate the patient for possible cause of her nausea, vomiting, and abdominal pain. There are 4 elements of HPI: location (abdomen), duration (2 days), context (intake-tube placement 2010), and associated signs and symptoms (constipation) for a level 4 or comprehensive HPI. Six systems were reviewed: constitutional (denies fever or chills), cardiovascular (denies chest pain), respiratory (denies shortness of breath), gastrointestinal (on tube feedings, denies change in bowel movements, denies melena, GERD), and genitourinary (denies dysuria), and endocrine (diabetic) for a level 3, detailed ROS. The PFSH includes: past (hypertension, diabetic gastroparesis), family (no GI problems) and social (does not smoke or drink) for a level 4 or complete PFSH. A comprehensive HPI, detailed ROS and comprehensive PFSH make this a level 3 detailed history.

The examination consists of 4 constitutional elements (temperature, pulse, blood pressure, general appearance) that count as 1 OS. The BAs that were examined include neck, abdomen, and all 4 extremities for a total of 6 BAs. A total of 6 additional OSs, ophthalmologic (PERRL, extraocular motions intact), otolaryngologic (oropharynx benign, mucous membranes moist), cardiovascular (regular rate and rhythm, S1, S2 normal), respiratory (clear to auscultation bilaterally), gastrointestinal (no hepatosplenomegaly or mass), and neurologic (intact) were examined. This is a total of 6 BAs and 7 OSs; however, only OSs count when assigning a comprehensive level. When recounting, there are 7 OSs for a level 3, or detailed examination.

The MDM has a Level 4 or extensive diagnosis/management options (surgical consult called for surgery), level 3 or moderate data were reviewed (labs, x-ray, reviewed x-rays), and the patient has level 4 or high risk (may have biliary obstruction, evaluation for small bowel obstruction/possible surgery) that makes this a level 4 or high MDM.

The detailed history, detailed level examination and high medical decision making make this consult 99253.

ICD-9-CM: The first diagnosis under the physician's impression states that these symptoms could represent diabetic gastroparesis, which is also known as delayed gastric emptying due to paralysis of the stomach muscles. This patient already has a gastrostromy for feedings for diabetic gastroparesis, which may be causing the problems 250.60 [536.3]. The Index indicates that 250.60 is listed before the gastroparesis, 536.3. A definitive diagnosis has not been made; therefore, report the symptoms nausea, with vomiting (787.01) and abdominal pain (789.00). The fifth digit on abdominal pain (789.00) is "0" for unspecified abdominal pain because no further indication of location was documented. Also reported is the elevated transaminase (790.4). The diabetes is reported as indicated above 250.60, 536.3. She is also on long-term methadone for pain control as well as Duragesic, which could be causing the ileus (V58.69). The patient is also status gastrostomy (V44.2) and status long-term insulin use (V58.67).

ICD-10-CM: The first diagnosis under the physician's impression states that these symptoms could represent diabetic gastroparesis, which is also known as delayed gastric emptying due to paralysis of the stomach muscles. This patient already has a gastrostromy for feedings for diabetic gastroparesis, which may be causing the problems E11.43. A definitive diagnosis has not been made; therefore, report the symptoms nausea, with vomiting (R11.2) and abdominal pain (R10.9). Also reported is the elevated transaminase level (R74.0). She is also on long-term methadone for pain management as well as Duragesic, which could be causing the ileus (Z79.891). The patient is also status gastrostomy (Z93.1) and status long-term insulin use (Z79.4).

HISTORY ELEMENTS	Documented
HISTORY OF PRESENT ILLNESS (HPI)	
1. Location (site on body)	X
2. Quality (characteristic: throbbing, sharp)	
3. Severity (1/10 or how intense)	
4. Duration* (how long for problem or episode)	X
5. Timing (when it occurs)	
6. Context (under what circumstances does it occur)	X
7. Modifying factors (what makes it better or worse)	
8. Associated signs and symptoms (what else is happening when it occurs)	X
*Duration not in CPT as HPI Element TOTAL	4
LEVEL	4

REVIEW OF SYSTEMS (ROS)	Documented
1. Constitutional (e.g., weight loss, fever)	X
2. Ophthalmologic (eyes)	
3. Otolaryngologic (ears, nose, mouth, throat)	
4. Cardiovascular	X
5. Respiratory	X
6. Gastrointestinal	X
7. Genitourinary	X
8. Musculoskeletal	
9. Integumentary (skin and/or breasts)	
10. Neurological	
11. Psychiatric	
12. Endocrine	X
13. Hematologic/Lymphatic	
14. Allergic/Immunologic	
TOTAL	6
LEVEL	3

PAST, FAMILY, AND/OR SOCIAL HISTORY (PFSH)	Documented
1. Past illness, operations, injuries, treatments, and current medications	X
2. Family medical history for heredity and risk	X
3. Social activities, both past and present	X
TOTAL	3
LEVEL	4

History Level	1	2	3	4
	Problem Focused	Expanded Problem Focused	Detailed	Comprehensive
HPI	Brief 1-3	Brief 1-3	Extended 4+	Extended 4+
ROS	None	Problem Pertinent 1	Extended 2-9	Complete 10+
PFSH	None	None	Pertinent 1	Complete 2-3
			HISTORY LEVEL	3

EXAMINATION ELEMENTS	Documented
CONSTITUTIONAL (OS)	
• Blood pressure, sitting	
• Blood pressure, lying	X
• Pulse	X
• Respirations	
• Temperature	X
• Height	
• Weight	
• General appearance	X
(Counts as only 1) NUMBER	1

BODY AREAS (BA)	Documented
1. Head (including face)	
2. Neck	X
3. Chest (including breasts and axillae)	
4. Abdomen	X
5. Genitalia, groin, buttocks	
6. Back (including spine)	
7. Each extremity	XXXX
NUMBER	6

ORGAN SYSTEMS (OS)	Documented
1. Ophthalmologic (eyes)	X
2. Otolaryngologic (ears, nose, mouth, throat)	X
3. Cardiovascular	X
4. Respiratory	X
5. Gastrointestinal	X
6. Genitourinary	
7. Musculoskeletal	
8. Integumentary (skin)	
9. Neurologic	X
10. Psychiatric	
11. Hematologic/Lymphatic/Immunologic	
NUMBER	6
TOTAL BA/OS	13/7

Exam Level	1	2	3	4
	Problem Focused	Expanded Problem Focused	Detailed	Comprehensive
	Limited to affected BA/OS	Limited to affected BA/OS & other related OS(s)	Extended of affected BA(s) & other related OS(s)	General multi-system (OSs only)
# of OS or BA	1	2-7 limited	2-7 extended	8+
			EXAMINATION LEVEL	3

MDM ELEMENTS	Documented
# OF DIAGNOSIS/MANAGEMENT OPTIONS	
1. Minimal	
2. Limited	
3. Multiple	
4. Extensive	X
LEVEL	4
AMOUNT AND/OR COMPLEXITY OF DATA TO REVIEW	Documented
1. Minimal/None	
2. Limited	
3. Moderate	X
4. Extensive	
LEVEL	3
RISK OF COMPLICATION OR DEATH IF NOT TREATED	Documented
1. Minimal	
2. Low	
3. Moderate	
4. High	X
LEVEL	4

MDM*	1	2	3	4
	Straightforward	Low	Moderate	High
Number of DX or management options	Minimal	Limited	Multiple	Extensive
Amount and/or complexity of data	Minimal/None	Limited	Moderate	Extensive
Risks	Minimal	Low	Moderate	High
			MDM LEVEL	4

*To qualify for a given type of MDM complexity, 2 of 3 elements in the table must be met or exceeded.

History: Detailed
Examination: Detailed
MDM: High
Number of Key Components: 3 of 3
Code: 99253

PRACTICE 5, EMERGENCY DEPARTMENT SERVICES

Practice 5, Report A

ICD-9-CM

Rationale:

A. **This is the correct answer. Using the acuity sheet, this is an ED encounter (99284), and the highest level of service was the administration of intravenous (IV) medications, level 4, point 10. 789.09 is assigned to report the abdominal pain with fifth digit "9" to indicate other specified site, because patient's complaint and examination indicate upper abdominal, diffuse and right upper quadrant. The nausea is reported with 787.02 and the diarrhea with 787.91. Note that the viral syndrome (079.99) is not reported because provider indicated this as "probable" diagnosis and probable diagnoses are not reported in the outpatient setting. Also not reported are asthma, hypertension, depression, migraines, esophageal reflux, or arthritis, because none of these conditions were treated or were documented to affect treatment.**

B. This choice is incorrect. 99285 requires a level of service as indicated on the acuity sheet, and the highest level of service in this case was level 4, point 10, administration of IV medication. The diagnosis is also incorrect as 789.00 reports abdominal pain of an unspecified site and the report indicated upper abdominal pain (fifth digit "9"). 079.99, viral syndrome, is incorrect because the diagnostic statement indicated the viral syndrome was a probable diagnosis. Also missing from this selection is the nausea reported with 787.02 and the diarrhea reported with 787.91.

C. This choice is incorrect. 99283 is too low a level of service because level 4, point 10 specifies administration of an IV medication and the documentation in this case indicated that level of service. Also documented was the level 3, point 4 service of prescription medication administration, but code selection should always be the highest code available that is supported by the provider's documentation or the service is undercoded. Diagnosis of 789.00 (abdominal pain, unspecified site) is incorrect, because the documentation indicates specific points of pain, 789.09. Also missing from this selection is the nausea reported with 787.02 and the diarrhea reported with 787.91.

D. This choice is incorrect. Although 99284 is correct with 789.09 (abdominal pain, other specified site), 079.99 (unspecified viral infection) is not reported because it is documented as "probable," and probable diagnoses are not reported in the outpatient setting. Also missing from this selection is the nausea reported with 787.02 and the diarrhea reported with 787.91.

ICD-10-CM

Rationale:

A. **This is the correct answer. Using the acuity sheet, this is an ED encounter (99284), and the highest level of service was the administration of intravenous (IV) medications, level 4, point 10. R10.10 is assigned to report the upper abdominal pain with fifth character 0 to indicate other specified site, because patient's complaint and examination indicate upper abdominal, diffuse and right upper quadrant. The nausea is reported with R11.0 and the diarrhea with R19.7. Note that the viral syndrome (B97.89) is not reported because provider indicated this as "probable" diagnosis and probable diagnoses are not reported in the**

outpatient setting. Also not reported are asthma, hypertension, depression, migraines, esophageal reflux, or arthritis, because none of these conditions were treated or were documented to affect treatment.

B. This choice is incorrect. 99285 requires a level of service as indicated on the acuity sheet, and the highest level of service in this case was level 4, point 10, administration of IV medication. The diagnosis is also incorrect as R10.9 reports abdominal pain of an unspecified site and the report indicated upper abdominal pain (fifth character "0"). B97.89, viral syndrome, is incorrect because the diagnostic statement indicated the viral syndrome was a probable diagnosis. Also missing from this selection is the nausea reported with R10.12 and the diarrhea reported with R19.7.

C. This choice is incorrect. 99283 is too low a level of service because level 4, point 10 specifies administration of an IV medication and the documentation in this case indicated that level of service. Also documented was the level 3, point 4 service of prescription medication administration, but code selection should always be the highest code available that is supported by the provider's documentation or the service is undercoded. Diagnosis of R10.9 (abdominal pain, unspecified site) is incorrect, because the documentation indicates specific points of pain, R10.10. Also missing from this selection is the nausea reported with R10.12 and the diarrhea reported with R19.7.

D. This choice is incorrect. Although 99284 is correct with R10.10 (abdominal pain, other specified site), B97.89 (unspecified viral infection) is not reported because it is documented as "probable," and probable diagnoses are not reported in the outpatient setting. Also missing from this selection is the nausea reported with R10.12 and the diarrhea reported with R19.7.

Practice 5, Report B

Professional Services: 99283 (Evaluation and Management, Emergency Department)

ICD-9-CM: 845.00 (Sprain, strain, ankle), E885.2 (Fall/falling, from, off, skateboard)

ICD-10-CM: S96.402A (Sprain, ankle, left), V00.131A (Fall/falling, from, off, skateboard)

Rationale: The patient presents to the emergency room complaining of ankle pain due to a fall. Using the ED acuity sheet, the highest level of service is level 3, point 3, x-ray of one area, reported with 99283.

ICD-9-CM: The ankle was not fractured, but sprained (845.00). The external cause of the injury was a fall from a skateboard (E885.2).

ICD-10-CM: The left ankle was not fractured, but sprained (S96.402A). The external cause of the injury was a fall from a skateboard (V00.131A). The seventh character "A" indicates the initial encounter.

PRACTICE 6, CRITICAL CARE SERVICES

Practice 6, Report A

ICD-9-CM

Rationale:

A. This choice is incorrect. 99291 is correct for the critical care service, based on time documented. Diagnosis 806.00 (fracture, C1-C4 with unspecified spinal cord injury) is incorrect because there is no documentation of spinal cord injury. Diagnosis E888.8 is not reported because there is no clear documentation of what happened and the injury was likely the result of a medical condition (syncopal episode) versus an "accident." 780.09 (other alteration of consciousness) is incorrect because the documentation indicates syncope (780.2).

B. This choice is incorrect. 99221 reports an initial hospital service. When critical care is part of the initial visit by the same provider, the work for the admission is "bundled" into the critical care service code and not reported separately. E888.8 is not reported because there is no clear documentation of what happened, and the injury was likely the result of a medical condition (syncopal episode) versus an "accident." The remaining diagnoses are correct.

C. **Is the correct answer. Only 99291 can be assigned because the nonspecific statement of "Total critical care time did exceed 30 minutes" was the only documentation. 805.04 is the correct code for a closed cervical 4 fracture without any indication of spinal cord injury; 780.2 is correct for the syncope because there is no further information available. An E code is not assigned because the fracture was a result of the fall from the syncope, not an actual accident.**

D. This choice is incorrect. 99221 is for an initial hospital service. When critical care is part of the initial visit by the same provider, the work for the admission is "bundled" into the critical care service code and not separately reported. Diagnosis coding is correct.

ICD-10-CM

Rationale:

A. This choice is incorrect. 99291 is correct for the critical care service, based on time documented. Diagnosis S12.300A, S14.104A (fracture, fourth cervical vertebra with unspecified spinal cord injury) is incorrect because there is no documentation of spinal cord injury. R40.0 (other alteration of consciousness) is incorrect because the documentation indicates syncope (R55).

B. This choice is incorrect. 99221 reports an initial hospital service. When critical care is part of the initial visit by the same provider, the work for the admission is "bundled" into the critical care service code and not reported separately.

C. **Is the correct answer. Only 99291 can be assigned because the nonspecific statement of "Total critical care time did exceed 30 minutes" was the only documentation.**

   S12.300A is the correct code for a closed cervical (4th cervical) fracture without any indication of spinal cord injury. The default for a fracture is "displaced" if not otherwise specified. R55 is correct for the syncope because there is no further information available. An external cause code is not assigned because the fracture was a result of the fall from the syncope, not an actual accident.

D. This choice is incorrect. 99221 is for an initial hospital service. When critical care is part of the initial visit by the same provider, the work for the admission is "bundled" into the critical care service code and not separately reported. Diagnosis coding is correct.

Practice 6, Report B

Professional Services: 99291 (Evaluation and Management, Critical Care)

ICD-9-CM: 780.97 (Change(s) [of], [mental], status/NEC), 465.9 (Infection/ infective/infected, respiratory, upper, [acute], [infectious], NEC), 458.9 (Hypotension), 599.0 (Urosepsis), 412 (Infarct/infarction, myocardium/ myocardial, healed or old, currently presenting no symptoms), V10.51 (History [of], malignant neoplasm, bladder), V58.61 (Long-term [current] drug use, anticoagulants), E888.9 (Index to External Causes, Fall/falling, same level NEC), E849.7 (Index to External Causes, Accident, occurring (at) (in), home)

ICD-10-CM: R41.82 (Alteration [of], mental status). J06.9 (Infection/infected/ infective, respiratory, upper [acute] NOS), I95.9 (Hypotension), N39.0 (Urine, pus in), I25.2 (Infarct/infarction, myocardium/myocardial, old), Z85.51 (History [of], malignant neoplasm, bladder), Z79.01 (Long-term [current] drug use, anticoagulants), W18.30XA (Fall/falling, same level), Y92.199 (Accident, occurring (at) (in), home, (other specified residential institution)

Rationale: This is a critical care service, which is based on the time spent with the patient, not the usual key components. At the end of the documentation it states that the physician spent 30 minutes of critical care time on the patient. When billing for critical care, the table in the E/M section of your CPT manual is helpful. The table indicates that for 30-74 minutes code 99291 is to be assigned.

ICD-9-CM: The patient presents with an altered level of consciousness, 780.97. On further testing he was found to have urosepsis, 599.0, an upper respiratory infection, 465.9, and hypotension, 458.9. We are not given the cause of the hypotension but it responded to fluid; therefore, it could have been from the infection or fluid volume. Do not report 796.3 (Hypotension, transient), because it was treated with fluids. The patient also has a history of bladder cancer, V10.51 and long-term use of anticoagulants, V58.61. The instructions at the beginning of the E code chapter in the ICD-9-CM direct the coder to assign E codes to identify the cause of the injury. In this case, the patient was at home (E849.7) when he fell (E888.9).

ICD-10-CM: The patient presents with an altered level of consciousness, R41.82. On further testing he was found to have urosepsis, N39.0, an upper respiratory infection, J06.9, and hypotension, I95.9. We are not given the cause of the hypotension but it responded to fluid; therefore, it could have been from the infection or fluid volume. Do not report R03.1 (Hypotension, transient), because it was treated with fluids. The patient also has a history of bladder cancer, Z85.51 and long-term use of anticoagulants, Z79.01. The external cause codes are reported with W18.30XA (fall, same level, unspecified) and Y92.199 (place of occurrence, home).

PRACTICE 7, NURSING FACILITY SERVICES

Practice 7, Report A

ICD-9-CM

Rationale:

A. This choice is incorrect because 296.90 reports an unspecified episodic mood disorder when a bipolar disorder was documented (296.80). 333.82, orofacial dyskinesia should be 333.85 for orofacial dyskinesia due to drugs. The other codes are correct.

B. This choice is incorrect because 99308 is for a subsequent nursing facility service requiring expanded problem focused history and exam with a low MDM. Two of three key components are required and the expanded problem focused history, detailed exam, and moderate MDM documented support a higher level code (99309). Diagnosis 401.9 is incorrect, because the documentation did not indicate unspecified hypertension. 333.82, orofacial dyskinesia should be 333.85 for orofacial dyskinesia due to drugs. The other diagnoses are correct.

C. This choice is incorrect because 99336 is for an established patient service in a domiciliary, rest home, or custodial care setting and this patient is a resident in a nursing home. 296.90 (unspecified episodic mood disorder) is incorrect because a bipolar disorder was documented and is reported with 296.80. 969.3 is incorrect because there is no current "poisoning" from a medication documented. The correct code is 333.85 (tardive dyskinesia due to drugs). The remaining codes are correct.

D. Is the correct answer. 99309 is correct because the patient is a resident in a nursing home and this is a subsequent service. As a subsequent service, 2 of 3 key components are required to select a level of service. The documentation supports an interval history, a detailed exam, and moderate MDM. 784.0 reports the headaches; 296.80 reports unspecified bipolar disorder; 401.1 reports benign hypertension; 333.85 reports tardive dyskinesia due to drugs and requires the corresponding E code, E939.3, to indicate the cause of condition as adverse effects of antidepressants. Note that the Tabular note under 333.82 (Orofacial dyskinesia) excludes: orofacial dyskinesia due to drugs. Also reported is 788.30 for the urinary incontinence.

ICD-10-CM

Rationale:

A. This choice is incorrect because F39 reports an unspecified episodic mood disorder when a bipolar disorder was documented (F31.9). G24.4, orofacial dyskinesia should be G24.01 for orofacial dyskinesia due to drugs. The other codes are correct.

B. This choice is incorrect because 99308 is for a subsequent nursing facility service requiring expanded problem focused history and exam with a low MDM. Two of three key components are required and the expanded problem focused history, detailed exam, and moderate MDM documented support a higher level code (99309). Diagnosis I10 is correct, as it reports unspecified and benign. 333.82, orofacial dyskinesia should be G24.01 for orofacial dyskinesia due to drugs. The other diagnoses are correct.

C. This choice is incorrect because 99336 is for an established patient service in a domiciliary, rest home, or custodial care setting and this patient is a resident in a nursing home. F39 (unspecified episodic mood disorder) is incorrect because a bipolar disorder was documented and is reported with F31.9. T43.011A is incorrect because there is no current "poisoning" from a medication documented. The correct code is G24.01 (tardive dyskinesia, due to drugs). The remaining codes are correct.

D. Is the correct answer. 99309 is correct because the patient is a resident in a nursing home and this is a subsequent service. As a subsequent service, 2 of 3 key components are required to select a level of service. The documentation supports an interval history, a detailed exam, and moderate MDM. R51 reports the headaches; F31.9 reports unspecified bipolar disorder; I10 reports benign hypertension; G24.01 reports tardive dyskinesia due to drugs. Note that the Tabular note under G24.2 (Orofacial dyskinesia) excludes: orofacial dyskinesia due to drugs. Also reported is R32 for the urinary incontinence.)

Practice 7, Report B

Professional Services: 99308 (Evaluation and Management, Nursing Facility, Subsequent Care)

ICD-9-CM: 331.0 (Alzheimer's, dementia, with behavioral disturbance), 294.11 (Dementia, with behavioral disturbance)

ICD-10-CM: G30.9 (Alzheimer's, dementia, with behavioral disturbance), F02.81 (Dementia, with behavioral disturbance)

Rationale: The first line of the note states that this is a routine nursing facility service, which indicates this is an established patient. The only element of the HPI is the statement about frequent combative behavior for a level 1 of problem focused HPI. The ROS consisted of constitutional (no fever, chills), cardiovascular (no chest pain), and respiratory (no shortness of breath), and psychiatric (wanders off) for a level 3, or detailed ROS. The PFSH includes past (dementia) for a level 3 or detailed PFSH. The problem focused HPI, detailed ROS and detailed PFSH make this a problem focused history.

The examination consisted of only one constitutional element (general appearance—well-developed, well-nourished), so this would qualify as a 1 OS. Only 2 BAs were examined, the head (normocephalic and atraumatic) and neck (supple). OSs include: respiratory (clear to auscultation) for a total of 4 BAs/OSs, which constitute a level 2 or expanded problem focused level examination.

The MDM consisted of a level 3 or multiple number of diagnosis/management options (Alzheimer's, combative behavior, advanced directives), level 1 or minimal or no data to review, and level 2 or low risk decision making (patient clinically stable, one chronic disease, for a level 2 MDM.).

A problem focused interval history, expanded problem focused examination, and low complexity MDM qualifies as 99308.

ICD-9-CM: The documentation indicates the diagnosis of Alzheimer's (331.0). The patient is also experiencing behavior disturbances (294.11). The Index indicates 331.0 followed by 294.11 in slanted brackets, indicating that 294.11 is to be reported after 331.0.

ICD-10-CM: The documentation indicates the diagnosis of Disease, Alzheimer's (G30.9). The patient is also experiencing behavior disturbances (F02.81). The Index indicates G30.9 followed by F02.81 in slanted brackets, indicating that F02.81 is to be reported after G30.9.

HISTORY ELEMENTS	Documented
HISTORY OF PRESENT ILLNESS (HPI)	
1. Location (site on body)	
2. Quality (characteristic: throbbing, sharp)	
3. Severity (1/10 or how intense)	
4. Duration* (how long for problem or episode)	X
5. Timing (when it occurs)	
6. Context (under what circumstances does it occur)	
7. Modifying factors (what makes it better or worse)	
8. Associated signs and symptoms (what else is happening when it occurs)	

*Duration not in CPT as HPI Element	TOTAL	1
	LEVEL	1

REVIEW OF SYSTEMS (ROS)	Documented
1. Constitutional (e.g., weight loss, fever)	X
2. Ophthalmologic (eyes)	
3. Otolaryngologic (ears, nose, mouth, throat)	
4. Cardiovascular	X
5. Respiratory	X
6. Gastrointestinal	
7. Genitourinary	
8. Musculoskeletal	
9. Integumentary (skin and/or breasts)	
10. Neurological	
11. Psychiatric	X
12. Endocrine	
13. Hematologic/Lymphatic	
14. Allergic/Immunologic	

	TOTAL	4
	LEVEL	3

PAST, FAMILY, AND/OR SOCIAL HISTORY (PFSH)	Documented
1. Past illness, operations, injuries, treatments, and current medications	X
2. Family medical history for heredity and risk	
3. Social activities, both past and present	

	TOTAL	1
	LEVEL	3

History Level	1 Problem Focused	2 Expanded Problem Focused	3 Detailed	4 Comprehensive
HPI	Brief 1-3	Brief 1-3	Extended 4+	Extended 4+
ROS	None	Problem Pertinent 1	Extended 2-9	Complete 10+
PFSH	None	None	Pertinent 1	Complete 2-3
			HISTORY LEVEL	1

EXAMINATION ELEMENTS	Documented
CONSTITUTIONAL (OS)	
• Blood pressure, sitting	
• Blood pressure, lying	
• Pulse	
• Respirations	
• Temperature	
• Height	
• Weight	
• General appearance	X

(Counts as only 1) NUMBER	1

BODY AREAS (BA)	Documented
1. Head (including face)	X
2. Neck	X
3. Chest (including breasts and axillae)	
4. Abdomen	
5. Genitalia, groin, buttocks	
6. Back (including spine)	
7. Each extremity	

	NUMBER	2

ORGAN SYSTEMS (OS)	Documented
1. Ophthalmologic (eyes)	
2. Otolaryngologic (ears, nose, mouth, throat)	
3. Cardiovascular	
4. Respiratory	X
5. Gastrointestinal	
6. Genitourinary	
7. Musculoskeletal	
8. Integumentary (skin)	
9. Neurologic	
10. Psychiatric	
11. Hematologic/Lymphatic/Immunologic	

	NUMBER	1
	TOTAL BA/OS	4

Exam Level	1 Problem Focused	2 Expanded Problem Focused	3 Detailed	4 Comprehensive
	Limited to affected BA/OS	Limited to affected BA/OS & other related OS(s)	Extended of affected BA(s) & other related OS(s)	General multi-system (OSs only)
# of OS or BA	1	2-7 limited	2-7 extended	8+
			EXAMINATION LEVEL	2

MDM ELEMENTS	Documented
# OF DIAGNOSIS/MANAGEMENT OPTIONS	
1. Minimal	
2. Limited	
3. Multiple	X
4. Extensive	

	LEVEL	3

AMOUNT AND/OR COMPLEXITY OF DATA TO REVIEW	Documented
1. Minimal/None	X
2. Limited	
3. Moderate	
4. Extensive	

	LEVEL	1

RISK OF COMPLICATION OR DEATH IF NOT TREATED	Documented
1. Minimal	
2. Low	X
3. Moderate	
4. High	

	LEVEL	2

MDM*	1 Straightforward	2 Low	3 Moderate	4 High
Number of DX or management options	Minimal	Limited	Multiple	Extensive
Amount and/or complexity of data	Minimal/None	Limited	Moderate	Extensive
Risks	Minimal	Low	Moderate	High
			MDM LEVEL	2

*To qualify for a given type of MDM complexity, 2 of 3 elements in the table must be met or exceeded.

History: Problem Focused interval

Examination: Expanded Problem Focused

MDM: Low

Number of Key Components: 2 of 3

Code: 99308

PRACTICE 8, DOMICILIARY, REST HOME (E.G., BOARDING HOME), OR CUSTODIAL CARE SERVICES, AND DOMICILIARY, REST HOME (E.G., ASSISTED LIVING FACILITY), OR HOME CARE PLAN OVERSIGHT SERVICES (99324-99340)

Practice 8, Report A

ICD-9-CM

Rationale:

A. This is the correct choice because this is an established patient in a custodial care facility. The documentation supports an EPF interval history, a PF exam, and low complexity MDM. This category requires 2 out of 3 key elements to assign a code; therefore, the correct code is 99335. The diagnosis correctly reported is a rash (782.1).

B. Incorrect choice because 99307 is for an established patient in a nursing facility not a custodial care facility. The diagnosis 307.42 for idiopathic insomnia is incorrect.

C. Incorrect choice because 99347 is for an established patient home service, not a custodial care center. The diagnosis 307.42 for idiopathic insomnia is incorrect.

D. Incorrect diagnosis code of 780.52 because the sleep disturbance noted is not being treated or addressed in the care plan, so it is not reported. The diagnosis correctly reported is a rash (782.1). 99325 is incorrect because it is for a new patient and this patient is established.

ICD-10-CM

Rationale:

A. This is the correct choice because this is an established patient in a custodial care facility. The documentation supports an EPF interval history, a PF exam, and low complexity MDM. This category requires 2 out of 3 key elements to assign a code; therefore, the correct code is 99335. The diagnosis correctly reported is a rash (R21).

B. Incorrect choice because 99307 is for an established patient in a nursing facility, not a custodial care facility. The diagnosis F51.01 for idiopathic insomnia is incorrect.

C. Incorrect choice because 99347 is for an established patient home service, not a custodial care center. The diagnosis F51.01 for idiopathic insomnia is incorrect.

D. Incorrect diagnosis code of G47.00 because the sleep disturbance noted is not being treated or addressed in the care plan, so it is not reported. The diagnosis correctly reported is a rash (R21). 99325 is incorrect because it is for a new patient and this patient is established.

Practice 8, Report B

Professional Services: 99336 (Evaluation and Management, Domiciliary or Rest Home, Established Patient)

ICD-9-CM: 599.0 (Infection/infected/infective [urinary] tract NEC), V44.59 (Status, cystotomy)

ICD-10-CM: N39.0 (Infection/infected/infective, urinary [tract]), Z93.59 (Status, cystostomy, specified NEC)

Rationale: This service is an established patient service at the rest home where the patient resides. The HPI consists of: location (urinary system), quality (painful), severity (5 out of 10), and associated signs and symptoms (fever, abdominal pain) for a level 4 or comprehensive HPI. The ROS includes: constitutional (eating fair but skipping meals, denies weight loss), cardiovascular (suprapubic catheter due to urinary retention), psychiatric (confused), and respiratory (denies SOB) for a level 3 or detailed ROS. The history consisted of the patient's past medical history (urinary retention) and social history (resides in a rest home) for a level 4 or complete PFSH. Level selection of history must match all three areas to qualify for level selection. This documentation contained comprehensive HPI, detailed ROS, and a comprehensive PFSH for level 3 or detailed interval history.

The examination consisted of vitals and general appearance which constitutes 1 OS, 5 BAs, including the abdomen and all 4 extremities and 3 OSs, cardiovascular (regular without murmur), respiratory (diminished breath sounds with mild crackles at both bases), and integumentary (color is pink), for a total of 9 BAs/OSs; however, only OSs can count for a comprehensive examination. Recounting without the BAs, there is a total of 4 OSs, making this a level 3 or detailed examination.

The MDM entailed level 3 or multiple diagnosis/management options (new problem), level 1 or minimal data as none were reviewed, and level 3 or moderate risk (prescription drug management). This is a level 3 or moderate MDM.

A detailed interval history, detailed examination, and moderate MDM are assigned 99336.

ICD-9-CM: The diagnosis is UTI, reported with 599.0. The fever and abdominal pain would not be reported because they are symptoms of the UTI. V44.59 is reported to indicate the status of the suprapubic catheter, because the status is related to the organ system being treated. The Index lists V44.50, which is an unspecified cystostomy. Other cystostomy (V44.59) is correct as we know this is a suprapubic cystostomy.

ICD-10-CM: The diagnosis is UTI, reported with N39.0. The fever and abdominal pain would not be reported because they are symptoms of the UTI. Z93.59 is reported to indicate the status of the suprapubic catheter, because the status is related to the organ system being treated. The Index lists Z93.50, which is an unspecified cystostomy. Specified cystostomy (Z93.59) is correct as we know this is a suprapubic cystostomy.

HISTORY ELEMENTS	Documented
HISTORY OF PRESENT ILLNESS (HPI)	
1. Location (site on body)	X
2. Quality (characteristic: throbbing, sharp)	X
3. Severity (1/10 or how intense)	X
4. Duration* (how long for problem or episode)	
5. Timing (when it occurs)	
6. Context (under what circumstances does it occur)	
7. Modifying factors (what makes it better or worse)	
8. Associated signs and symptoms (what else is happening when it occurs)	X
*Duration not in CPT as HPI Element TOTAL	4
LEVEL	4

REVIEW OF SYSTEMS (ROS)	Documented
1. Constitutional (e.g., weight loss, fever)	X
2. Ophthalmologic (eyes)	
3. Otolaryngologic (ears, nose, mouth, throat)	
4. Cardiovascular	X
5. Respiratory	X
6. Gastrointestinal	
7. Genitourinary	
8. Musculoskeletal	
9. Integumentary (skin and/or breasts)	
10. Neurological	
11. Psychiatric	X
12. Endocrine	
13. Hematologic/Lymphatic	
14. Allergic/Immunologic	
TOTAL	4
LEVEL	3

PAST, FAMILY, AND/OR SOCIAL HISTORY (PFSH)	Documented
1. Past illness, operations, injuries, treatments, and current medications	X
2. Family medical history for heredity and risk	
3. Social activities, both past and present	X
TOTAL	2
LEVEL	4

History Level		1	2	3	4
		Problem Focused	Expanded Problem Focused	Detailed	Comprehensive
HPI		Brief 1-3	Brief 1-3	Extended 4+	Extended 4+
ROS		None	Problem Pertinent 1	Extended 2-9	Complete 10+
PFSH		None	None	Pertinent 1	Complete 2-3
				HISTORY LEVEL	3

EXAMINATION ELEMENTS	Documented
CONSTITUTIONAL (OS)	
• Blood pressure, sitting	
• Blood pressure, lying	X
• Pulse	
• Respirations	
• Temperature	
• Height	
• Weight	
• General appearance	X
(Counts as only 1) NUMBER	1

BODY AREAS (BA)	Documented
1. Head (including face)	
2. Neck	
3. Chest (including breasts and axillae)	
4. Abdomen	X
5. Genitalia, groin, buttocks	
6. Back (including spine)	
7. Each extremity	XXXX
NUMBER	5

ORGAN SYSTEMS (OS)	Documented
1. Ophthalmologic (eyes)	
2. Otolaryngologic (ears, nose, mouth, throat)	
3. Cardiovascular	X
4. Respiratory	X
5. Gastrointestinal	
6. Genitourinary	
7. Musculoskeletal	
8. Integumentary (skin)	X
9. Neurologic	
10. Psychiatric	
11. Hematologic/Lymphatic/Immunologic	
NUMBER	3
TOTAL BA/OS	9/4

Exam Level	1	2	3	4
	Problem Focused	Expanded Problem Focused	Detailed	Comprehensive
	Limited to affected BA/OS	Limited to affected BA/OS & other related OS(s)	Extended of affected BA(s) & other related OS(s)	General multi-system (OSs only)
# of OS or BA	1	2-7 limited	2-7 extended	8+
			EXAMINATION LEVEL	3

MDM ELEMENTS	Documented
# OF DIAGNOSIS/MANAGEMENT OPTIONS	
1. Minimal	
2. Limited	
3. Multiple	X
4. Extensive	
LEVEL	3
AMOUNT AND/OR COMPLEXITY OF DATA TO REVIEW	Documented
1. Minimal/None	X
2. Limited	
3. Moderate	
4. Extensive	
LEVEL	1
RISK OF COMPLICATION OR DEATH IF NOT TREATED	Documented
1. Minimal	
2. Low	
3. Moderate	X
4. High	
LEVEL	3

MDM*		1	2	3	4
		Straightforward	Low	Moderate	High
Number of DX or management options		Minimal	Limited	Multiple	Extensive
Amount and/or complexity of data		Minimal/None	Limited	Moderate	Extensive
Risks		Minimal	Low	Moderate	High
				MDM LEVEL	3

*To qualify for a given type of MDM complexity, 2 of 3 elements in the table must be met or exceeded.

History: Detailed interval
Examination: Detailed
MDM: Moderate
Number of Key Components: 2 of 3
Code: 99336

PRACTICE 9, HOME SERVICES

Practice 9, Report A

ICD-9-CM

Rationale:

A. This is an incorrect choice because 99343 is a new patient home visit rather than an established patient home visit. Diagnosis code 491.0 (chronic bronchitis) is incorrect because documentation did not specify acute or chronic. The osteoarthritis (715.90), decubiti of sacrum (707.03), decubiti of hip (707.04) and pitting edema (782.3) were correctly reported.

B. This is an incorrect choice because 99343 is a new patient home visit rather than an established patient home visit. Diagnosis codes are correct based on the documentation in the report as bronchitis (490), osteoarthritis (715.90), and pitting edema (782.3). Multiple decubiti of unspecified site (707.00) is incorrect as sacrum and hip are mentioned as the sites of decubiti (782.3).

C. This is the correct choice because 99349 is a home service for an established patient for a detailed history, detailed level examination and moderate MDM. ICD-9-CM: Diagnosis codes are correct based on the documentation in the report as bronchitis (490), osteoarthritis (715.90), decubitus of sacrum (707.03) decubitus of hip (707.04), and pitting edema (782.3).

D. This is an incorrect choice because the bronchitis was not documented as acute or chronic (491.0) and as such should be reported with 490. The osteoarthritis (715.90) and pitting edema (782.3) were correctly reported. Multiple decubiti of unspecified site (707.00) is incorrect as we are told the decubiti are of the sacrum (707.03) and the hip (707.04). 99349 is correct for an established patient home service.

ICD-10-CM

Rationale:

A. This is an incorrect choice because 99343 is a new patient home visit rather than an established patient home visit. Diagnosis code J41.0 (chronic bronchitis) is incorrect because documentation did not specify acute or chronic. The osteoarthritis (M19.90), decubiti of the sacrum (L89.159), decubiti of hip (L89.209) and pitting edema (R60.0) were correctly reported.

B. This is an incorrect choice because 99343 is a new patient home visit rather than an established patient home visit. Diagnosis codes are correct based on the documentation in the report as bronchitis (J40), osteoarthritis (M19.90), and pitting edema (R60.0). Multiple decubiti of unspecified site (L89.90) is incorrect as sacrum and hip are mentioned as the sites of decubiti.

C. This is the correct choice because 99349 is a home service for an established patient for a detailed history, detailed level examination and moderate MDM. Diagnosis codes are correct based on the documentation in the report as bronchitis (J40), osteoarthritis (M19.90) decubitus of sacrum, unspecified stage (L89.159), decubitus of hip (L89.209), and pitting edema (R60.0).

D. This is an incorrect choice because the bronchitis was not documented as acute or chronic (J41.0) and as such should be reported with J40. The osteoarthritis (M19.90), and pitting edema (R60.0) were correctly reported. Multiple decubiti of unspecified site (L89.90) is incorrect as we are told the decubiti are of the sacrum (L89.159) and the hip (L89.209). 99349 is correct for an established patient home service.

Practice 9, Report B

Professional Services: 99349 (Evaluation and Management, Home Services)

ICD-9-CM: 490 (Bronchitis), 428.0 (Failure/failed, heart, congestive), 332.0 (Parkinsonism [primary])

ICD-10-CM: J40 (Bronchitis), I50.9 (Failure/failed, heart, congestive), G20 (Parkinsonism [primary])

Rationale: This is a home service, which is based on whether the patient is new or established and the key components.

The HPI consists of 4 elements: location (lung), quality (productive), duration (since Monday), and modifying factor (Robitussin AC). This qualifies as a level 4 or comprehensive HPI. The patient was not able to answer questions for the ROS due to his condition so this would then qualify for a level 4 or comprehensive ROS. The PFSH includes: past (osteoarthritis, Parkinson's) for a level 3 or detailed history. This documentation contains a comprehensive HPI, a comprehensive ROS and a detailed PFSH for a level 3 or detailed interval history.

The examination contains 3 constitutional elements of blood pressure, respirations, and temperature that qualify as 1 OS. The BAs examined are head (normocephalic, atraumatic), and all 4 extremities, for a total of 5 BAs. Only 3 OSs were examined: cardiovascular (RRR), respiratory (few basilar rales, otherwise clear) and gastrointestinal (abdomen benign, no masses or tenderness). The total of 9 BAs/OSs makes this a comprehensive examination; however, only OSs count toward a comprehensive examination. Recounting without BAs, there are 4 OSs, making this a level 3 or detailed examination. The MDM contains a level 3 or multiple number of diagnosis and management options (CHF, Parkinson's, cough), level 1 or no data to review (none reviewed) and level 3 or moderate risk (medication management, management of two or more chronic illnesses). This qualifies as a level 3 or moderate MDM.

The detailed history, detailed examination and moderate MDM make this home visit 99349.

ICD-9-CM: The primary diagnosis for this home service is the bronchitis (490). The cough is not reported as according to Section II.A. of the Official Guidelines for Coding and Reporting, symptoms (such as the cough) are not reported when a more definitive diagnosis has been established (bronchitis). The patient also has CHF (428.0) and primary Parkinson's disease (332.0). The diagnosis osteoarthritis (715.90) is not necessarily reported as it was not treated.

ICD-10-CM: The primary diagnosis for this home service is bronchitis (J40). The cough is not reported as according to Section.II.A. of the Official Guidelines for Coding and Reporting, symptoms (such as the cough) are not reported when a more definitive diagnosis has been established (bronchitis). The patient also has CHF (I50.9) and primary Parkinson's disease (G20). The diagnosis osteoarthritis (M19.90) is not necessarily reported as it was not treated.

HISTORY ELEMENTS	Documented
HISTORY OF PRESENT ILLNESS (HPI)	
1. Location (site on body)	✗
2. Quality (characteristic: throbbing, sharp)	✗
3. Severity (1/10 or how intense)	
4. Duration* (how long for problem or episode)	✗
5. Timing (when it occurs)	
6. Context (under what circumstances does it occur)	
7. Modifying factors (what makes it better or worse)	✗
8. Associated signs and symptoms (what else is happening when it occurs)	
*Duration not in CPT as HPI Element TOTAL	4
LEVEL	4

REVIEW OF SYSTEMS (ROS)	Documented
1. Constitutional (e.g., weight loss, fever)	
2. Ophthalmologic (eyes)	
3. Otolaryngologic (ears, nose, mouth, throat)	
4. Cardiovascular	
5. Respiratory	
6. Gastrointestinal	
7. Genitourinary	
8. Musculoskeletal	
9. Integumentary (skin and/or breasts)	
10. Neurological	
11. Psychiatric	
12. Endocrine	
13. Hematologic/Lymphatic	
14. Allergic/Immunologic	
TOTAL	Unobtainable
LEVEL	4

PAST, FAMILY, AND/OR SOCIAL HISTORY (PFSH)	Documented
1. Past illness, operations, injuries, treatments, and current medications	✗
2. Family medical history for heredity and risk	
3. Social activities, both past and present	
TOTAL	1
LEVEL	3

History Level	1	2	3	4
	Problem Focused	Expanded Problem Focused	Detailed	Comprehensive
HPI	Brief 1-3	Brief 1-3	Extended 4+	Extended 4+
ROS	None	Problem Pertinent 1	Extended 2-9	Complete 10+
PFSH	None	None	Pertinent 1	Complete 2-3
			HISTORY LEVEL	3

EXAMINATION ELEMENTS	Documented
CONSTITUTIONAL (OS)	
• Blood pressure, sitting	
• Blood pressure, lying	✗
• Pulse	
• Respirations	✗
• Temperature	✗
• Height	
• Weight	
• General appearance	
(Counts as only 1) NUMBER	1

BODY AREAS (BA)	Documented
1. Head (including face)	✗
2. Neck	
3. Chest (including breasts and axillae)	
4. Abdomen	
5. Genitalia, groin, buttocks	
6. Back (including spine)	
7. Each extremity	✗✗✗✗
NUMBER	5

ORGAN SYSTEMS (OS)	Documented
1. Ophthalmologic (eyes)	
2. Otolaryngologic (ears, nose, mouth, throat)	
3. Cardiovascular	✗
4. Respiratory	✗
5. Gastrointestinal	✗
6. Genitourinary	
7. Musculoskeletal	
8. Integumentary (skin)	
9. Neurologic	
10. Psychiatric	
11. Hematologic/Lymphatic/Immunologic	
NUMBER	3
TOTAL BA/OS	9/4

Exam Level	1	2	3	4
	Problem Focused	Expanded Problem Focused	Detailed	Comprehensive
	Limited to affected BA/OS	Limited to affected BA/OS & other related OS(s)	Extended of affected BA(s) & other related OS(s)	General multi-system (OSs only)
# of OS or BA	1	2-7 limited	2-7 extended	8+
			EXAMINATION LEVEL	3

MDM ELEMENTS	Documented
# OF DIAGNOSIS/MANAGEMENT OPTIONS	
1. Minimal	
2. Limited	
3. Multiple	✗
4. Extensive	
LEVEL	3
AMOUNT AND/OR COMPLEXITY OF DATA TO REVIEW	Documented
1. Minimal/None	✗
2. Limited	
3. Moderate	
4. Extensive	
LEVEL	1
RISK OF COMPLICATION OR DEATH IF NOT TREATED	Documented
1. Minimal	
2. Low	
3. Moderate	✗
4. High	
LEVEL	3

MDM*	1	2	3	4
	Straightforward	Low	Moderate	High
Number of DX or management options	Minimal	Limited	Multiple	Extensive
Amount and/or complexity of data	Minimal/None	Limited	Moderate	Extensive
Risks	Minimal	Low	Moderate	High
			MDM LEVEL	3

*To qualify for a given type of MDM complexity, 2 of 3 elements in the table must be met or exceeded.

History: Detailed interval

Examination: Detailed

MDM: Moderate

Number of Key Components: 2 of 3

Code: 99349

PRACTICE 10A, PROLONGED SERVICES WITH OR WITHOUT DIRECT PATIENT CONTACT (99354-99359)

Practice 10A, Report A

ICD-9-CM

Rationale:

A. This is the correct choice because the documentation supported a comprehensive history and exam with a moderate complexity of MDM. As an established patient, 2 of 3 key components are required for determining a level of service, so this service qualifies for 99215. The additional 40 minutes are reported with the prolonged service code 99354, which is direct face-to-face care of a patient in an outpatient setting. The diagnosis is reported with 403.90, hypertensive kidney disease, even though the report did not state that there was a correlation between the hypertension and kidney disease. The Guidelines (Section I.C.9.a.2.) direct the coder to assume a causal relationship between the two conditions and report a 403 code rather than 401.9 (hypertension). Also to be reported is the stage of the kidney disease, which in this case is 585.9, unspecified CKD. The history of present illness indicates that the patient was started on an Advair inhaler but by another physician, and there is no documentation that this physician treated the breathing problem, and as such the condition is not reported. V45.89, Other postprocedural status, is correct to report the previous renal artery stenting. This patient also is a diabetic, which certainly can impact the renovascular disease. The Index indicates 250.40 [583.81], which instructs you to list 583.81 for diabetic nephropathy after 250.40. The fifth digit "0" is assigned to 250.40 as there is no mention of uncontrolled diabetes. The type of renal failure is already noted. V58.67 is also reported for long-term insulin use.

B. This is an incorrect choice because the level of service is too low and no prolonged service code is reported. Diagnosis coding is incorrect as the type of renal failure is not noted. Also the diabetes is not reported.

C. This is an incorrect choice because the level of service is too low and the code 99358 is for non-direct face-to-face care. Also incorrect are 401.9 and 585.9 to report the hypertension and chronic kidney disease because according to the Guidelines (Section I.C.9.a.2.) the coder is to assign a 403 category code to report kidney disease and renal failure by assuming a causal relationship between the two. The 440.1 is incorrect because the renal artery stenosis has already been stented.

D. This is an incorrect choice because of 401.9 and 585.9 reporting the hypertension and chronic kidney disease. According to the Guidelines (Section I.C.9.a.2.), you are to assign a 403 category code to report kidney disease and renal failure by assuming a causal relationship between the two. The V45.89 is correct; however, the diabetes with nephropathy is missing. The CPT coding is correct.

ICD-10-CM

Rationale:

A. This is the correct choice because the documentation supported a comprehensive history and exam with a moderate complexity of MDM. As an established patient, 2 of 3 key components are required for determining a level of service, so this service qualifies for 99215. The additional 40 minutes are reported with the prolonged service code 99354, which is direct face-to-face care of a patient in an outpatient setting.

    The diagnosis is reported with I12.9, hypertensive kidney disease, even though the report did not state that there was a correlation between the hypertension and kidney disease the Guidelines (Section I.C.9.a.2.) direct the coder to assume a causal relationship between the two conditions and report a I12 code rather than I10 (hypertension). Also to be reported is the stage of the kidney disease, which in this case is N18.9, unspecified CKD. The history of present illness indicates that the patient was started on an Advair inhaler but by another physician, and there is no documentation that this physician treated the breathing problem, and as such the condition is not reported. Z98.89, Other postprocedural status, is correct to report the previous renal artery stenting. This patient also is a diabetic, which certainly can impact the renovascular disease. The diabetic nephropathy is reported with E11.22. Z79.4 is also reported for long-term insulin use.

B. This is an incorrect choice because the level of service is too low and no prolonged service code is reported. Diagnosis coding is incorrect as the type of renal failure is not noted. Also the diabetes is not reported.

C. This is an incorrect choice because the level of service is too low and the code 99358 is for non-direct face-to-face care. Also incorrect are I10 and N18.9 to report the hypertension and chronic kidney disease because according to the Guidelines (Section I.C.7.a.3.), the coder is to assign a I12 category code to report kidney disease and renal failure by assuming a causal relationship between the two. The I70.1 is incorrect because the renal artery stenosis has already been stented.

D. This is an incorrect choice because of I10 and N18.9 reporting the hypertension and chronic kidney disease. According to the Guidelines (Section I.C.7.a.3.), you are to assign a I12 category code to report kidney disease and renal failure by assuming a causal relationship between the two. Z98.89 is correct; however, the diabetes with nephropathy is missing (E11.22). The CPT coding is correct.

Practice 10A, Report B

Professional Services: 99233 (Evaluation and Management, Hospital), 99356 (Evaluation and Management, Prolonged Services), 99357 × 2 (Evaluation and Management, Prolonged Services)

    ICD-9-CM: 584.9 (Failure/failed, renal, acute), 599.60 (Uropathy, obstructive), 585.9 (Failure/failed, renal, chronic), 591 (Hydronephrosis), 276.1 (Hyponatremia), 276.69 (Overload, fluid)

    ICD-10-CM: N17.9 (Failure/failed, renal, acute), N13.9 (Obstructive, urinary), N18.9 (Failure/failed, renal, chronic), N13.30 (Hydronephrosis, unspecified), E87.1 (Hyponatremia), E87.70 (Fluid, overload)

Rationale: This is a document that represents prolonged service of care. When reporting for prolonged services an E/M code from the accurate subcategory is first selected using the key components of the documentation. The time allotted for that E/M level is subtracted from the total time of the service and the remaining time is reported with a prolonged service code. Prolonged service codes are add-on codes; therefore, never reported alone.

This patient is acutely ill and is being followed for his acute renal failure. There are 4 elements of HPI: location (kidney), quality (worsening), severity (acute), and associated signs and symptoms (bloody urine) for a level 4 or comprehensive HPI. Only two systems were reviewed, cardiovascular (no chest pain) and respiratory (no shortness of breath), for a level 3 or detailed ROS. The documentation included only the past history (chronic renal failure) element of PFSH for a level 3 or detailed PFSH. A comprehensive HPI, detailed ROS, and detailed PFSH qualify as a level 3 or detailed interval history.

The constitutional examination consisted of 3 elements, blood pressure (lying down), pulse, and temperature, to qualify as 1 OS. No BAs were examined. Two OSs were examined, cardiovascular (no edema) and respiratory (lungs are clear), for a total of 2 OSs. The exam performed on this patient entailed 3 OSs and qualifies as a level 3 or detailed examination.

Level 4 or extensive diagnosis/management options (acute renal failure, obstructive uropathy, possible dialysis), level 2 or limited data were reviewed (labs), and the level 4 or high risk (need for surgery), which make this level 4 or high MDM.

The detailed history, detailed examination and high MDM make the subsequent hospital visit 99233; only 2 of the 3 elements of history, examination and MDM are required.

This code is allotted 35 minutes. At the end of this documentation it states that 2 hours and 25 minutes were spent with the patient. The total in minutes is 145 minutes. Subtract the 35 minutes for the E/M code 99233, which leaves 110 minutes for prolonged services. The prolonged services are categorized by either direct contact or without direct contact. The direct codes are further divided by whether the service took place in an outpatient or inpatient setting. The prolonged service codes that accompany 99233 are 99356 for the first 74 minutes of prolonged time and 99357 × 2 for the additional 36 minutes. The prolonged Services table in your CPT manual is a good tool to aid in code selection for time.

ICD-9-CM: The patient is being evaluated for acute renal failure (584.9). The other diagnoses are obstructive uropathy (599.60), chronic renal failure (585.9), hydronephrosis (591), hyponatremia (276.1) and fluid overload (276.69). All of these diagnoses would be assigned because all are being treated and each may affect the others.

ICD-10-CM: The patient is being evaluated for acute renal failure (N17.9). The other diagnoses are obstructive uropathy (N13.9), chronic renal failure (N18.9), hydronephrosis (N13.30), hyponatremia (E87.1) and fluid overload (E87.70). All of these diagnoses would be assigned because all are being treated and each may affect the others.

Practice 10A, Report B

HISTORY ELEMENTS	Documented
HISTORY OF PRESENT ILLNESS (HPI)	
1. Location (site on body)	X
2. Quality (characteristic: throbbing, sharp)	X
3. Severity (1/10 or how intense)	X
4. Duration* (how long for problem or episode)	
5. Timing (when it occurs)	
6. Context (under what circumstances does it occur)	
7. Modifying factors (what makes it better or worse)	
8. Associated signs and symptoms (what else is happening when it occurs)	X
*Duration not in CPT as HPI Element TOTAL	4
LEVEL	4

REVIEW OF SYSTEMS (ROS)	Documented
1. Constitutional (e.g., weight loss, fever)	
2. Ophthalmologic (eyes)	
3. Otolaryngologic (ears, nose, mouth, throat)	
4. Cardiovascular	X
5. Respiratory	X
6. Gastrointestinal	
7. Genitourinary	
8. Musculoskeletal	
9. Integumentary (skin and/or breasts)	
10. Neurological	
11. Psychiatric	
12. Endocrine	
13. Hematologic/Lymphatic	
14. Allergic/Immunologic	
TOTAL	2
LEVEL	3

PAST, FAMILY, AND/OR SOCIAL HISTORY (PFSH)	Documented
1. Past illness, operations, injuries, treatments, and current medications	X
2. Family medical history for heredity and risk	
3. Social activities, both past and present	
TOTAL	1
LEVEL	3

History Level	1	2	3	4
	Problem Focused	Expanded Problem Focused	Detailed	Comprehensive
HPI	Brief 1-3	Brief 1-3	Extended 4+	Extended 4+
ROS	None	Problem Pertinent 1	Extended 2-9	Complete 10+
PFSH	None	None	Pertinent 1	Complete 2-3
			HISTORY LEVEL	3

EXAMINATION ELEMENTS	Documented
CONSTITUTIONAL (OS)	
• Blood pressure, sitting	
• Blood pressure, lying	X
• Pulse	X
• Respirations	
• Temperature	X
• Height	
• Weight	
• General appearance	
(Counts as only 1) NUMBER	1

BODY AREAS (BA)	Documented
1. Head (including face)	
2. Neck	
3. Chest (including breasts and axillae)	
4. Abdomen	
5. Genitalia, groin, buttocks	
6. Back (including spine)	
7. Each extremity	
NUMBER	0

ORGAN SYSTEMS (OS)	Documented
1. Ophthalmologic (eyes)	
2. Otolaryngologic (ears, nose, mouth, throat)	
3. Cardiovascular	X
4. Respiratory	X
5. Gastrointestinal	
6. Genitourinary	
7. Musculoskeletal	
8. Integumentary (skin)	
9. Neurologic	
10. Psychiatric	
11. Hematologic/Lymphatic/Immunologic	
NUMBER	2
TOTAL BA/OS	3

Exam Level	1	2	3	4
	Problem Focused	Expanded Problem Focused	Detailed	Comprehensive
	Limited to affected BA/OS	Limited to affected BA/OS & other related OS(s)	Extended of affected BA(s) & other related OS(s)	General multi-system (OSs only)
# of OS or BA	1	2-7 limited	2-7 extended	8+
			EXAMINATION LEVEL	3

MDM ELEMENTS	Documented
# OF DIAGNOSIS/MANAGEMENT OPTIONS	
1. Minimal	
2. Limited	
3. Multiple	
4. Extensive	X
LEVEL	4
AMOUNT AND/OR COMPLEXITY OF DATA TO REVIEW	Documented
1. Minimal/None	
2. Limited	X
3. Moderate	
4. Extensive	
LEVEL	2
RISK OF COMPLICATION OR DEATH IF NOT TREATED	Documented
1. Minimal	
2. Low	
3. Moderate	
4. High	X
LEVEL	4

MDM*	1	2	3	4
	Straightforward	Low	Moderate	High
Number of DX or management options	Minimal	Limited	Multiple	Extensive
Amount and/or complexity of data	Minimal/None	Limited	Moderate	Extensive
Risks	Minimal	Low	Moderate	High
			MDM LEVEL	4

*To qualify for a given type of MDM complexity, 2 of 3 elements in the table must be met or exceeded.

History: Detailed interval
Examination: Detailed
MDM: High
Number of Key Components: 2 of 3
Code: 99233, 99356, 99357 x 2

PRACTICE 10B, STANDBY SERVICES

Practice 10B, Report A

Rationale:

A. Correct because the total time of standby was 25 minutes. The 6 minutes on the telephone regarding another patient cannot be included in the standby time. Per guidelines, standby time of less than 30 minutes cannot be separately reported.

B. Incorrect because the total time was less than 30 minutes, so no code would be assigned.

C. Incorrect because modifier -80 indicates assistant at surgery and the provider was not scrubbed or assisting in the surgery.

D. Incorrect because modifier -52 cannot be appended to an E/M service and the service cannot be reported as it was less than 30 minutes.

Practice 10B, Report B

Professional Services: 99360 × 3 (Evaluation and Management, Standby Services)

ICD-9-CM: 656.81 (Distress, fetal, affecting management of pregnancy or childbirth

ICD-10-CM: O77.9 (Stress, fetal, complicating pregnancy)

Rationale: This is a document that represents standby services. There is only one code in this subcategory, and it is reported in units depending on the length of standby time. The requirements for this code are as follows, the standby service must be requested by another physician, no direct contact is made with the patient, and the physician standing by cannot be providing care to any other patient during that time. If the standby time is less than 30 minutes, the time is not reported. Unlike some of the other E/M codes, the unit of time for standby services must be a full 30 minutes. It is very important to read and understand the guidelines that precede this subcategory before assigning the code.

This documentation indicates 1 hour and 40 minutes of standby or 100 minutes, requested by the patient's OB/GYN physician, due to increased fetal distress. 99360 is assigned with 3 units (×3), for 90 minutes of the 100 minutes spent in standby. The extra 10 minutes cannot be reported because it is not a full 30 minutes.

ICD-9-CM: The diagnosis is the reason the attending physician requested the physician to standby. In this case, the standby was requested for fetal distress that was affecting the management of childbirth 656.81. The fifth digit of "1" is assigned because the physician was present until the patient delivered.

ICD-10-CM: The diagnosis is the reason the attending physician requested the physician to standby. In this case, the standby was requested for fetal distress that was affecting the management of childbirth, O77.9.

PRACTICE 11A, CASE MANAGEMENT SERVICES (99363-99368)

Practice 11A, Report A

ICD-9-CM

Rationale:

A. This choice is incorrect because V66.7 is for an encounter for palliative care and the patient was not seen during this service. V65.49 is appropriate for counseling the family on the options for care. The remaining diagnosis codes are correct. The CPT code is correct.

B. This choice is incorrect because 99367 is reported for a conference in which neither the patient nor the family are present. Diagnosis codes are correct.

C. This choice is incorrect because 99368 is reported for a team conference in which neither the family nor patient attend and a nonphysician leads the team. V66.7 is incorrect because it is for an encounter for palliative care and the patient was not seen during this service. V65.49 is appropriate for counseling the family on the options for care. The remaining diagnosis codes are correct.

D. This is the correct choice with both the diagnoses and service code correct. ICD-9-CM V65.49 reports consulting, which was the primary reason for the service. The patient's diagnoses are stomach cancer (primary) 151.9, secondary lung cancer (197.0), congestive heart failure (428.0), and chronic interstitial pneumonia (515).

ICD-10-CM

Rationale:

A. This choice is incorrect because Z51.5 is for an encounter for palliative care and the patient was not seen during this service. Z71.89 is appropriate for counseling the family on the options for care. The remaining diagnosis codes are correct. The CPT code is correct.

B. This choice is incorrect because 99367 is reported for a conference in which neither the patient nor the family are present. Diagnosis codes are correct.

C. This choice is incorrect because 99368 is reported for a team conference in which neither the family nor patient attend and a nonphysician leads the team. Z51.5 is incorrect because it is for an encounter for palliative care and the patient was not seen during this service. Z71.89 is appropriate for counseling the family on the options for care. The remaining diagnosis codes are correct.

D. This is the correct choice with both the diagnoses and service code correct. Z71.89 reports consulting, which was the primary reason for the service. The patient's diagnoses are stomach cancer (primary) C16.9, secondary lung cancer (C78.00), congestive heart failure (I50.9), and chronic interstitial pneumonia (J84.10).

Practice 11A, Report B

Professional Services: 99367 (Evaluation and Management, Case Management Services)

ICD-9-CM: 583.9 (Nephritis), 585.6 (Disease/diseased, renal, end-stage), V49.75 (Absence, leg, below knee), V45.11 (Status, dialysis)

ICD-10-CM: N05.9 (Nephritis), N18.6 (Disease/diseased, end stage renal [ESRD]), Z89.519 (Absence, extremity, lower, below knee), Z99.2 (Status, dialysis)

Rationale: Case management is when the physician is responsible for the direct care of the patient and for coordinating the care and needs of the patient with other health care services. 99367 is correct to assign because the time spent was 60 minutes and no family was present.

ICD-9-CM: The diagnoses are nephritis (583.9), end stage renal disease (585.6), the patient's postoperative amputation status (V49.75), and the renal dialysis status (V45.11).

ICD-10-CM: The diagnoses are nephritis (N05.9), end stage renal disease (N18.6), the patient's postoperative amputation status (Z89.519), and the renal dialysis status (Z99.2)

PRACTICE 11B, ANTICOAGULANT MANAGEMENT

Practice 11B, Report A

Rationale:

A. Is correct because it reports a 90-day period of anticoagulant management with 99363 and the minimum of 8 INR measurements was met.

B. This choice is incorrect because although it reports 99363 correctly for the initial 90 days of management, 99364 should not be reported.

C. This choice is incorrect because it reports a subsequent 90 days with 99364 and this patient service was an initial 90 days of management.

D. This choice is incorrect because it reports a subsequent 90 days with 99364 and initial 90 days with 99363.

Practice 11B, Report B

Professional Services: 99364 (Anticoagulant Management)

ICD-9-CM: 453.42 (Embolism, vein, lower extremity, deep, acute, distal [lower leg])

ICD-10-CM: I82.4Z3 (Embolism, vein, lower extremity, distal, deep)

Rationale: This code is correct because it reports a subsequent 90 days of anticoagulant management that contained at least 3 INR measurements.

ICD-9-CM: 453.42 reports deep vein thrombosis of the lower leg.

ICD-10-CM: Code I82.4Z3 reports bilateral deep vein thrombosis of the lower legs.

PRACTICE 12, CARE PLAN OVERSIGHT SERVICES

Practice 12, Report A

ICD-9-CM

Rationale:

A. Incorrect because a medical team conference was not provided. Care Plan Oversight service (99380) is correct. Diagnosis coding is correct.

B. **Correct because all the diagnosis and service coding are correct. The physician for whom services are being reported is not the physician in charge of chemotherapy administration; the patient's gynecologist is overseeing that treatment. This physician is providing a care plan oversight for the patient's total care. When the patient presents for chemotherapy, the gynecologist would report the chemotherapy encounter code V58.11. The patient's diagnoses are primary ovarian cancer (183.0), neoplasm-related pain (338.3), and edema (782.3).**

C. Incorrect because 99308 is a subsequent nursing facility care service, and in this scenario the provider is managing the plan by telephone and is not present at the facility. The diagnosis coding is correct except for V58.11. This physician is providing a care plan oversight for the patient's total care. When the patient presents for chemotherapy, the gynecologist would report the chemotherapy encounter code V58.11.

D. Incorrect because the diagnosis for pain management and edema are missing and they should be reported because these conditions are being managed. This physician is providing a care plan oversight for the patient's total care. When the patient presents for chemotherapy, the gynecologist would report the chemotherapy encounter code V58.11. The CPT code is correct.

ICD-10-CM

Rationale:

A. Incorrect because a medical team conference was not provided. Care Plan Oversight service (99380) is correct. Diagnosis coding is correct.

B. **Correct because all the diagnosis and service coding are correct. The physician for whom services are being reported is not the physician in charge of chemotherapy administration; the patient's gynecologist is overseeing that treatment. This physician is providing a care plan oversight for the patient's total care. When the patient presents for chemotherapy, the gynecologist would report the chemotherapy encounter code Z51.11. The patient's diagnoses are primary ovarian cancer (C56.9), neoplasm-related pain (G89.3), and edema (R60.0).**

C. Incorrect because 99308 is a subsequent nursing facility care service, and in this scenario the provider is managing the plan by telephone and is not present at the facility. The diagnosis coding is correct except for Z51.11. This physician is providing a care plan oversight for the patient's total care. When the patient presents for chemotherapy, the gynecologist would report the chemotherapy encounter code Z51.11.

D. Incorrect because the diagnosis for pain management and edema are missing and they should be reported because these conditions are being managed. This physician is providing a care plan oversight for the patient's total care. When the patient presents for chemotherapy, the gynecologist would report the chemotherapy encounter code Z51.11. The CPT code is correct.

Practice 12, Report B

Professional Services: 99378 (Evaluation and Management, Care Plan Oversight Services)

ICD-9-CM: 162.5 (Neoplasm, lung, lower lobe, Malignant, Primary), 338.3 (Pain[s], neoplasm related)

ICD-10-CM: C34.30 (Neoplasm, lung, lower lobe, Malignant Primary), G89.3 (Pain[s], neoplasm related)

Rationale: Care plan oversight services reflect a supervisory role of the physician over the patient's care. The patient is not present when the physician is performing the service. Codes entail development or revision of a care plan, review of reports of patient status, communication with other health care professionals, and review of any lab or tests that may have been performed. These codes may only be reported once for every 30-day period. Codes are divided by whether the patient is receiving care from a home health agency, hospice, or a nursing facility. The codes are further categorized based on time spent in care plan oversight. 99378 is the correct code to report this service because the patient is receiving hospice care and the documented time was longer than 30 minutes.

ICD-9-CM: The diagnoses are lower lobe lung cancer (162.5) and pain due to the malignancy (338.3).

ICD-10-CM: The diagnoses are lower lobe lung cancer (C34.30) and pain due to the malignancy (G89.3).

PRACTICE 13, PREVENTIVE MEDICINE SERVICES

Practice 13, Report A

ICD-9-CM

Rationale:

A. Correct because this is a yearly physical examination of a 43-year-old established patient. 99396 is a preventive medicine code for an established patient between the ages of 40 and 64 years. The diagnoses are V70.0 (Routine medical exam), V72.31 (Routine GYN exam) for the health check-up, and V76.47 (Pap). No other diagnoses are reported because the patient was not treated at this time for her weight gain or depression.

B. Incorrect because 99213 is an E/M code for an office service for an established patient reported for the diagnosis of a new problem or follow-up care of an existing problem, not for yearly physicals. The diagnosis code 783.1, weight gain, is not reported because it was not treated during this evaluation.

C. Incorrect because 99386 is a new patient preventive medicine service and this is an established patient. The diagnoses of weight gain (783.1) and depression (311) are not reported because they were not treated by this physician.

D. Incorrect because the age range for this code is 18-39 years and this patient is 43 years old.

ICD-10-CM

Rationale:

A. Correct because this is a yearly physical examination of a 43-year-old established patient. 99396 is a preventive medicine code for an established patient between the ages of 40 and 64 years. The diagnoses are Z00.00 (Routine medical exam), Z01.419 (Routine GYN exam, without abnormal findings) for the health check-up, and Z12.72 (Pap). No other diagnoses are reported because the patient was not treated at this time for her weight gain or depression.

B. Incorrect because 99213 is an E/M code for an office service for an established patient reported for the diagnosis of a new problem or follow-up care of an existing problem, not for yearly physicals. The diagnosis code R63.5, weight gain, is not reported because it was not treated during this evaluation.

C. Incorrect because 99386 is a new patient preventive medicine service and this is an established patient. The diagnoses of weight gain (R63.5) and depression (F32.9) are not reported because they were not treated by this physician.

D. Incorrect because the age range for this code is 18-39 years and this patient is 43 years old.

Practice 13, Report B

Professional Services: 99396 (Evaluation and Management, Preventive Services)

ICD-9-CM: V70.0 (Checkup, health), V72.31 (Gynecological examination), V76.47 (Screening, vaginal), 305.1 (Abuse, tobacco)

ICD-10-CM: Z00.00 (Checkup, health), Z01.419 (Gynecological examination), Z12.72 (Screening, vaginal), F17.200 (Abuse, tobacco)

Rationale: Preventive medicine services are for physicals. Codes are selected based on patient age—unlike other E/M codes that are based on time or key components. Codes are further divided by whether the patient is new or established.

This documentation is of a 44-year-old established patient. The correct code for the preventive medicine service is 99396. 99406 is not reported since the physician did not document the amount of time spent discussing the tobacco cessation.

ICD-9-CM: The assessment contains 3 diagnoses, yearly physical performed today, gynecological exam, and tobacco abuse. When coding the diagnosis on preventive examinations the first code assigned would be V70.0 for the health checkup followed by the codes to report the gynecological exam and Pap. Only code the other diagnoses if there is an indication in the plan that these diagnoses are going to be treated or followed up. The physician is recommending smoking cessation, so the abuse of tobacco, 305.1, could be reported. It is important to familiarize yourself with the guidelines that precede the preventive medicine category because these guidelines explain the requirements for reporting both a preventive medicine code and an E/M service on the same day.

ICD-10-CM: The assessment contains 3 diagnoses, yearly physical performed today, gynecological exam, and tobacco abuse. When coding the diagnosis on preventive examinations the first code assigned would be Z00.0 for the health checkup followed by the codes to report the gynecological exam and Pap. Only code the other diagnoses if there is an indication in the plan that these diagnoses are going to be treated or followed up. The physician is recommending smoking cessation, so the abuse of tobacco, F17.200, could be reported. It is important to familiarize yourself with the guidelines that precede the preventive medicine category because these guidelines explain the requirements for reporting both a preventive medicine code and an E/M service on the same day.

PRACTICE 14, NON-FACE-TO-FACE SERVICES; SPECIAL E/M SERVICES; AND OTHER E/M SERVICES

Practice 14, Report A

ICD-9-CM

Rationale:

A. Incorrect because diagnoses 846.8 and E819.9 are for current injuries, rather than late effects. The CPT code is correct because special evaluation management services report basic life and/or disability evaluations or work-related medical disability evaluations. This evaluation is for disability resulting from an automobile accident. The treating physician is performing the evaluation. Diagnosis codes 723.1 (neck pain) and 724.2 (back pain) are correct because these represent the residual effects of the previous injury. 99455 is correct because the evaluation was performed by the treating physician, as indicated by the statement "Patient will continue with prescribed chronic pain management regimen…"

B. Incorrect because 99456 is for evaluation by other than treating physician, which was not the case in this scenario. Diagnosis coding is correct except code 338.21 (chronic pain) is missing.

C. Incorrect because 99456 is for evaluation by other than treating physician, which was not the case in this scenario. The diagnoses 846.8 and E819.9 are for current injuries, rather than late effects. Diagnosis codes 723.1 (neck pain) and 724.2 (back pain) are correct because they report the residual effects of previous injury. Code 338.21 (chronic pain) is missing.

D. Correct, because 99455 reports the evaluation performed by the treating physician, as indicated by the statement "Patient will continue with prescribed chronic pain management regimen…" Diagnosis codes 723.1 (neck pain) and 724.2 (back pain) are correct because they report the residual effects of previous injury. Code 338.21 is assigned to report the chronic pain (see Section I.C.6.a. of the Guidelines). Diagnoses 905.7 (Late effect of sprain and strain without mention of tendon injury) and E929.0 (Index to External Causes, Late effect of accident, specified NEC) are for the late effects of previously sustained injury.

ICD-10-CM

Rationale:

A. Incorrect because diagnoses S33.8XXA and V89.2XXA are for current injuries, rather than late effects. The CPT code is correct because special evaluation management services report basic life and/or disability evaluations or work-related medical disability evaluations. This evaluation is for disability resulting from an automobile accident. The treating physician is performing the evaluation. Diagnosis codes M54.2 (neck pain) and M54.5 (back pain) are correct because these represent the residual effects of the previous injury. 99455 is correct because the evaluation was performed by the treating physician, as indicated by the statement "Patient will continue with prescribed chronic pain management regimen…"

B. Incorrect because 99456 is for evaluation by other than treating physician, which was not the case in this scenario. Diagnosis coding is correct except code G89.21 (chronic pain) is missing.

C. Incorrect because 99456 is for evaluation by other than treating physician, which was not the case in this scenario. The diagnoses S33.8XXA and V89.2XXA are for current injuries, rather than late effects. Diagnosis codes

M54.2 (neck pain) and M54.5 (back pain) are correct because they report the residual effects of previous injury. Code G89.21 (chronic pain) is missing.

D. Correct, because 99455 reports the evaluation performed by the treating physician, as indicated by the statement "Patient will continue with prescribed chronic pain management regimen..." Diagnosis codes M54.2 (neck pain) and M54.5 (back pain) are correct because they report the residual effects of previous injury. Code G89.21 is assigned to report the chronic pain (see Section I.C.6.b. of the Guidelines). Diagnoses S33.8XXS (Late effect of sprain and strain injury) and X58.XXXS (External Cause Index, Late effect of accident, specified NEC) are for the late effects of previously sustained injury.

Practice 14, Report B

Professional Services: 99455 (Evaluation and Management, Insurance Examination)

ICD-9-CM: 354.0 (Syndrome, carpal tunnel); 338.21 (Pain[s], chronic, due to trauma)

ICD-10-CM: G56.00 (Syndrome, carpal tunnel); G89.21 (Pain[s], chronic, due to trauma)

Rationale: Special evaluation management services are for basic life and/or disability evaluations or work-related medical disability evaluations. This evaluation is for disability resulting from a work-related injury. The treating physician is performing the evaluation and correctly reporting the service with 99455.

ICD-9-CM: The diagnoses are carpal tunnel syndrome (354.0) and chronic pain due to trauma (338.21).

ICD-10-CM: The diagnoses are carpal tunnel syndrome, unspecified upper limb (G56.00) and chronic pain due to trauma (G89.21).

PRACTICE 15, NEWBORN CARE SERVICES

Practice 15, Report A

ICD-9-CM

Rationale:

A. Incorrect because diagnosis **V30.1** is for an infant born outside of the hospital. This infant was born in the hospital as evidenced by the exact time of birth noted and the APGAR scores reported. Diagnosis **779.31** is not reported because "disorganized suck" alone in a newborn is not indicative of a feeding disorder. It is noted that once the infant is able to suck, 10-20 cc are taken per feeding. CPT **99463** is correct.

B. Incorrect because **99234** is reported for observation and discharge on the same date. Although the baby was admitted and discharged on the same day, **99234** is incorrect because there is a code for newborn admitted and discharged on the same date, which is more appropriate for the patient involved. Diagnosis **V30.1** is incorrect because it is for an infant born outside of the hospital. This infant was born in the hospital as evidenced by the exact time of birth noted and the APGAR scores reported.

C. Incorrect because **99234** is reported for observation and discharge on the same date. Although the baby was admitted and discharged on the same day, **99234** is incorrect because there is a code for newborn admitted and discharged on the same date, which is more appropriate for the patient involved. Diagnosis **779.31** is not reported because "disorganized suck" alone in a newborn is not indicative of a feeding disorder. It is noted that once the infant is able to suck, 10-20 cc are taken per feeding. Diagnosis **V30.00** is correct.

D. Correct because 99463 correctly reports the admission and discharge of a normal newborn on the same date.

   ICD-9-CM: Diagnosis V30.00 is correct because it reports a single liveborn infant, born in a hospital without mention of cesarean section.

ICD-10-CM

Rationale:

A. Incorrect because diagnosis **Z38.1** is for an infant born outside of the hospital. This infant was born in the hospital as evidenced by the exact time of birth noted and the APGAR scores reported. Diagnosis **P92.2** is not reported because "disorganized suck" alone in a newborn is not indicative of a feeding disorder. It is noted that once the infant is able to suck, 10-20 cc are taken per feeding. CPT **99463** is correct.

B. Incorrect because **99234** is reported for observation and discharge on the same date. Although the baby was admitted and discharged on the same day, **99234** is incorrect because there is a code for newborn admitted and discharged on the same date, which is more appropriate for the patient involved. Diagnosis **Z38.1** is incorrect because it is for an infant born outside of the hospital. This infant was born in the hospital as evidenced by the exact time of birth noted and the APGAR scores reported.

C. Incorrect because **99234** is reported for observation and discharge on the same date. Although the baby was admitted and discharged on the same day, **99234** is incorrect because there is a code for newborn admitted and discharged on the same date, which is more appropriate for the patient involved. Diagnosis **P92.2** is not reported because "disorganized suck" alone in a newborn is not indicative of a feeding disorder. It is noted that once the infant is able to suck, 10-20 cc are taken per feeding. Diagnosis V30.00 is correct.

D. Correct because 99463 correctly reports the admission and discharge of a normal newborn on the same date. Diagnosis code Z38.00 is correct because it reports a single liveborn infant, born in a hospital without mention of cesarean section.

Practice 15, Report B

Professional Services: 99462 (Evaluation and Management, Newborn Care)
ICD-9-CM: 767.19 (Birth, injury, scalp)
ICD-10-CM: P12.3 (Bruise, scalp, due to birth injury, newborn)

Rationale: The patient is a normal newborn, born in the hospital with a multiple day stay. CPT 99462 is reported for the subsequent hospital care of the newborn, per day. There are no elements or key components to be considered when assigning this code.

ICD-9-CM: Diagnosis 767.19 is still reported because the condition is re-evaluated on examination ("exam is unchanged"). Note that diagnosis code V30.00 is not reported for services other than the initial admission (see newborn guidelines, Section I.C.15.b).

ICD-10-CM: Diagnosis P12.3 is still reported because the condition is re-evaluated on examination ("exam is unchanged"). Note that diagnosis code Z38.00 is not reported for services other than the initial admission (see newborn Guidelines, Section I.C.16.a.2.).

PRACTICE 16, OTHER

Practice 16A, Report A

Rationale:

A. Incorrect because the critical care time at the initial facility is reported separately as the report states this was a "critical care patient" and $1^1/_2$ hours was spent with this patient prior to transport. The transport time is not reported correctly as it should be 99479, 99467.

B. Incorrect because the multiple units for 99467 is incorrect.

C. Incorrect because the critical care time at the initial facility is not reported. The transport time is incorrectly reported.

D. **Correct. One and one-half hours of critical care time were spent at the initial facility prior to transport. The report states "critical care patient"; therefore, the patient was registered in the initial facility. Code 99291 reports 30-74 minutes of critical care, and 99292 reports additional blocks of time up to 30 minutes. The total initial facility time was 90 minutes. The remaining time (90-75 = 15 minutes) of 15 minutes is reported with 99292. The transport time was 2 hours; therefore, report 99466 (30-74 minutes) and 99467 (75-120 minutes = 45 minutes = 1 unit). Code 99467 represents each additional 30 minutes. Fifteen minutes remain; therefore, the 15 minutes is not reported. The correct answer is 99291, 99292, 99466, and 99467.**

Practice 16A, Report B

Professional Services: 99466 (Evaluation and Management, Pediatric Interfacility Transport); 99467 × 2 (Evaluation and Management, Pediatric Interfacility Transport)

ICD-9-CM: 949.0 (Burn, unspecified), 785.50 (Shock), E924.0 (Index to External Causes, Burning/burns, hot, liquid)

ICD-10-CM: T30.0 (Burn, unspecified), R57.9 (Shock), X12.XXXA (External Cause Index, Burn, hot, liquid)

Rationale: This documentation is very vague. You should discuss with the physician the need for more detailed documentation to ensure proper coding and achievement of the highest level of specificity.

The time given in this documentation is 2 hours and 40 minutes, or 160 minutes. 99466 is reported for the first 30-74 minutes. 99467 is an add-on code and is reported in conjunction with 99466 to report each additional 30 minutes of time after the first 74 minutes. The additional time after the first 74 minutes is 86 minutes or 99467 × 2. The remaining 26 minutes is not reported because it is less than the 30 minutes required. No audit form is needed when assigning codes from this subcategory because the codes are time-based and not based on key components.

ICD-9-CM: This is an 18-month-old who was burned by hot liquid and went into shock. The body area and severity of the burn are not specified in this documentation. The diagnoses are reported as 949.0 (Burn) and shock (785.50). An E code is assigned to report a burn due to hot liquid, E924.0.

ICD-10-CM: This is an 18-month-old who was burned and went into shock. The body area and severity of the burn are not specified in this documentation. Neither is the cause of the burn. The diagnoses are reported as T30.0 (Burn) and shock (R57.9). An external cause code is assigned to report a burn due to hot liquid, X12.XXXA.

220

Practice 16B, Report A

ICD-9-CM

Rationale:

A. Incorrect because there is no indication that the neonatal intensive care physician was the surgeon. Critical care providers do not generally perform surgical procedures, other than those necessary to maintain the patient's viability, such as intubation.

B. Incorrect because the patient is in the NICU (Neonatal Intensive Care Unit) and vitals are being monitored continuously. This is not a subsequent hospital service reported with 99231. Also incorrect in this selection is the diagnosis code of 764.09, Light for date, because there is no indication of the birthweight. V45.89 reports a surgical status for the hernia repair, when this admission was for the surgery and none of the conditions were documented to be a result of surgery. Code 550.10 to report the inguinal hernia is correct.

C. This is the correct choice because the infant weighed 4696 grams and is 2 months and 1 week of age. This was a subsequent care indicated by the title of the report "Progress Note" and the content of the note indicating previous studies and care; therefore, the service is reported with 99480. The service 99480 is appropriate as the infant does not require pediatric critical care per day service; however, he does require intensive observation and monitoring of perfusion.

   The patient was admitted for repair of a unilateral incarcerated inguinal hernia (550.10) and developed acute postsurgical status (486) pneumonia and bradycardia (427.89).

D. Incorrect because V45.89 reports a for the hernia repair, when this admission was for the surgery and none of the conditions were documented to be a result of surgery. The remaining codes are correct.

ICD-10-CM

Rationale:

A. Incorrect because there is no indication that the neonatal intensive care physician was the surgeon. Critical care providers do not generally perform surgical procedures, other than those necessary to maintain the patient's viability, such as intubation.

B. Incorrect because the patient is in the NICU (Neonatal Intensive Care Unit) and vitals are being monitored continuously. This is not a subsequent hospital service reported with 99231. Z98.89 reports a surgical status for the hernia repair, when this admission was for the surgery and none of the conditions were documented to be a result of surgery. Code K40.30 to report the inguinal hernia is correct.

C. This is the correct choice because the infant weighed 4696 grams and is 2 months and 1 week of age. This was a subsequent care indicated by the title of the report "Progress Note" and the content of the note indicating previous studies and care; therefore, the service is reported with 99480. The service 99480 is appropriate as the infant does not require pediatric critical care per day service; however, he does require intensive observation and monitoring of perfusion. The patient was admitted for repair of a unilateral incarcerated inguinal hernia (K40.30) and developed acute pneumonia (J18.9) and bradycardia (R00.1).

D. Incorrect because Z98.89 reports a postsurgical status for the hernia repair, when this admission was for the surgery and none of the conditions were documented to be a result of surgery. The remaining codes are correct.

Practice 16B, Report B

Professional Services: 99479 (Evaluation and Management, Low Birthweight Infant)

ICD-9-CM: 765.10 (Premature, birth NEC); 765.24 (Newborn, gestation, 27–28 completed weeks)

ICD-10-CM: P07.10 (Low, birthweight, [2499 grams or less]); P07.26 (Immaturity, gestational age, 27 weeks completed)

Rationale: Codes 99478, 99479, and 99480 report physician services on days other than the day of admit, for infants of very low birthweight (VLBW) (infants weighing less than 1500 grams), low birthweight (LBW) (1500-2500 grams), or normal weight (2501-5000 grams) who do not meet the definition of critically ill but still require intensive services. These infants are recovering. Code selection depends on the weight of the infant. The infant in this documentation is 2100 grams with stable respiratory status. The correct code to assign is 99479.

ICD-9-CM: The patient is a premature underweight infant (765.10 with a 5th digit of "0" to represent the birthweight of the infant) delivered at **27 weeks gestation (765.24).** The birthweight of the infant is not given; therefore, the 5th digit "0" for unspecified is reported. The current weight is 2100 grams; however, that is 55 days after birth. Coding guidelines for code range 765.xx also indicate to "use additional code for weeks of gestation (765.20-765.29).

ICD-10-CM: The patient is a premature underweight infant (P07.10 with a fifth digit of "0" to represent the birthweight of the infant) delivered at **27 weeks gestation (P07.26).** The birthweight of the infant is not given; therefore, the 5th character "0" for unspecified is reported. The current weight is 2100 grams; however, that is 55 days after birth.

Examination Answers

Examination, Report 1

Professional Services: 99304 (Evaluation and Management, Nursing Facility, Initial Care)

ICD-9-CM: 331.0 (Alzheimer's, disease or sclerosis), 294.11 (Dementia, due to or associated with condition(s) classified elsewhere, with behavioral disturbance), 332.0 (Parkinsonism [primary]), 250.70 (Disease, vascular, peripheral [occlusive], in [with], diabetes mellitus), 443.81 (Angiopathy), (Diabetes/diabetic, type II or unspecified type not stated as uncontrolled), 414.01 (Arteriosclerosis/ arteriosclerotic, native coronary artery), 412 (History of, myocardial infarction), 788.30 (Urine/urinary, incontinence), 706.3 (Seborrhea/seborrheic), 702.0 (Keratosis, actinic), V45.82 (Status, angioplasty, percutaneous transluminal coronary), V58.67 (Long-term [current] drug use, insulin)

ICD-10-CM: G30.9 (Alzheimer's, see Disease, Alzheimer's), G20 (Parkinsonism (idiopathic) (primary), E11.51 (Diabetes, type 2, with, peripheral angiopathy), I25.10 (Disease, arteriosclerotic, heart, coronary), I25.2 (History, personal, myocardial infarction (old), R32 (Incontinence, urinary), L21.9 (Seborrhea), L57.0 (Keratosis, actinic), Z98.61 (Status, angioplasty, coronary artery), Z79.4 (Long-term [current] use of, insulin).

Rationale: The first line of the note states that this is a nursing facility admission. This is reported as an initial service in the nursing facility and would be reported in the range of (99304-99306).

The history contained 4 elements of HPI: location (brain), severity (worsened), duration (Parkinson's 10 years), and associated signs and symptoms (inappropriate behavior) for a level 4 or comprehensive HPI. A detailed ROS that consists of cardiovascular (intermittent edema), respiratory (no paroxysmal nocturnal dyspnea), gastrointestinal (no nausea, vomiting, melena), genitourinary (incontinent), musculoskeletal (frequent falls, no fractures), endocrine (diabetes type II), psychiatric (sundowning), and neurological (impaired balance). Although the patient has Alzheimer's, the physician does not state the condition prevented him from obtaining a complete ROS. The PFSH includes past (MI 6 years ago, medications), family (mother and father died in 70's, other not known), and social (lived at home with wife until now, cigarette and alcohol abuse in past). All 3 elements of PFSH are stated for a level 4 or comprehensive PFSH. A comprehensive HPI, detailed ROS and comprehensive PFSH make this a detailed history.

The examination consisted of only one constitutional element (general appearance) considered 1 OS. A total of 5 BAs were examined: head (normocephalic with male pattern baldness, face symmetrical), neck (supple), abdomen (round) and lower extremities (pitting edema). The 10 OSs examined are ophthalmologic (no papilledema), otolaryngologic (mucous membranes moist, many absent teeth), cardiovascular (no bruits noted, RRR, faint ejection murmur), respiratory (dry crackles in right lower lobe), gastrointestinal (liver, spleen, kidneys not palpable), genitourinary (uncircumcised), integumentary (some actinic keratoses), neurologic (deep tendon reflexes hypoactive), psychiatric (not capable of making decisions), and lymphatic (lymphadenopathy not evident in neck/supraclavicular region) for a total of 16 BAs/OSs. BAs are not counted for the comprehensive exam. Recounting without the BAs, there was 1 constitutional element (which counts as an OS) and 10 OSs for a total of 11 OSs, which is a level 4 or comprehensive examination.

The MDM consisted of level 4 or an extensive number of diagnosis/ management options (Alzheimer's, Parkinson's, diabetes, ASHD, incontinence, PVD), level 3 or moderate data to review (labs, PT evaluation, Glucoscan monitors), and level 4 or high risk (no code status, poor prognosis), making this high MDM.

A detailed history, comprehensive examination and high MDM qualify as 99304. If the ROS had contained 2 more elements, this documentation would have qualified for a higher level.

ICD-9-CM: The patient has Alzheimer's (331.0). The ICD-9-CM Index shows Alzheimer's with behavioral disturbance as 331.0 [294.11], which indicates that 294.11 must follow 331.0. The patient also has primary Parkinson's (332.0). The other listed diagnoses are reported because they may impact the management of this patient while he is in the nursing home. These include: diabetes type II (250.70, 453.81). The patient is diabetic with vascular disease; therefore, 250.70 and 453.81 are reported instead of 250.00, 443.9. Peripheral vascular disease is not necessary as it is already reported with 250.70 and 453.81, arteriosclerotic heart disease, native artery (414.01), history of an MI (412), urinary incontinence (788.30), seborrhea (706.3), actinic keratosis (702.0). Status, angioplasty, percutaneous transluminal coronary (V45.82), Long-term [current] drug use, insulin (V58.67).

ICD-10-CM: The patient has Alzheimer's (G30.9). The ICD-10-CM Index shows Alzheimer's (see Disease, Alzheimer's), with behavioral disturbance G30.9 [F02.81] which indicates that F02.81 must follow G30.9. The patient also has primary Parkinson's (G20). The other listed diagnoses are reported because they may impact the management of this patient while he is in the nursing home. These include: diabetes type II, with diabetic peripheral angiography, without gangrene (E11.51), arteriosclerotic heart disease, native artery, without angina pectoris (I25.10), history of an old MI (I25.2), incontinence urinary (R32), seborrhea (L21.9), keratosis, actinic (L57.0). Status, angioplasty, coronary artery (Z98.61), Long-term [current] use of, insulin (Z79.4).

Examination 1, Report 1

HISTORY ELEMENTS	Documented
HISTORY OF PRESENT ILLNESS (HPI)	
1. Location (site on body)	X
2. Quality (characteristic: throbbing, sharp)	
3. Severity (1/10 or how intense)	X
4. Duration* (how long for problem or episode)	X
5. Timing (when it occurs)	
6. Context (under what circumstances does it occur)	
7. Modifying factors (what makes it better or worse)	
8. Associated signs and symptoms (what else is happening when it occurs)	X
*Duration not in CPT as HPI Element TOTAL	4
LEVEL	4

REVIEW OF SYSTEMS (ROS)	Documented
1. Constitutional (e.g., weight loss, fever)	
2. Ophthalmologic (eyes)	
3. Otolaryngologic (ears, nose, mouth, throat)	
4. Cardiovascular	X
5. Respiratory	X
6. Gastrointestinal	X
7. Genitourinary	X
8. Musculoskeletal	X
9. Integumentary (skin and/or breasts)	
10. Neurological	X
11. Psychiatric	X
12. Endocrine	X
13. Hematologic/Lymphatic	
14. Allergic/Immunologic	
TOTAL	8
LEVEL	3

PAST, FAMILY, AND/OR SOCIAL HISTORY (PFSH)	Documented
1. Past illness, operations, injuries, treatments, and current medications	X
2. Family medical history for heredity and risk	X
3. Social activities, both past and present	X
TOTAL	3
LEVEL	4

History Level		1	2	3	4
		Problem Focused	Expanded Problem Focused	Detailed	Comprehensive
HPI		Brief 1-3	Brief 1-3	Extended 4+	Extended 4+
ROS		None	Problem Pertinent 1	Extended 2-9	Complete 10+
PFSH		None	None	Pertinent 1	Complete 2-3
				HISTORY LEVEL	3

EXAMINATION ELEMENTS	Documented
CONSTITUTIONAL (OS)	
• Blood pressure, sitting	
• Blood pressure, lying	
• Pulse	
• Respirations	
• Temperature	
• Height	
• Weight	
• General appearance	X
(Counts as only 1) NUMBER	1
BODY AREAS (BA)	Documented
1. Head (including face)	X
2. Neck	X
3. Chest (including breasts and axillae)	
4. Abdomen	X
5. Genitalia, groin, buttocks	
6. Back (including spine)	
7. Each extremity	XX
NUMBER	5
ORGAN SYSTEMS (OS)	Documented
1. Ophthalmologic (eyes)	X
2. Otolaryngologic (ears, nose, mouth, throat)	X
3. Cardiovascular	X
4. Respiratory	X
5. Gastrointestinal	X
6. Genitourinary	X
7. Musculoskeletal	
8. Integumentary (skin)	X
9. Neurologic	X
10. Psychiatric	X
11. Hematologic/Lymphatic/Immunologic	X
NUMBER	10
TOTAL BA/OS	16/11

Exam Level	1	2	3	4
	Problem Focused	Expanded Problem Focused	Detailed	Comprehensive
	Limited to affected BA/OS	Limited to affected BA/OS & other related OS(s)	Extended of affected BA(s) & other related OS(s)	General multi-system (OSs only)
# of OS or BA	1	2-7 limited	2-7 extended	8+
			EXAMINATION LEVEL	4

MDM ELEMENTS	Documented
# OF DIAGNOSIS/MANAGEMENT OPTIONS	
1. Minimal	
2. Limited	
3. Multiple	
4. Extensive	X
LEVEL	4
AMOUNT AND/OR COMPLEXITY OF DATA TO REVIEW	Documented
1. Minimal/None	
2. Limited	
3. Moderate	X
4. Extensive	
LEVEL	3
RISK OF COMPLICATION OR DEATH IF NOT TREATED	Documented
1. Minimal	
2. Low	
3. Moderate	
4. High	X
LEVEL	4

MDM*		1	2	3	4
		Straightforward	Low	Moderate	High
Number of DX or management options		Minimal	Limited	Multiple	Extensive
Amount and/or complexity of data		Minimal/None	Limited	Moderate	Extensive
Risks		Minimal	Low	Moderate	High
				MDM LEVEL	4

*To qualify for a given type of MDM complexity, 2 of 3 elements in the table must be met or exceeded.

History: Detailed

Examination: Comprehensive

MDM: High

Number of Key Components: 3 of 3

Code: 99304

Examination, Report 2

Professional Services: 99243 (Evaluation and Management, Consultation, Hospital)

ICD-9-CM: V72.81 (Examination, preoperative, cardiovascular), 794.39 (Findings, abnormal, without diagnosis, stress test), 414.01 (Arteriosclerosis/arteriosclerotic, coronary [artery]), V45.81 (Status [post], coronary artery bypass or shunt), 786.50 (Pain, chest)

ICD-10-CM: Z01.810 (Examination, preprocedure, cardiovascular), R94.39 (Findings, without diagnosis, abnormal, stress test), I25.10 (Arteriosclerosis/arteriosclerotic, coronary [artery]), Z95.1 (Status [post], aortocoronary artery bypass), R07.9 (Pain, chest)

Rationale: The patient has been admitted to observation after an abnormal exercise tolerance test. Pre-op consultation was requested by Dr. Cardiologist for left heart catheterization. There are 4 elements of HPI: location (heart), duration (August), context (exercise), associated signs and symptoms (fatigue) for a level 4, or comprehensive, HPI. The ROS consisted of only 2 systems: cardiovascular (intermittent chest pain) and respiratory (dyspnea), for a level 3 or detailed ROS. The documentation included the past history (CABG) for a level 3 or detailed PFSH. The level 3 history was based on a comprehensive HPI, detailed ROS, and detailed PFSH.

The examination consisted of 5 constitutional elements, blood pressure (lying down), pulse, respirations, temperature, and general appearance. This qualifies as 1 OS. A total of 2 BAs were examined, including head (unremarkable) and abdomen (benign). A total of 5 OSs were examined including ophthalmologic (unremarkable), otolaryngologic (unremarkable), cardiovascular (regular rate), respiratory (clear), and psychiatric (mood congruent, affect appropriate). There was a total of 8 BAs/OSs; however, only OSs count for a comprehensive examination. Recounting without the BAs, there are 6 OSs, making this a level 3 or detailed examination.

Level 4 or extensive diagnosis/management options (ASHD with coronary artery bypass, abnormal stress test), level 3 or moderate data were reviewed (old records for stress tests results, labs), and the patient has high risk (cardiac catheterization, known heart problems), a level 4. This a level 4 or high MDM.

A detailed history, a detailed level examination, and high MDM make this consult 99243.

ICD-9-CM: The primary diagnosis is the preoperative cardiovascular examination (V72.81), followed by the reason for the cardiac catherization, which is the abnormal cardiac function study (794.30) based on imaging that showed an ejection fraction of 45%. The findings of the examination are listed last, which is the coronary arteriosclerosis (414.01), with the fifth digit of "1" to indicate native coronary artery. The *Coding Clinic* states that if unspecified, the default is the native coronary artery. Report also the status post bypass (V45.81). *The Official Guidelines for Coding and Reporting*, Section IV.N., for preoperative evaluation state to sequence first a code from category V72.8, assign the condition to describe the reason for the surgery, then list findings.

ICD-10-CM: The primary diagnosis is the preoperative cardiovascular examination (Z01.810), followed by the reason for the cardiac catheterization, which is the abnormal cardiac function study (R94.39) based on imaging that showed an ejection fraction of 45%. The findings of the examination are listed last, which is the coronary arteriosclerosis, without angina pectoris (I25.10). Report also the status post bypass (Z95.1). Code also the chest pain (R07.9).

HISTORY ELEMENTS	Documented
HISTORY OF PRESENT ILLNESS (HPI)	
1. Location (site on body)	X
2. Quality (characteristic: throbbing, sharp)	
3. Severity (1/10 or how intense)	
4. Duration* (how long for problem or episode)	X
5. Timing (when it occurs)	
6. Context (under what circumstances does it occur)	X
7. Modifying factors (what makes it better or worse)	
8. Associated signs and symptoms (what else is happening when it occurs)	X
*Duration not in CPT as HPI Element TOTAL	4
LEVEL	4

REVIEW OF SYSTEMS (ROS)	Documented
1. Constitutional (e.g., weight loss, fever)	
2. Ophthalmologic (eyes)	
3. Otolaryngologic (ears, nose, mouth, throat)	
4. Cardiovascular	X
5. Respiratory	X
6. Gastrointestinal	
7. Genitourinary	
8. Musculoskeletal	
9. Integumentary (skin and/or breasts)	
10. Neurological	
11. Psychiatric	
12. Endocrine	
13. Hematologic/Lymphatic	
14. Allergic/Immunologic	
TOTAL	2
LEVEL	3

PAST, FAMILY, AND/OR SOCIAL HISTORY (PFSH)	Documented
1. Past illness, operations, injuries, treatments, and current medications	X
2. Family medical history for heredity and risk	
3. Social activities, both past and present	
TOTAL	1
LEVEL	3

History Level		1	2	3	4
		Problem Focused	Expanded Problem Focused	Detailed	Comprehensive
HPI		Brief 1-3	Brief 1-3	Extended 4+	Extended 4+
ROS		None	Problem Pertinent 1	Extended 2-9	Complete 10+
PFSH		None	None	Pertinent 1	Complete 2-3
				HISTORY LEVEL	3

EXAMINATION ELEMENTS	Documented
CONSTITUTIONAL (OS)	
• Blood pressure, sitting	
• Blood pressure, lying	X
• Pulse	X
• Respirations	X
• Temperature	X
• Height	
• Weight	
• General appearance	X
(Counts as only 1) NUMBER	1

BODY AREAS (BA)	Documented
1. Head (including face)	X
2. Neck	
3. Chest (including breasts and axillae)	
4. Abdomen	X
5. Genitalia, groin, buttocks	
6. Back (including spine)	
7. Each extremity	
NUMBER	2

ORGAN SYSTEMS (OS)	Documented
1. Ophthalmologic (eyes)	X
2. Otolaryngologic (ears, nose, mouth, throat)	X
3. Cardiovascular	X
4. Respiratory	X
5. Gastrointestinal	
6. Genitourinary	
7. Musculoskeletal	
8. Integumentary (skin)	
9. Neurologic	
10. Psychiatric	X
11. Hematologic/Lymphatic/Immunologic	
NUMBER	5
TOTAL BA/OS	8/6

Exam Level	1	2	3	4
	Problem Focused	Expanded Problem Focused	Detailed	Comprehensive
	Limited to affected BA/OS	Limited to affected BA/OS & other related OS(s)	Extended of affected BA(s) & other related OS(s)	General multi-system (OSs only)
# of OS or BA	1	2-7 limited	2-7 extended	8+
			EXAMINATION LEVEL	3

MDM ELEMENTS	Documented
# OF DIAGNOSIS/MANAGEMENT OPTIONS	
1. Minimal	
2. Limited	
3. Multiple	
4. Extensive	X
LEVEL	4

AMOUNT AND/OR COMPLEXITY OF DATA TO REVIEW	Documented
1. Minimal/None	
2. Limited	
3. Moderate	X
4. Extensive	
LEVEL	3

RISK OF COMPLICATION OR DEATH IF NOT TREATED	Documented
1. Minimal	
2. Low	
3. Moderate	
4. High	X
LEVEL	4

MDM*	1	2	3	4
	Straightforward	Low	Moderate	High
Number of DX or management options	Minimal	Limited	Multiple	Extensive
Amount and/or complexity of data	Minimal/None	Limited	Moderate	Extensive
Risks	Minimal	Low	Moderate	High
			MDM LEVEL	4

*To qualify for a given type of MDM complexity, 2 of 3 elements in the table must be met or exceeded.

History: Detailed
Examination: Detailed
MDM: High
Number of Key Components: 3 of 3
Code: 99243

Examination, Report 3

Professional Services: 99203 (Evaluation and Management, New patient encounter)

ICD-9-CM: 836.1 (Tear/torn, meniscus, lateral), 836.0 (Tear/torn, meniscus, medial, posterior horn), 715.16 (Osteoarthrosis, primary, lower leg), 401.9 (Hypertension/hypertensive, unspecified), 736.42 (Genu, varum [acquired]), 414.01 (Arteriosclerosis/arteriosclerotic, coronary artery), 272.0 (Hypercholesterolemia), V58.61 (Long-term [current] drug use, anticoagulants)

ICD-10-CM: S83.281A (Tear/torn, meniscus, lateral, specified type) right knee, S83.241A (Tear/torn, meniscus, medial, specified type) right knee, M17.11 (Osteoarthrosis, see also Osteoarthritis, primary, knee), I10 (Hypertension/ hypertensive, unspecified), M21.161 (Genu, yarum [acquired]) right knee, I25.10 (Arteriosclerosis/arteriosclerotic, coronary artery, without angina pectoris), E78.0 (Hypercholesterolemia, pure), Z79.01 (Long-term [current] drug therapy (use of), anticoagulants)

Rationale: The physician has been asked to evaluate the patient and render an opinion regarding the knee pain. There are 4 elements of HPI: location (right knee), duration (a few months), context (getting out of the truck when he felt a pop), and associated signs and symptoms (buckling) for a level 4 or comprehensive HPI. Five systems were reviewed: otolaryngologic (no tinnitus or vertigo), cardiovascular (positive for coronary disease, occasional chest pain), GI (GERD, no change in bowel habits), GU (no frequency, dysuria, hematuria), and neurological (no seizure disorder) and the physician documented the remainder of the ROS was negative for a level 4, comprehensive ROS. The PFSH includes the past history (hypertension, medications, surgeries) for a level 3 or detailed PFSH. All 3 elements of history must qualify for level selection. The HPI is comprehensive, the ROS is comprehensive, and the PFSH qualifies as detailed; therefore, this is a detailed or level 3 history.

The examination consisted of 7 constitutional elements for 1 OS. The only BAs examined were the 2 lower extremities. The BA of extremities is not counted as it is included in the musculoskeletal system. A total of 2 OSs: musculoskeletal (genu varus deformity of the right knee with atrophy of his right quadriceps) and neurologic (negative McMurray's) were examined. This is a total of 3 OSs. This qualifies as a level 3 or detailed examination.

Level 4 or extensive diagnosis/management options (valgus deformity, torn meniscus, CAD, requesting medical clearance, Coumadin), level 2 or limited data were reviewed (x-rays, CT), and the patient has high risk (level 4) (surgery, on anticoagulants). This a level 4 or high MDM.

The detailed history, detailed examination and high MDM make the visit 99203. This is a new patient initial encounter.

Modifier -57 is not appended to 99203 (Medicare does not accept consultation codes (99241-99245), because the documentation indicates the patient first needs medical clearance and to discontinue taking his Coumadin 1 to 2 days prior to the procedure. Modifier -57 is only assigned when the E/M was performed the day of or the day before the major procedure.

ICD-9-CM: During the course of the consultation the patient was diagnosed with lateral (836.1) and medial (836.0) meniscus tear. We know the tears are acute not degenerative because the report states they occurred 2 weeks ago. The documentation indicates the patient has degenerative joint disease and when referencing the index of the ICD-9-CM under the main term "Degeneration, joint disease," you are directed to "see Osteoarthrosis." Osteoarthrosis of the knee, primary, which is considered part of the lower leg, is reported with 715.16 (see the Tabular at the beginning of Chapter 13, Diseases of the Muscoloskeletal

System and Connective Tissues, which indicates the 5th digit "6" includes the knee). The report does state primary osteoarthritis; therefore, 715.16 is reported. 401.9 reports the essential hypertension. Also noted on review of the x-rays was genu varus deformity (bow legged) of the right knee (736.42). The coronary artery disease (414.0) and hypercholesterolemia (272.0) are also reported as they affect the management of this case. According to the *Coding Clinic*, when the type of coronary vessel atherosclerosis is not documented, default to native vessel (414.01). Assign long-term use of anticoagulants (V58.61) as this is addressed in the report.

ICD-10-CM: During the course of the visit the patient was diagnosed with lateral (S83.281A) and medical (S83.214A) meniscus tear, initial encounter. We know the tears are acute not degenerative because the report states they occurred 2 weeks ago. The documentation indicates the patient has degenerative joint disease and when referencing the Index of the ICD-10-CM under the main term "Osteoarthrosis" (Osteoarthritis, primary) of the right knee, is reported with M17.11. I10 reports the essential hypertension. Also noted on review of the x-rays was genu varus deformity (bow legged) of the right knee (M21.161). The coronary artery disease, without angina (I25.10) and pure hypercholesterolemia (E78.0) are also reported as they affect the management of this case. Assign long-term use of anticoagulants (Z79.01) as this was addressed in the report.

HISTORY ELEMENTS	Documented
HISTORY OF PRESENT ILLNESS (HPI)	
1. Location (site on body)	X
2. Quality (characteristic: throbbing, sharp)	
3. Severity (1/10 or how intense)	
4. Duration* (how long for problem or episode)	X
5. Timing (when it occurs)	
6. Context (under what circumstances does it occur)	X
7. Modifying factors (what makes it better or worse)	
8. Associated signs and symptoms (what else is happening when it occurs)	X
*Duration not in CPT as HPI Element TOTAL	4
LEVEL	4

REVIEW OF SYSTEMS (ROS)	Documented
1. Constitutional (e.g., weight loss, fever)	X
2. Ophthalmologic (eyes)	X
3. Otolaryngologic (ears, nose, mouth, throat)	X
4. Cardiovascular	X
5. Respiratory	X
6. Gastrointestinal	X
7. Genitourinary	X
8. Musculoskeletal	X
9. Integumentary (skin and/or breasts)	X
10. Neurological	X
11. Psychiatric	X
12. Endocrine	X
13. Hematologic/Lymphatic	X
14. Allergic/Immunologic	X
TOTAL	14
LEVEL	4

PAST, FAMILY, AND/OR SOCIAL HISTORY (PFSH)	Documented
1. Past illness, operations, injuries, treatments, and current medications	X
2. Family medical history for heredity and risk	
3. Social activities, both past and present	
TOTAL	1
LEVEL	3

History Level	1	2	3	4
	Problem Focused	Expanded Problem Focused	Detailed	Comprehensive
HPI	Brief 1-3	Brief 1-3	Extended 4+	Extended 4+
ROS	None	Problem Pertinent 1	Extended 2-9	Complete 10+
PFSH	None	None	Pertinent 1	Complete 2-3
			HISTORY LEVEL	3

EXAMINATION ELEMENTS	Documented
CONSTITUTIONAL (OS)	
• Blood pressure, sitting	
• Blood pressure, lying	X
• Pulse	X
• Respirations	X
• Temperature	X
• Height	X
• Weight	X
• General appearance	X
(Counts as only 1) NUMBER	1

BODY AREAS (BA)	Documented
1. Head (including face)	
2. Neck	
3. Chest (including breasts and axillae)	
4. Abdomen	
5. Genitalia, groin, buttocks	
6. Back (including spine)	
7. Each extremity	
NUMBER	0

ORGAN SYSTEMS (OS)	Documented
1. Ophthalmologic (eyes)	
2. Otolaryngologic (ears, nose, mouth, throat)	
3. Cardiovascular	
4. Respiratory	
5. Gastrointestinal	
6. Genitourinary	
7. Musculoskeletal	X
8. Integumentary (skin)	
9. Neurologic	X
10. Psychiatric	
11. Hematologic/Lymphatic/Immunologic	
NUMBER	2
TOTAL BA/OS	3

Exam Level	1	2	3	4
	Problem Focused	Expanded Problem Focused	Detailed	Comprehensive
	Limited to affected BA/OS	Limited to affected BA/OS & other related OS(s)	Extended of affected BA(s) & other related OS(s)	General multi-system (OSs only)
# of OS or BA	1	2-7 limited	2-7 extended	8+
			EXAMINATION LEVEL	3

MDM ELEMENTS	Documented
# OF DIAGNOSIS/MANAGEMENT OPTIONS	
1. Minimal	
2. Limited	
3. Multiple	
4. Extensive	X
LEVEL	4
AMOUNT AND/OR COMPLEXITY OF DATA TO REVIEW	Documented
1. Minimal/None	
2. Limited	X
3. Moderate	
4. Extensive	
LEVEL	2
RISK OF COMPLICATION OR DEATH IF NOT TREATED	Documented
1. Minimal	
2. Low	
3. Moderate	
4. High	X
LEVEL	4

MDM*	1	2	3	4
	Straightforward	Low	Moderate	High
Number of DX or management options	Minimal	Limited	Multiple	Extensive
Amount and/or complexity of data	Minimal/None	Limited	Moderate	Extensive
Risks	Minimal	Low	Moderate	High
			MDM LEVEL	4

*To qualify for a given type of MDM complexity, 2 of 3 elements in the table must be met or exceeded.

History: Detailed
Examination: Detailed
MDM: High
Number of Key Components: 3 of 3
Code: 99203

Examination, Report 4

Professional Services: 99282 (Evaluation and Management, Emergency Department)
ICD-9-CM: 462 (Pharyngitis)
ICD-10-CM: J02.9 (Pharyngitis)

Rationale: The HPI includes: location (throat), quality (sore), duration (5-7 days), and associated signs and symptoms (generalized aches) for a level 4 or comprehensive HPI. The ROS includes: constitutional (no fever, fatigue, no weight loss), otolaryngologic (some fullness in ears), respiratory (no SOB), and integumentary (no rash) for a level 3 or detailed ROS. The PFSH includes past (bipolar disorder) and social (does not smoke, occasional alcohol) history for a level 4 or comprehensive PFSH. The comprehensive HPI, detailed ROS and comprehensive PFSH make this a level 3, detailed history.

The examination includes BP, respirations, and afebrile for 1 OS. Other OSs include: otolaryngologic (clear tympanic membranes, oropharynx slight erythema), lymphatic (cervical lymphadenopathy), cardiovascular (heart regular), and respiratory (clear to auscultation) for a total of 5 OSs, making this a level 3 or detailed examination.

The diagnoses/treatment options meet level 3 or moderate (new patient, pharyngitis); the data reviewed are level 2 or limited. The risk is low (acute uncomplicated illness, over-the-counter medication) making this a level 2 or low MDM.

The detailed history, detailed level examination and low MDM make this Emergency Department visit 99282.

ICD-9-CM: The patient was diagnosed with pharyngitis (462). The patient also has bipolar disorder; however, it is not reported as it is not being treated and does not affect the outcome of the patient's diagnosis.

ICD-10-CM: The patient was diagnosed with pharyngitis (J02.9). The patient also has bipolar disorder; however, it is not reported as it is not being treated and does not affect the outcome.

HISTORY ELEMENTS	Documented
HISTORY OF PRESENT ILLNESS (HPI)	
1. Location (site on body)	X
2. Quality (characteristic: throbbing, sharp)	X
3. Severity (1/10 or how intense)	
4. Duration* (how long for problem or episode)	X
5. Timing (when it occurs)	
6. Context (under what circumstances does it occur)	
7. Modifying factors (what makes it better or worse)	
8. Associated signs and symptoms (what else is happening when it occurs)	X
*Duration not in CPT as HPI Element TOTAL	4
LEVEL	4

REVIEW OF SYSTEMS (ROS)	Documented
1. Constitutional (e.g., weight loss, fever)	X
2. Ophthalmologic (eyes)	
3. Otolaryngologic (ears, nose, mouth, throat)	X
4. Cardiovascular	
5. Respiratory	X
6. Gastrointestinal	
7. Genitourinary	
8. Musculoskeletal	
9. Integumentary (skin and/or breasts)	X
10. Neurological	
11. Psychiatric	
12. Endocrine	
13. Hematologic/Lymphatic	
14. Allergic/Immunologic	
TOTAL	4
LEVEL	3

PAST, FAMILY, AND/OR SOCIAL HISTORY (PFSH)	Documented
1. Past illness, operations, injuries, treatments, and current medications	X
2. Family medical history for heredity and risk	
3. Social activities, both past and present	X
TOTAL	2
LEVEL	4

History Level	1	2	3	4
	Problem Focused	Expanded Problem Focused	Detailed	Comprehensive
HPI	Brief 1-3	Brief 1-3	Extended 4+	Extended 4+
ROS	None	Problem Pertinent 1	Extended 2-9	Complete 10+
PFSH	None	None	Pertinent 1	Complete 2-3
			HISTORY LEVEL	3

EXAMINATION ELEMENTS	Documented
CONSTITUTIONAL (OS)	
• Blood pressure, sitting	
• Blood pressure, lying	X
• Pulse	
• Respirations	X
• Temperature	X
• Height	
• Weight	
• General appearance	
(Counts as only 1) NUMBER	1

BODY AREAS (BA)	Documented
1. Head (including face)	
2. Neck	
3. Chest (including breasts and axillae)	
4. Abdomen	
5. Genitalia, groin, buttocks	
6. Back (including spine)	
7. Each extremity	
NUMBER	0

ORGAN SYSTEMS (OS)	Documented
1. Ophthalmologic (eyes)	
2. Otolaryngologic (ears, nose, mouth, throat)	X
3. Cardiovascular	X
4. Respiratory	X
5. Gastrointestinal	
6. Genitourinary	
7. Musculoskeletal	
8. Integumentary (skin)	
9. Neurologic	
10. Psychiatric	
11. Hematologic/Lymphatic/Immunologic	X
NUMBER	4
TOTAL BA/OS	5

Exam Level	1	2	3	4
	Problem Focused	Expanded Problem Focused	Detailed	Comprehensive
	Limited to affected BA/OS	Limited to affected BA/OS & other related OS(s)	Extended of affected BA(s) & other related OS(s)	General multi-system (OSs only)
# of OS or BA	1	2-7 limited	2-7 extended	8+
			EXAMINATION LEVEL	3

MDM ELEMENTS	Documented
# OF DIAGNOSIS/MANAGEMENT OPTIONS	
1. Minimal	
2. Limited	
3. Multiple	X
4. Extensive	
LEVEL	3
AMOUNT AND/OR COMPLEXITY OF DATA TO REVIEW	Documented
1. Minimal/None	
2. Limited	X
3. Moderate	
4. Extensive	
LEVEL	2
RISK OF COMPLICATION OR DEATH IF NOT TREATED	Documented
1. Minimal	
2. Low	X
3. Moderate	
4. High	
LEVEL	2

MDM*		1	2	3	4
		Straightforward	Low	Moderate	High
Number of DX or management options		Minimal	Limited	Multiple	Extensive
Amount and/or complexity of data		Minimal/None	Limited	Moderate	Extensive
Risks		Minimal	Low	Moderate	High
				MDM LEVEL	2

*To qualify for a given type of MDM complexity, 2 of 3 elements in the table must be met or exceeded.

History: Detailed

Examination: Detailed

MDM: Low

Number of Key Components: 3 of 3

Code: 99282

Examination, Report 5

Professional Services: 99291 (Evaluation and Management, Critical Care), 99292 (Evaluation and Management, Critical Care)

ICD-9-CM: 486 (Pneumonia), 584.9 (Failure/failed, renal, acute), 410.91 (Infarct/infarction, myocardium/myocardial, initial episode), 799.02 (Hypoxemia), 790.99 (Findings, abnormal, without diagnosis, BNP NEC), 780.97 (Change(s) [of], mental [status] NEC)

ICD-10-CM: J18.9 (Pneumonia), N17.9 (Failure/failed, renal, acute), I21.3 (Infarct/infarction, myocardium/myocardial,), R09.02 (Hypoxemia), R79.89 (Findings, abnormal, without diagnosis, BNP), R41.82 (Change(s) [of], mental [status] NEC)

Rationale: This is a critical care service, which is based on the time spent with the patient, not the usual key components. At the end of the documentation it states that the physician spent 90 minutes of critical care time with this patient. When billing for critical care, the table in the E/M section of your CPT is helpful. The Critical Care Table indicates that for 75-104 minutes report 99291 and 99292.

ICD-9-CM: The patient presents with acute mental status changes (780.97). On further testing the following was found: acute renal failure (584.9), acute MI, (410.91), pneumonia (486), and hypoxemia (799.0). The patient was also found to have elevated BNP (790.99). B-type Natriuretic Peptide is a lab (83880) that is performed on plasma of the blood that aids in diagnosing the degree of CHF. The elevated troponins (796.9) are not necessary to report as myocardial infarction is the definitive diagnosis. The patient presented with acute mental status changes, which could be due to a number of definitive diagnoses such as acute renal failure, pneumonia, hypoxemia, and the acute MI. The physician listed "acute febrile illness/acute mental status changes"; therefore, a symptom and not necessarily reported.

ICD-10-CM: The patient presents with acute mental status changes (R41.82). On further testing the following was found: acute renal failure (N17.9), acute MI (I21.3), pneumonia (J18.9), and hypoxemia, (R09.02). The patient was also found to have elevated BNP (R79.89). B-type Natriuretic Peptide is a lab (83880) that is performed on plasma that aids in diagnosing the degree of CHF. The elevated troponins are not necessary to report as myocardial infarction is the definitive diagnosis. The patient presented with acute mental status changes, which could be due to a number of definitive diagnoses such as acute renal failure, pneumonia, hypoxemia, and the acute MI. The physician listed "acute febrile illness/acute mental status changes"; therefore, a symptom and not necessarily reported.

Examination, Report 6

Professional Services: 99349 (Evaluation and Management, Home Services)

ICD-9-CM: 496 (Disease/diseased, pulmonary, obstructive diffuse [chronic]), 332.0 (Parkinsonism), 715.16 (Osteoarthrosis, localized, primary), 300.00 (Anxiety)

ICD-10-CM: J44.9 (Disease/diseased, pulmonary, chronic obstructive), G20 (Parkinsonism (idiopathic) (primary)), M17.0 (Osteoarthrosis, see also Osteoarthritis, knee, bilateral), F41.9 (Anxiety)

Rationale: This is a home service, which is based on whether the patient is new or established and the key components.

The HPI consisted of 4 elements, location (lung), context (has gotten over episode of pneumonia), modifying factors (nebulizer), and associated signs and symptoms (coughing spells). This qualifies as a level 4 or comprehensive HPI. The ROS includes: constitutional (good appetite), cardiovascular (edema), and psychiatric (anxiety) for a level 3 or detailed, ROS. The PFSH contained the past (Parkinson's) and social (lives at home with wife) history of the patient for a level 4 or comprehensive PFSH. This documentation contains a comprehensive HPI, a detailed ROS, and a comprehensive PFSH for a level 3 or detailed interval history.

The examination contains 4 constitutional elements (blood pressure (lying), pulse, respirations, and general appearance) that qualify as 1 OS. The BAs examined are all 4 extremities (demonstrate no edema) for a total of 4 BAs. Only 4 OSs were examined: cardiovascular (demonstrates regular rate and rhythm), respiratory (no wheezes rales or rhonchi), gastrointestinal (abdomen soft, benign, no masses or tenderness), and psychiatric (somewhat lethargic today). The total of 9 BAs/OSs is a level 4 or comprehensive examination; however, only OSs count for a comprehensive examination. Recounting without the BAs, there are 5 OSs, which makes this a level 3 or detailed examination.

The MDM contains level 3 or multiple diagnosis and management options (COPD, Parkinson's, osteoarthritis), level 1 or minimal data (no data reviewed), and moderate risk (2 or more stable chronic illnesses). This qualifies as a level 3 or moderate MDM.

The detailed interval history, detailed level examination and moderate MDM make this home visit 99349.

ICD-9-CM: The diagnoses for this home service are COPD (496), Parkinson's disease (332.0) and severe primary osteoarthritis of the knees (715.16). Although the Parkinson's and osteoarthritis were not directly addressed, the physician states that he will continue his current therapy. Also, the patient is only up in a chair twice a week, and he is checked for pressure ulcers. Also noted is the patient's anxiety (300.00), which is treated with Xanax with good relief.

ICD-10-CM: The diagnoses for this home service are COPD (J44.9), Parkinson's disease (G20) and severe primary osteoarthritis of the knees (M17.0). Although the Parkinson's and osteoarthritis were not directly addressed, the physician states that he will continue his current therapy. Also, the patient is only up in a chair twice a week, and he is checked for pressure ulcers. Also noted is the patient's anxiety (F41.9), which is treated with Xanax with good relief.

HISTORY ELEMENTS	Documented
HISTORY OF PRESENT ILLNESS (HPI)	
1. Location (site on body)	X
2. Quality (characteristic: throbbing, sharp)	
3. Severity (1/10 or how intense)	
4. Duration* (how long for problem or episode)	
5. Timing (when it occurs)	
6. Context (under what circumstances does it occur)	X
7. Modifying factors (what makes it better or worse)	X
8. Associated signs and symptoms (what else is happening when it occurs)	X
*Duration not in CPT as HPI Element TOTAL	4
LEVEL	4

REVIEW OF SYSTEMS (ROS)	Documented
1. Constitutional (e.g., weight loss, fever)	X
2. Ophthalmologic (eyes)	
3. Otolaryngologic (ears, nose, mouth, throat)	
4. Cardiovascular	X
5. Respiratory	
6. Gastrointestinal	
7. Genitourinary	
8. Musculoskeletal	
9. Integumentary (skin and/or breasts)	
10. Neurological	
11. Psychiatric	X
12. Endocrine	
13. Hematologic/Lymphatic	
14. Allergic/Immunologic	
TOTAL	3
LEVEL	3

PAST, FAMILY, AND/OR SOCIAL HISTORY (PFSH)	Documented
1. Past illness, operations, injuries, treatments, and current medications	X
2. Family medical history for heredity and risk	
3. Social activities, both past and present	X
TOTAL	2
LEVEL	4

History Level		1 Problem Focused	2 Expanded Problem Focused	3 Detailed	4 Comprehensive
HPI		Brief 1-3	Brief 1-3	Extended 4+	Extended 4+
ROS		None	Problem Pertinent 1	Extended 2-9	Complete 10+
PFSH		None	None	Pertinent 1	Complete 2-3
HISTORY LEVEL					3

EXAMINATION ELEMENTS	Documented
CONSTITUTIONAL (OS)	
• Blood pressure, sitting	
• Blood pressure, lying	X
• Pulse	X
• Respirations	X
• Temperature	
• Height	
• Weight	
• General appearance	X
(Counts as only 1) NUMBER	1

BODY AREAS (BA)	Documented
1. Head (including face)	
2. Neck	
3. Chest (including breasts and axillae)	
4. Abdomen	
5. Genitalia, groin, buttocks	
6. Back (including spine)	
7. Each extremity	XXXX
NUMBER	4

ORGAN SYSTEMS (OS)	Documented
1. Ophthalmologic (eyes)	
2. Otolaryngologic (ears, nose, mouth, throat)	
3. Cardiovascular	X
4. Respiratory	X
5. Gastrointestinal	X
6. Genitourinary	
7. Musculoskeletal	
8. Integumentary (skin)	
9. Neurologic	
10. Psychiatric	X
11. Hematologic/Lymphatic/Immunologic	
NUMBER	4
TOTAL BA/OS	9/5

Exam Level	1 Problem Focused	2 Expanded Problem Focused	3 Detailed	4 Comprehensive
	Limited to affected BA/OS	Limited to affected BA/OS & other related OS(s)	Extended of affected BA(s) & other related OS(s)	General multi-system (OSs only)
# of OS or BA	1	2-7 limited	2-7 extended	8+
EXAMINATION LEVEL				3

MDM ELEMENTS	Documented
# OF DIAGNOSIS/MANAGEMENT OPTIONS	
1. Minimal	
2. Limited	
3. Multiple	X
4. Extensive	
LEVEL	3
AMOUNT AND/OR COMPLEXITY OF DATA TO REVIEW	Documented
1. Minimal/None	X
2. Limited	
3. Moderate	
4. Extensive	
LEVEL	1
RISK OF COMPLICATION OR DEATH IF NOT TREATED	Documented
1. Minimal	
2. Low	
3. Moderate	X
4. High	
LEVEL	3

MDM*		1 Straightforward	2 Low	3 Moderate	4 High
Number of DX or management options		Minimal	Limited	Multiple	Extensive
Amount and/or complexity of data		Minimal/None	Limited	Moderate	Extensive
Risks		Minimal	Low	Moderate	High
MDM LEVEL					3

*To qualify for a given type of MDM complexity, 2 of 3 elements in the table must be met or exceeded.

History: Detailed interval
Examination: Detailed
MDM: Moderate
Number of Key Components: 2 of 3
Code: 99349

Examination, Report 7

Professional Services: 99233 (Evaluation and Management, Hospital), 99356 (Evaluation and Management, Prolonged Services)

ICD-9-CM: 423.9 (Effusion, pericardium pericardial), 584.9 (Failure, renal, acute), 276.1 (Hyponatremia), 275.41 (Hypocalcemia), 288.60 (Leukocytosis), 599.0 (Infection/infected/infective, urinary (tract) NEC), 280.0 (Anemia, due to blood loss [chronic]), 790.5 (Findings, abnormal, without diagnosis, liver function test)

ICD-10-CM: I31.3 (Effusion, pericardium, pericardial noninflammatory), N17.9 (Failure, renal, acute), E87.1 (Hyponatremia), E83.51 (Hypocalcemia), D72.829 (Leukocytosis), N39.0 (Infection/infected/infective, urinary [tract] NEC), D50.0 (Anemia, due to blood loss [chronic], R79.89 (Findings, abnormal, without diagnosis, liver function test)

Rationale: This is a document that represents prolonged service of care. The time allotted for E/M service is subtracted from the total time of the service and the remaining time is reported with prolonged service codes. Prolonged service codes are add-on codes and are only reported in addition to another code.

This patient is acutely ill with acute renal failure and now has developed a pericardial effusion, which is an accumulation of fluid in the pericardial sac that surrounds the heart. The HPI includes: location (heart), quality (improved - hyponatremia, improving, acute renal failure improving), modifying factors (6 units of fresh frozen plasma), and associated signs and symptoms (tired) for a level 4 or comprehensive HPI. The ROS included 3 organ systems reviewed: genitourinary (making adequate amounts of urine), cardiovascular (some chest pressure but no chest pain), respiratory (on 3 liters per nasal cannula) for a level 3 or detailed ROS. PFSH includes social (wife with patient) a level 3 or detailed PFSH. A comprehensive HPI, detailed ROS and detailed PFSH make this a level 3 or detailed history.

The examination consisted of general appearance (no apparent distress), blood pressure (in 130 range), and respiration (saturation in high 90s) for 1 OS. The abdomen (nontender) is the only BA examined and 3 OSs were examined: cardiovascular (slight generalized edema), respiratory (good air entry bilaterally, few crackles), and integumentary (IJ tunneled dialysis catheter), for a total of 5 BAs/OSs. The exam qualifies as a level 3 or detailed examination.

There are extensive or level 4 diagnosis/management options (pericardial effusion, acute renal failure, plan for blood transfusion for anemia, urinary infection), level 3 or moderate data were reviewed (labs and speaking with cardiologist on plan for pericardial effusion), and the patient has a level 4 or high risk (surgery for pericardial effusion "without tamponade, yet") making this level 4 or high MDM.

The detailed history, detailed level examination, and high MDM make this subsequent hospital service 99233. This code is allotted 35 minutes. At the end of this report it states that 1 hour and 55 minutes were spent with the patient. The total in minutes is 115 minutes. Subtract the 35 minutes included in the initial code 99233, which leaves 80 minutes of time to report as prolonged services. The prolonged services are categorized by either direct contact or without direct contact. The direct face-to-face codes are further categorized by whether the service took place in an outpatient or inpatient setting. The prolonged service code to report with 99233 is 99356 for the first 30-74 minutes of prolonged service time in the inpatient setting. The remaining 20 minutes is not reported. The Prolonged Service Table in your CPT is a good tool to aid in code selection.

ICD-9-CM: The patient has the acute problem of pericardial effusion (423.9). The other diagnoses impacting the management of this patient are: acute renal failure (584.9), hyponatremia (276.1), hypocalcemia (275.41), leukocytosis (288.60), UTI (599.0), anemia due to blood loss (280.0) and an abnormal liver function test (790.5). All of these diagnoses are being treated. The report does not state acute blood loss; therefore, 280.0 is reported.

ICD-10-CM: The patient has the acute problem of pericardial effusion (I31.3). The other diagnoses impacting the management of this patient are: acute renal failure (N17.9), hyponatremia (E87.1), hypocalcemia (E83.51), leukocytosis (D72.829), UTI (N39.0), anemia due to blood loss (D50.0) and an abnormal liver function test (R79.89). All of these diagnoses are being treated. The report does not state acute blood loss; therefore, D50.0 is reported.

HISTORY ELEMENTS	Documented
HISTORY OF PRESENT ILLNESS (HPI)	
1. Location (site on body)	✗
2. Quality (characteristic: throbbing, sharp)	✗
3. Severity (1/10 or how intense)	
4. Duration* (how long for problem or episode)	
5. Timing (when it occurs)	
6. Context (under what circumstances does it occur)	
7. Modifying factors (what makes it better or worse)	✗
8. Associated signs and symptoms (what else is happening when it occurs)	✗
*Duration not in CPT as HPI Element TOTAL	4
LEVEL	4

REVIEW OF SYSTEMS (ROS)	Documented
1. Constitutional (e.g., weight loss, fever)	
2. Ophthalmologic (eyes)	
3. Otolaryngologic (ears, nose, mouth, throat)	
4. Cardiovascular	✗
5. Respiratory	✗
6. Gastrointestinal	
7. Genitourinary	✗
8. Musculoskeletal	
9. Integumentary (skin and/or breasts)	
10. Neurological	
11. Psychiatric	
12. Endocrine	
13. Hematologic/Lymphatic	
14. Allergic/Immunologic	
TOTAL	3
LEVEL	3

PAST, FAMILY, AND/OR SOCIAL HISTORY (PFSH)	Documented
1. Past illness, operations, injuries, treatments, and current medications	
2. Family medical history for heredity and risk	
3. Social activities, both past and present	✗
TOTAL	1
LEVEL	3

History Level		1	2	3	4
		Problem Focused	Expanded Problem Focused	Detailed	Comprehensive
HPI		Brief 1-3	Brief 1-3	Extended 4+	Extended 4+
ROS		None	Problem Pertinent 1	Extended 2-9	Complete 10+
PFSH		None	None	Pertinent 1	Complete 2-3
HISTORY LEVEL					3

EXAMINATION ELEMENTS	Documented
CONSTITUTIONAL (OS)	
• Blood pressure, sitting	
• Blood pressure, lying	✗
• Pulse	
• Respirations	✗
• Temperature	
• Height	
• Weight	
• General appearance	✗
(Counts as only 1) NUMBER	1

BODY AREAS (BA)	Documented
1. Head (including face)	
2. Neck	
3. Chest (including breasts and axillae)	
4. Abdomen	✗
5. Genitalia, groin, buttocks	
6. Back (including spine)	
7. Each extremity	
NUMBER	1

ORGAN SYSTEMS (OS)	Documented
1. Ophthalmologic (eyes)	
2. Otolaryngologic (ears, nose, mouth, throat)	
3. Cardiovascular	✗
4. Respiratory	✗
5. Gastrointestinal	
6. Genitourinary	
7. Musculoskeletal	
8. Integumentary (skin)	✗
9. Neurologic	
10. Psychiatric	
11. Hematologic/Lymphatic/Immunologic	
NUMBER	3
TOTAL BA/OS	5

Exam Level	1	2	3	4
	Problem Focused	Expanded Problem Focused	Detailed	Comprehensive
	Limited to affected BA/OS	Limited to affected BA/OS & other related OS(s)	Extended of affected BA(s) & other related OS(s)	General multi-system (OSs only)
# of OS or BA	1	2-7 limited	2-7 extended	8+
EXAMINATION LEVEL				3

MDM ELEMENTS	Documented
# OF DIAGNOSIS/MANAGEMENT OPTIONS	
1. Minimal	
2. Limited	
3. Multiple	
4. Extensive	✗
LEVEL	4
AMOUNT AND/OR COMPLEXITY OF DATA TO REVIEW	Documented
1. Minimal/None	
2. Limited	
3. Moderate	✗
4. Extensive	
LEVEL	3
RISK OF COMPLICATION OR DEATH IF NOT TREATED	Documented
1. Minimal	
2. Low	
3. Moderate	
4. High	✗
LEVEL	4

MDM*	1	2	3	4
	Straightforward	Low	Moderate	High
Number of DX or management options	Minimal	Limited	Multiple	Extensive
Amount and/or complexity of data	Minimal/None	Limited	Moderate	Extensive
Risks	Minimal	Low	Moderate	High
MDM LEVEL				4

*To qualify for a given type of MDM complexity, 2 of 3 elements in the table must be met or exceeded.

History: Detailed interval

Examination: Detailed

MDM: High

Number of Key Components: 2 of 3

Code: 99233, 99356

Examination, Report 8

Professional Services: 99360 (Evaluation and Management, Standby Services)
   ICD-9-CM: 724.02 (Stenosis, spinal, lumbar, lumbosacral)
   ICD-10-CM: M48.07 (Stenosis, spinal, lumbosacral region)

Rationale: This is a document that represents standby services for which there is only one code—99360. The code is reported in units depending on the time the physician provides standby service. The standby must be requested by another physician and documented in the patient record. No face-to-face contact was made with the patient, and the physician standing by was not providing care to any other patient during the standby time. If the standby time is less than 30 minutes, the service is not reported. Unlike some of the other E/M codes, the unit of time for standby services must be a full 30 minutes. It is very important to read and understand the guidelines in the CPT that apply to standby service.

   The time reported was 8:45 AM to 9:25 AM, or 40 minutes of standby time requested by the neurosurgeon. Code 99360 is reported for 30 of the 40 minutes. The extra 10 minutes cannot be reported because it is not a full 30 minutes. Prior to reporting this, check for documentation in the patient's record for the request for this service.

   ICD-9-CM: The diagnosis is the reason the physician was asked to stand by. In this case it was the reason for the surgery, lumbar stenosis (724.02).

   ICD-10-CM: The diagnosis is the reason the physician was asked to stand by. In this case it was the reason for the surgery, lumbar stenosis (M48.07).

Examination, Report 9

Professional Services: 99367 (Evaluation and Management, Case Management Services)
   ICD-9-CM: 786.2 (Cough), 793.19 (Findings, abnormal, without diagnosis, radiologic, lung)
   ICD-10-CM: R05 (Cough), R91.8 (Abnormal, diagnostic imaging, lung)

Rationale: Case management is a process in which the physician responsible for the direct care of the patient coordinates the care of the patient with other health care services to meet the needs of the patient. These services may be provided by means of a medical team conference. The code description for 99367 states without the patient present in a conference that lasted 30 minutes or more.

   ICD-9-CM: The diagnoses are cough (786.2) and abnormal chest x-ray (793.19).

   ICD-10-CM: The diagnoses are cough (R05) and abnormal chest x-ray (R91.8).

Examination, Report 10

Professional Services: 99395 (Evaluation and Management, Preventive Services)

ICD-9-CM: V70.0 (Checkup, health), V72.31 (Gynecological, examination), 623.8 (Bleeding, vagina, vaginal)

ICD-10-CM: Z00.0 (Examination, general, routine), Z01.411 (Gynecological, examination), N93.9 (Bleeding, vagina, vaginal (abnormal)

Rationale: Preventive medicine services are for timely evaluations and yearly physicals. Codes are selected by patient age, unlike other E/M codes that are selected by time or key components. Codes are further categorized by whether the patient is new or established.

This documentation is of an established patient who is 39 years old. The correct code for the preventive medicine service is 99395.

ICD-9-CM: The assessment contains 3 diagnoses: gynecologic examination with pap, vaginal tenderness and slight vaginal bleeding, and health maintenance issues. When reporting the diagnosis on preventive examinations the first-listed diagnosis is for the health checkup (V70.0) followed by the gynecological exam (V72.31). Report other diagnoses if there is an indication in the plan that a condition will be treated or followed up on. The Premarin cream was prescribed to decrease vaginal bleeding (623.8). It is important to familiarize yourself with the guidelines that precede the preventive medicine codes in the CPT because they explain the requirements for reporting a preventive medicine code and an E/M service on the same day.

ICD-10-CM: The assessment contains 3 diagnoses: gynecologic examination with pap, vaginal tenderness and slight vaginal bleeding, and health maintenance issues. When reporting the diagnosis on preventive examinations the first listed diagnosis is for the health checkup (Z00.00) followed by the gynecological exam (Z01.411). Report other diagnoses if there is an indication in the plan that they will be treated or followed up on. The Premarin cream was prescribed to decrease vaginal bleeding (N93.9). It is important to familiarize yourself with the guidelines that precede the preventive medicine codes in the CPT because they explain the requirements for reporting a preventive medicine code and an E/M service on the same day.

Examination, Report 11

Professional Services: 99450 (Evaluation and Management, Basic Life and/or Disability Evaluation Services)

ICD-9-CM: V70.3 (Examination, medical (for), insurance certification), V77.99 (Screening, metabolic disorder NEC), V81.6 (Screening, disease or disorder, genitourinary condition NEC)

ICD-10-CM: Z02.6 (Examination, medical, insurance purposes), Z13.228 (Screening, metabolic errors, inborn), Z13.89 (Screening, disease or disorder, genitourinary condition NEC)

Rationale: Special evaluation management services are for basic life and/or disability evaluations or work-related medical disability evaluations. This evaluation is a life insurance examination. The correct code is 99450.

ICD-9-CM: The diagnosis is a V code to indicate that this was an insurance evaluation (V70.3). The notes following the heading for V70 indicate "Use additional code(s) to identify any special screening examinations performed (V73.0-V82.9)."

ICD-10-CM: The diagnosis is a V code to indicate that this was an insurance evaluation (Z02.6). Screening for metabolic disorder will map to code (Z13.288). Screening for genitourinary conditions maps to code Z13.89.

Examination, Report 12

Professional Services: 99480 (Evaluation and Management, Low Birthweight Infant)

ICD-9-CM: V21.30 (Status, low birthweight), 550.90 (Hernia/hernial, inguinal, unilateral or unspecified), V45.89 (Status [post], postoperative NEC)

ICD-10-CM: P07.10 (Low birthweight), K40.90 (Hernia/hernial, inguinal, unilateral or unspecified), Z98.89 (Status [post], postoperative [postprocedure])

Rationale: Codes 99478, 99479, and 99480 report physician services on days other than the day of admission for infants of VLBW (infants weighing less than 1500 grams), LBW (1500-2500 grams), or normal weight (2501-5000 grams) who are not critically ill but do still require intensive services. These infants are recovering. Code selection depends on the weight of the infant. The infant in this report is 4725 grams now working on increasing weight, reported with 99480.

ICD-9-CM: The patient is still in NICU for low birth weight; therefore, the first-listed diagnosis is V21.30 (Status, low birth weight). We do not know the weight at birth; therefore, the unspecified code is selected. The infant has a scrotal hernia (550.900) and is status post supraglottoplasty (V45.89). The Index for Hernia, scrotum, scrotal states - *see* Hernia inguinal.

ICD-10-CM: The patient is still in NICU for low birth weight; therefore, the first-listed diagnosis is P07.10 (Status, low birth weight). We do not know the weight at birth; therefore, the unspecified code is selected. The infant has a scrotal hernia (K40.90) and is status post supraglottoplasty (Z98.89). The Index for Hernia, scrotum, scrotal states - *see* Hernia inguinal.

Examination, Report 13

Professional Services: 99379 (Evaluation and Management, Care Plan Oversight Services)

ICD-9-CM: 585.46 (Disease/diseased, renal, end-stage), 496 (Disease, lung, obstructive [chronic] [COPD]), 331.0 (Alzheimer's, disease or sclerosis), V45.11 (Dialysis, renal, status only)

ICD-10-CM: N18.6 (Disease/diseased, renal, end-stage [failure]), J44.9 (Disease, lung, obstructive [chronic] [COPD], G30.9 [F02.80] (Disease, Alzheimer's, without behavioral disturbance), Z99.2 (Dialysis, renal, status only)

Rationale: Care plan oversight services reflect a supervisory role provided to the patient. The patient is not present when the physician is performing the service. Codes include development or revision of a care plan, review of reports of patient status, communication with other health care professionals, and review of any lab or tests that may have been performed. These codes may only be reported once for every 30-day period. Codes are divided by where the patient is residing—home health agency, hospice, or a nursing facility—and further divided based on time. Code 99379 is the correct CPT code for this documentation because the patient is in a skilled nursing facility and the time of service was less than 30 minutes.

ICD-9-CM: The diagnoses are ESRD (585.46), COPD (496), Alzheimer's (331.0), and V45.11 to report the dialysis status. The notes in the Tabular under 331.0 state "Use additional code, where applicable, to identify dementia: with behavioral disturbances (294.11); without behavioral disturbances (294.10)." In this case, the report does not provide this information; therefore, it is not reported.

ICD-10-CM: The diagnoses are ESRD (N18.6), COPD (J44.9), Alzheimer's (G30.9), [F02.80], and Z99.2 to report the dialysis status.

Examination, Report 14

Professional Services: 99340 (Evaluation and Management, Care Plan Oversight Services)

ICD-9-CM: 715.96 (Osteoarthritis/arthritic, lower leg), 492.8 (Emphysema), 285.9 (Anemia)

ICD-10-CM: M17.0 (Osteoarthritis, knee, bilateral), J43.9 (Emphysema), D64.9 (Anemia, unspecified)

Rationale: This is a care plan oversight service for a patient who resides in a rest home. The time involved in care plan oversight was 45 minutes during a 30-day period and an additional 38 minutes discussing this with family members. The total time was 83 minutes; therefore, the correct code is 99340. The description of the service in CPT includes telephone calls with family members; therefore, the 38 minutes is added to the 45 minutes of care plan oversight.

ICD-9-CM: The diagnoses are arthritis of the knees, which is reported as lower leg (715.96), emphysema (492.8), and anemia (285.9) as all these conditions were addressed.

ICD-10-CM: The diagnoses are osteoarthritis of the knees, primary (M17.0), emphysema (J43.9), and anemia (D64.9) as all these conditions were addressed.

Examination, Report 15

See audit form that follows this report.

Professional Services: 99204 (Evaluation and Management, Office and Other Outpatient)

ICD-9-CM: 719.45 (Pain(s), joint, hip), 786.2 (Cough), 787.1 (Heartburn), 305.10 (Addiction, nicotine, unspecified), 296.20 (Psychosis, depressive), 278.00 (Obesity), V85.34 (Body Mass Index (BMI), adult, 34.0–34.9)

ICD-10-CM: M25.551 (Pain(s), joint, hip, right), R05 (Cough), R12 (Heartburn), F17.200 (Addiction, nicotine, see Dependence, drug, nicotine), F32.9 (Psychosis, depressive, see Disorder, depressive), E66.9 (Obesity), Z68.34 (Body Mass Index (BMI), adult, 34.0–34.9)

Rationale: The patient is a new patient establishing with a physician. The HPI includes 5 elements: location (hip), duration (3 months), timing (constant), modifying factor (over-the-counter pain medication), and associated signs and symptoms (tingling) for a level 4 or comprehensive HPI. The ROS includes: constitutional (obesity), ophthalmologic (negative), otolaryngologic (negative), cardiovascular (negative), respiratory (nagging dry cough), gastrointestinal (heartburn), genitourinary (one kidney thought to be congenital), musculoskeletal (does not feel pain as much when walking), neurological (pain radiates to buttocks down to heel) and psychiatric (wants off Zoloft) for a total of 10 or a level 4 or comprehensive ROS. The PFSH includes: past (hysterectomy), family (mother has hypertension and heart problems with high cholesterol), and social (married, smokes) history were reviewed for a level 4 or comprehensive PFSH. The comprehensive HPI, comprehensive ROS, and comprehensive PFSH make this a level 4 or comprehensive history.

The examination includes blood pressure, pulse, weight, and general appearance for 1 OS. The BAs examined are: head (normocephalic), neck (supple, no jugular distension, no thyromegaly) for 2 BAs. The OSs examined included: ophthalmologic (pink conjunctivae, anicteric sclerae, PERRL), cardiovascular (normal rate and rhythm, no murmur/gallop), respiratory (no rales or wheezes), gastrointestinal (no organomegaly), musculoskeletal (straight-leg testing negative, pain on internal rotation of right hip joint), integumentary (warm and dry), and lymphatic (no cervical lymphadenopathy) for 7 OSs. This is a total of 10 BAs/OSs for a level 4 or comprehensive level examination; however, only OSs count for a comprehensive examination. Recounting without BAs, there are 8 OSs. This still counts as a comprehensive examination.

The MDM includes level 4 or extensive management options (hip pain, cough, wean off Zoloft, smoking), level 2 or limited data were reviewed (none), and the patient has level 3 or moderate risk (prescription management) for a level 3 or moderate MDM.

Because this is a new patient, 3 of the 3 key components must be met for level selection.

The comprehensive history, comprehensive level examination and moderate MDM make this new patient service 99204.

ICD-9-CM: The reason for the office service is to establish a new physician. The first condition listed in the assessment section of the report is the joint pain. When reporting joint pain do not reference the Index under "Pain, hip." Reference "Pain, joint, hip." The other diagnoses of cough (786.2), heartburn (787.1), and nicotine addiction (305.10) would also be reported. The patient also has a major depressive disorder (296.20), but when referencing this code in the Tabular of the ICD-9-CM you see "single episode or unspecified." The report does not specify; therefore, 296.20 is correct. The obesity (278.00) and body mass index of 34 (V85.34) are also reported.

ICD-10-CM: The first condition listed in the assessment section of the report is the joint pain. When reporting joint pain do not reference the Index under "Pain, hip." Reference "Pain, joint, hip" (M25.551). The other diagnoses are cough (R05), heartburn (R12), and nicotine addiction (F17.200). The patient also has a major depressive disorder (F32.9), but when referencing this code in the Tabular of the ICD-10-CM you see "single episode or unspecified." The report does not specify; therefore, F32.9 is correct. The obesity (E66.9) and body mass index of 34 (Z68.34) are also reported.

HISTORY ELEMENTS			Documented
HISTORY OF PRESENT ILLNESS (HPI)			
1. Location (site on body)			X
2. Quality (characteristic: throbbing, sharp)			
3. Severity (1/10 or how intense)			
4. Duration* (how long for problem or episode)			X
5. Timing (when it occurs)			X
6. Context (under what circumstances does it occur)			
7. Modifying factors (what makes it better or worse)			X
8. Associated signs and symptoms (what else is happening when it occurs)			X
*Duration not in CPT as HPI Element		TOTAL	5
		LEVEL	4

REVIEW OF SYSTEMS (ROS)			Documented
1. Constitutional (e.g., weight loss, fever)			X
2. Ophthalmologic (eyes)			X
3. Otolaryngologic (ears, nose, mouth, throat)			X
4. Cardiovascular			X
5. Respiratory			X
6. Gastrointestinal			X
7. Genitourinary			X
8. Musculoskeletal			X
9. Integumentary (skin and/or breasts)			
10. Neurological			X
11. Psychiatric			X
12. Endocrine			
13. Hematologic/Lymphatic			
14. Allergic/Immunologic			
		TOTAL	10
		LEVEL	4

PAST, FAMILY, AND/OR SOCIAL HISTORY (PFSH)			Documented
1. Past illness, operations, injuries, treatments, and current medications			X
2. Family medical history for heredity and risk			X
3. Social activities, both past and present			X
		TOTAL	3
		LEVEL	4

History Level	1	2	3	4
	Problem Focused	Expanded Problem Focused	Detailed	Comprehensive
HPI	Brief 1-3	Brief 1-3	Extended 4+	Extended 4+
ROS	None	Problem Pertinent 1	Extended 2-9	Complete 10+
PFSH	None	None	Pertinent 1	Complete 2-3
			HISTORY LEVEL	4

EXAMINATION ELEMENTS			Documented
CONSTITUTIONAL (OS)			
• Blood pressure, sitting			X
• Blood pressure, lying			
• Pulse			X
• Respirations			
• Temperature			
• Height			
• Weight			X
• General appearance			X
(Counts as only 1) NUMBER			1

BODY AREAS (BA)			Documented
1. Head (including face)			X
2. Neck			X
3. Chest (including breasts and axillae)			
4. Abdomen			
5. Genitalia, groin, buttocks			
6. Back (including spine)			
7. Each extremity			
		NUMBER	2

ORGAN SYSTEMS (OS)			Documented
1. Ophthalmologic (eyes)			X
2. Otolaryngologic (ears, nose, mouth, throat)			
3. Cardiovascular			X
4. Respiratory			X
5. Gastrointestinal			X
6. Genitourinary			
7. Musculoskeletal			X
8. Integumentary (skin)			X
9. Neurologic			
10. Psychiatric			
11. Hematologic/Lymphatic/Immunologic			X
		NUMBER	7
		TOTAL BA/OS	10/8

Exam Level	1	2	3	4
	Problem Focused	Expanded Problem Focused	Detailed	Comprehensive
	Limited to affected BA/OS	Limited to affected BA/OS & other related OS(s)	Extended of affected BA(s) & other related OS(s)	General multi-system (OSs only)
# of OS or BA	1	2-7 limited	2-7 extended	8+
			EXAMINATION LEVEL	4

MDM ELEMENTS			Documented
# OF DIAGNOSIS/MANAGEMENT OPTIONS			
1. Minimal			
2. Limited			
3. Multiple			
4. Extensive			X
		LEVEL	4

AMOUNT AND/OR COMPLEXITY OF DATA TO REVIEW			Documented
1. Minimal/None			
2. Limited			X
3. Moderate			
4. Extensive			
		LEVEL	2

RISK OF COMPLICATION OR DEATH IF NOT TREATED			Documented
1. Minimal			
2. Low			
3. Moderate			X
4. High			
		LEVEL	3

MDM*	1	2	3	4
	Straightforward	Low	Moderate	High
Number of DX or management options	Minimal	Limited	Multiple	Extensive
Amount and/or complexity of data	Minimal/None	Limited	Moderate	Extensive
Risks	Minimal	Low	Moderate	High
			MDM LEVEL	3

*To qualify for a given type of MDM complexity, 2 of 3 elements in the table must be met or exceeded.

History: Comprehensive

Examination: Comprehensive

MDM: Moderate

Number of Key Components: 3 of 3

Code: 99204

Examination, Report 16

See audit form that follows this report.

Professional Services: 99232 (Evaluation and Management, Hospital)

ICD-9-CM: 428.0 (Failure/failed, congestive); 424.1 (Stenosis, aortic [valve]), 585.9 (Failure/failed, renal, chronic), 276.69 (Overload fluid), V45.11 (Dialysis, renal, status only)

ICD-10-CM: I50.9 (Failure/failed, heart, congestive), I35.0 (Stenosis, aortic [valve], non-rheumatic), N18.9 (Failure/failed, renal, chronic), E87.70 (Overload fluid), Z99.2 (Dialysis, renal, status only)

Rationale: This is a subsequent hospital service progress note. The HPI consists of location (lung), severity (improved) and associated signs and symptoms (no orthopnea) for a level 2 or expanded problem focused HPI. The ROS is stated as complete and negative for a level 4 or comprehensive ROS. No elements of PFSH were performed for a level 2 or expanded problem focused PFSH. The interval history level for this progress note is level 2 or expanded problem focused.

The examination consisted of 3 constitutional elements (temperature, weight, and general appearance) for 1 OS. The BAs examined were head (unremarkable), neck (supple), abdomen (benign), and all 4 extremities (swelling has gone down) for 7 BAs. The OSs examined were ophthalmologic (unremarkable), otolaryngologic (unremarkable), and neurologic (intact and nonfocal) for 3 OSs. A total of 11 BAs/OSs were examined for a level 4 or comprehensive examination; however, BAs, do not count toward a comprehensive examination. Recounting without BAs, there are a total of 4 OSs, making this a level 3 or detailed examination.

The MDM consists of level 3 or multiple diagnosis/management options (blood sugar control, kidney function), level 1 or minimal data were reviewed (labs only), and level 3 or moderate risk (medication management) for a level 3 or moderate MDM.

The expanded problem focused history, detailed examination and moderate MDM make this subsequent hospital visit 99232.

ICD-9-CM: The diagnoses are congestive heart failure (428.0), aortic stenosis (424.1), unspecified chronic renal failure (585.9), fluid overload (276.69) and the dialysis status (V45.11).

ICD-10-CM: The diagnoses are congestive heart failure (I50.9), aortic stenosis (T35.0), unspecified chronic renal failure (N18.9), fluid overload (E87.70) and the dialysis status (Z99.2).

HISTORY ELEMENTS	Documented
HISTORY OF PRESENT ILLNESS (HPI)	
1. Location (site on body)	X
2. Quality (characteristic: throbbing, sharp)	
3. Severity (1/10 or how intense)	X
4. Duration* (how long for problem or episode)	
5. Timing (when it occurs)	
6. Context (under what circumstances does it occur)	
7. Modifying factors (what makes it better or worse)	
8. Associated signs and symptoms (what else is happening when it occurs)	X
*Duration not in CPT as HPI Element TOTAL	3
LEVEL	2

REVIEW OF SYSTEMS (ROS)	Documented
1. Constitutional (e.g., weight loss, fever)	X
2. Ophthalmologic (eyes)	X
3. Otolaryngologic (ears, nose, mouth, throat)	X
4. Cardiovascular	X
5. Respiratory	X
6. Gastrointestinal	X
7. Genitourinary	X
8. Musculoskeletal	X
9. Integumentary (skin and/or breasts)	X
10. Neurological	X
11. Psychiatric	X
12. Endocrine	X
13. Hematologic/Lymphatic	X
14. Allergic/Immunologic	X
TOTAL	14
LEVEL	4

PAST, FAMILY, AND/OR SOCIAL HISTORY (PFSH)	Documented
1. Past illness, operations, injuries, treatments, and current medications	
2. Family medical history for heredity and risk	
3. Social activities, both past and present	
TOTAL	0
LEVEL	2

History Level	1	2	3	4
	Problem Focused	Expanded Problem Focused	Detailed	Comprehensive
HPI	Brief 1-3	Brief 1-3	Extended 4+	Extended 4+
ROS	None	Problem Pertinent 1	Extended 2-9	Complete 10+
PFSH	None	None	Pertinent 1	Complete 2-3
			HISTORY LEVEL	2

EXAMINATION ELEMENTS	Documented
CONSTITUTIONAL (OS)	
• Blood pressure, sitting	
• Blood pressure, lying	
• Pulse	
• Respirations	
• Temperature	X
• Height	
• Weight	X
• General appearance	X
(Counts as only 1) NUMBER	1

BODY AREAS (BA)	Documented
1. Head (including face)	X
2. Neck	X
3. Chest (including breasts and axillae)	
4. Abdomen	X
5. Genitalia, groin, buttocks	
6. Back (including spine)	
7. Each extremity	XXXX
NUMBER	7

ORGAN SYSTEMS (OS)	Documented
1. Ophthalmologic (eyes)	X
2. Otolaryngologic (ears, nose, mouth, throat)	X
3. Cardiovascular	
4. Respiratory	
5. Gastrointestinal	
6. Genitourinary	
7. Musculoskeletal	
8. Integumentary (skin)	
9. Neurologic	X
10. Psychiatric	
11. Hematologic/Lymphatic/Immunologic	
NUMBER	3
TOTAL BA/OS	11/4

Exam Level	1	2	3	4
	Problem Focused	Expanded Problem Focused	Detailed	Comprehensive
	Limited to affected BA/OS	Limited to affected BA/OS & other related OS(s)	Extended of affected BA(s) & other related OS(s)	General multi-system (OSs only)
# of OS or BA	1	2-7 limited	2-7 extended	8+
			EXAMINATION LEVEL	3

MDM ELEMENTS	Documented
# OF DIAGNOSIS/MANAGEMENT OPTIONS	
1. Minimal	
2. Limited	
3. Multiple	X
4. Extensive	
LEVEL	3
AMOUNT AND/OR COMPLEXITY OF DATA TO REVIEW	Documented
1. Minimal/None	X
2. Limited	
3. Moderate	
4. Extensive	
LEVEL	1
RISK OF COMPLICATION OR DEATH IF NOT TREATED	Documented
1. Minimal	
2. Low	
3. Moderate	X
4. High	
LEVEL	3

MDM*	1	2	3	4
	Straightforward	Low	Moderate	High
Number of DX or management options	Minimal	Limited	Multiple	Extensive
Amount and/or complexity of data	Minimal/None	Limited	Moderate	Extensive
Risks	Minimal	Low	Moderate	High
			MDM LEVEL	3

*To qualify for a given type of MDM complexity, 2 of 3 elements in the table must be met or exceeded.

History: Expanded Problem Focused Interval
Examination: Detailed
MDM: Moderate
Number of Key Components: 2 of 3
Code: 99232

Examination, Report 17

Professional Services: 99291-25 (Evaluation and Management, Critical Care), 99288 (Evaluation and Management, Emergency Services)

ICD-9-CM: 427.5 (Arrest/arrested, cardiac), 994.8 (Shock, electric), 941.20 (Burn, head, second degree), 941.23 (Burn, lips, second degree), 947.0 (Burn, mouth), 948.00 (Burn, extent, less than 10%), E925.9 (Index to External Causes, Electric shock, electrocution [accidental])

ICD-10-CM: T75.4XXA (Electrocution, electric current), I46.8 (Arrest/arrested, cardiac), T20.29XA (Burn, head, second degree, multiple sites), T31.0 (Burn, extent, less than 10% body surface), W86.8XXA (Index to External Causes, Electric shock, see, Exposure, electric current)

Rationale: The report states that the child was admitted straight to NICU and he was prepped for transport and stabilized for air flight. This physician spent 70 minutes stabilizing this child. The notes in CPT under Inpatient Neonatal and Pediatric Critical Care state "When critical care services are provided to neonates or pediatric patients less than 6 years of age at two separate institutions by an individual from a different group on the same date of service, the individual from the referring institution should report their critical care services with the time-based critical care codes (99291, 99292) and the receiving institution should report the appropriate initial day of care code (99468, 99471, 99475) for the same date of service." In the case, 99291 is reported for 30-74 minutes of critical care and 99291 is reported for the remaining 15 minutes of critical care. Codes 99466 and 99467 report the attendance and face-to-face care during the transport of a critically ill or injured pediatric patient. This physician did not accompany the child on the air flight; therefore, 99466 and 99467 do not apply. The physician personally spoke to the transport team via two-way radio to instruct them on pulmonary and cardiac resuscitation when the patient went into cardiac arrest in flight; therefore, 99288 is reported. Modifier -25 is appended to 99291 and 99292 to indicate that this service was separate from the two-way radio physician direction of emergency medical systems (EMS) care, advanced life support.

ICD-9-CM: This is a 10-month-old male who went into cardiac arrest due to electrocution after chewing through an electrical cord. The primary and most serious diagnosis is the cardiac arrest (427.5). The nonfatal effects of electrocution are reported with 994.8; however, the notes in the Tabular below 994.8 states "Excludes electric burns" (940.0 - 949.5); therefore, it is not reported. The Index listing "Burn, electricity, electric current - see burn by site" directs you to the following codes: second degree burns of lower face (941.20), lips (941.23) and mouth (947.0). The total body surface area of less than 10% and with less than 10% 3rd degree burns is reported (948.00). The external cause of this injury is the electrical shock (E925.9).

ICD-10-CM: This is a 10-month-old male who went into cardiac arrest due to electrocution after chewing through an electrical cord. The cardiac arrest is (I46.8). A note under this code states: *Code first underlying condition.* The primary code is the electrocution and is reported with T75.4XXA; the Excludes 2 note in the Tabular below category T75 states "Excludes burns, electric" (T20-T31); therefore, it is reported with the burns as secondary diagnosis. The Index listing "Burn, electricity, electric current - see burn by site" directs you to the following codes: second degree burns of lower face, lips and mouth, multiple sites (T20.29XA). The total body surface area of less than 10% is reported (T31.0). The external cause of this injury is the electrical shock (W86.8XXA).

Examination 1, Report 18

See audit form that follows this report.

Professional Services: 99326 (Evaluation and Management, Domiciliary or Rest Home, New Patient)

    ICD-9-CM: 786.2 (Cough), 786.07 (Wheezing), 462 (Pharyngitis)

    ICD-10-CM: R05 (Cough), R06.2 (Wheezing), J02.9 (Pharyngitis)

Rationale: This service is a new patient service at the domiciliary home where the patient resides. The HPI consists of location (lung), quality (wheezing), duration (yesterday), and associated signs and symptoms (moderate cough) for a level 4 or comprehensive HPI or extended HPI. The ROS includes 4 systems: constitutional (very pleasant, weight has been stable), otolaryngologic (sore throat), respiratory (denies SOB) and lymphatic (glands in neck have been swollen) for a level 3 or detailed ROS. The PFSH indicates past (history of pneumonia) and social (resides in domiciliary care facility) history for a level 4 or comprehensive PFSH. The comprehensive HPI, detailed ROS and comprehensive PFSH make the history level 3 or detailed.

The examination consists of 4 constitutional items (blood pressure, pulse, respirations, and temperature) for 1 OS. A total of 5 BAs were examined including the abdomen (soft and nontender) and all extremities (extremities × 4 show no edema). Three OSs are examined: respiratory (lungs have wheezes throughout more accentuated in the upper airway), neurological (alert and oriented), and psychiatric (gets very upset when I attempt to elevate his head) for a total of 9 BAs/OSs for a level 4 or comprehensive examination; however, only OSs count toward a comprehensive examination. Recounting without BAs, there is 4 OSs, making this a level 3 or detailed examination.

The MDM entailed level 4 or extensive diagnosis/management options (possible pneumonia, further workup, new patient to examiner), limited or level 2 data were reviewed (chest x-ray ordered), and level 3 or moderate risk (medication management) for a level 3 or moderate MDM.

This is a new patient service; therefore, all three key components are required for the level selection. This documentation contains a detailed history, detailed examination, and moderate MDM for a new patient domiciliary service of 99326.

ICD-9-CM: This physician does not give us a definitive diagnosis and more testing is ordered to try to determine the cause of the patient's symptoms. In this case, the symptoms reported include cough (786.2), wheezing (786.07), and sore throat (462).

ICD-10-CM: This physician does not give us a definitive diagnosis and more testing is ordered to try to determine the cause of the patient's symptoms. In this case, the symptoms reported include cough (R05), wheezing (R06.2), and sore throat (J02.9).

HISTORY ELEMENTS	Documented
HISTORY OF PRESENT ILLNESS (HPI)	
1. Location (site on body)	X
2. Quality (characteristic: throbbing, sharp)	X
3. Severity (1/10 or how intense)	
4. Duration* (how long for problem or episode)	X
5. Timing (when it occurs)	
6. Context (under what circumstances does it occur)	
7. Modifying factors (what makes it better or worse)	
8. Associated signs and symptoms (what else is happening when it occurs)	X
*Duration not in CPT as HPI Element TOTAL	4
LEVEL	4

REVIEW OF SYSTEMS (ROS)	Documented
1. Constitutional (e.g., weight loss, fever)	X
2. Ophthalmologic (eyes)	
3. Otolaryngologic (ears, nose, mouth, throat)	X
4. Cardiovascular	
5. Respiratory	X
6. Gastrointestinal	
7. Genitourinary	
8. Musculoskeletal	
9. Integumentary (skin and/or breasts)	
10. Neurological	
11. Psychiatric	
12. Endocrine	
13. Hematologic/Lymphatic	X
14. Allergic/Immunologic	
TOTAL	4
LEVEL	3

PAST, FAMILY, AND/OR SOCIAL HISTORY (PFSH)	Documented
1. Past illness, operations, injuries, treatments, and current medications	X
2. Family medical history for heredity and risk	
3. Social activities, both past and present	X
TOTAL	2
LEVEL	4

History Level	1 Problem Focused	2 Expanded Problem Focused	3 Detailed	4 Comprehensive
HPI	Brief 1-3	Brief 1-3	Extended 4+	Extended 4+
ROS	None	Problem Pertinent 1	Extended 2-9	Complete 10+
PFSH	None	None	Pertinent 1	Complete 2-3
			HISTORY LEVEL	3

EXAMINATION ELEMENTS	Documented
CONSTITUTIONAL (OS)	
• Blood pressure, sitting	
• Blood pressure, lying	X
• Pulse	X
• Respirations	X
• Temperature	X
• Height	
• Weight	
• General appearance	
(Counts as only 1) NUMBER	1

BODY AREAS (BA)	Documented
1. Head (including face)	
2. Neck	
3. Chest (including breasts and axillae)	
4. Abdomen	X
5. Genitalia, groin, buttocks	
6. Back (including spine)	
7. Each extremity	XXXX
NUMBER	5

ORGAN SYSTEMS (OS)	Documented
1. Ophthalmologic (eyes)	
2. Otolaryngologic (ears, nose, mouth, throat)	
3. Cardiovascular	
4. Respiratory	X
5. Gastrointestinal	
6. Genitourinary	
7. Musculoskeletal	
8. Integumentary (skin)	
9. Neurologic	X
10. Psychiatric	X
11. Hematologic/Lymphatic/Immunologic	
NUMBER	3
TOTAL BA/OS	9/4

Exam Level	1 Problem Focused	2 Expanded Problem Focused	3 Detailed	4 Comprehensive
	Limited to affected BA/OS	Limited to affected BA/OS & other related OS(s)	Extended of affected BA(s) & other related OS(s)	General multi-system (OSs only)
# of OS or BA	1	2-7 limited	2-7 extended	8+
			EXAMINATION LEVEL	3

MDM ELEMENTS	Documented
# OF DIAGNOSIS/MANAGEMENT OPTIONS	
1. Minimal	
2. Limited	
3. Multiple	
4. Extensive	X
LEVEL	4
AMOUNT AND/OR COMPLEXITY OF DATA TO REVIEW	Documented
1. Minimal/None	
2. Limited	X
3. Moderate	
4. Extensive	
LEVEL	2
RISK OF COMPLICATION OR DEATH IF NOT TREATED	Documented
1. Minimal	
2. Low	
3. Moderate	X
4. High	
LEVEL	3

MDM*	1 Straightforward	2 Low	3 Moderate	4 High
Number of DX or management options	Minimal	Limited	Multiple	Extensive
Amount and/or complexity of data	Minimal/None	Limited	Moderate	Extensive
Risks	Minimal	Low	Moderate	High
			MDM LEVEL	3

*To qualify for a given type of MDM complexity, 2 of 3 elements in the table must be met or exceeded.

History: Detailed
Examination: Detailed
MDM: Moderate
Number of Key Components: 3 of 3
Code: 99326

E/M Audit Form

This Audit Form is based on the 1995 Documentation Guidelines for Evaluation and Management Services.

HISTORY ELEMENTS	Documented
HISTORY OF PRESENT ILLNESS (HPI)	
1. Location (site on body)	
2. Quality (characteristic: throbbing, sharp)	
3. Severity (1/10 or how intense)	
4. Duration* (how long for problem or episode)	
5. Timing (when it occurs)	
6. Context (under what circumstances does it occur)	
7. Modifying factors (what makes it better or worse)	
8. Associated signs and symptoms (what else is happening when it occurs)	
*Duration not in CPT as HPI Element — TOTAL	
LEVEL	

REVIEW OF SYSTEMS (ROS)	Documented
1. Constitutional (e.g., weight loss, fever)	
2. Ophthalmologic (eyes)	
3. Otolaryngologic (ears, nose, mouth, throat)	
4. Cardiovascular	
5. Respiratory	
6. Gastrointestinal	
7. Genitourinary	
8. Musculoskeletal	
9. Integumentary (skin and/or breasts)	
10. Neurological	
11. Psychiatric	
12. Endocrine	
13. Hematologic/Lymphatic	
14. Allergic/Immunologic	
TOTAL	
LEVEL	

PAST, FAMILY, AND/OR SOCIAL HISTORY (PFSH)	Documented
1. Past illness, operations, injuries, treatments, and current medications	
2. Family medical history for heredity and risk	
3. Social activities, both past and present	
TOTAL	
LEVEL	

History Level	1	2	3	4
	Problem Focused	Expanded Problem Focused	Detailed	Comprehensive
HPI	Brief 1-3	Brief 1-3	Extended 4+	Extended 4+
ROS	None	Problem Pertinent 1	Extended 2-9	Complete 10+
PFSH	None	None	Pertinent 1	Complete 2-3
HISTORY LEVEL				

EXAMINATION ELEMENTS	Documented
CONSTITUTIONAL (OS)	
• Blood pressure, sitting	
• Blood pressure, lying	
• Pulse	
• Respirations	
• Temperature	
• Height	
• Weight	
• General appearance	
(Counts as only 1) NUMBER	

BODY AREAS (BA)	Documented
1. Head (including face)	
2. Neck	
3. Chest (including breasts and axillae)	
4. Abdomen	
5. Genitalia, groin, buttocks	
6. Back (including spine)	
7. Each extremity	
NUMBER	

ORGAN SYSTEMS (OS)	Documented
1. Ophthalmologic (eyes)	
2. Otolaryngologic (ears, nose, mouth, throat)	
3. Cardiovascular	
4. Respiratory	
5. Gastrointestinal	
6. Genitourinary	
7. Musculoskeletal	
8. Integumentary (skin)	
9. Neurologic	
10. Psychiatric	
11. Hematologic/Lymphatic/Immunologic	
NUMBER	
TOTAL BA/OS	

Exam Level	1	2	3	4
	Problem Focused	Expanded Problem Focused	Detailed	Comprehensive
	Limited to affected BA/OS	Limited to affected BA/OS & other related OS(s)	Extended of affected BA(s) & other related OS(s)	General multi-system (OSs only)
# of OS or BA	1	2-7 limited	2-7 extended	8+
EXAMINATION LEVEL				

MDM ELEMENTS	Documented
# OF DIAGNOSIS/MANAGEMENT OPTIONS	
1. Minimal	
2. Limited	
3. Multiple	
4. Extensive	
LEVEL	

AMOUNT AND/OR COMPLEXITY OF DATA TO REVIEW	Documented
1. Minimal/None	
2. Limited	
3. Moderate	
4. Extensive	
LEVEL	

RISK OF COMPLICATION OR DEATH IF NOT TREATED	Documented
1. Minimal	
2. Low	
3. Moderate	
4. High	
LEVEL	

MDM*	1	2	3	4
	Straightforward	Low	Moderate	High
Number of DX or management options	Minimal	Limited	Multiple	Extensive
Amount and/or complexity of data	Minimal/None	Limited	Moderate	Extensive
Risks	Minimal	Low	Moderate	High
MDM LEVEL				

*To qualify for a given type of MDM complexity, 2 of 3 elements in the table must be met or exceeded.

History:

Examination:

MDM:

Number of Key Components:

Code:

HISTORY ELEMENTS	Documented
HISTORY OF PRESENT ILLNESS (HPI)	
1. Location (site on body)	
2. Quality (characteristic: throbbing, sharp)	
3. Severity (1/10 or how intense)	
4. Duration* (how long for problem or episode)	
5. Timing (when it occurs)	
6. Context (under what circumstances does it occur)	
7. Modifying factors (what makes it better or worse)	
8. Associated signs and symptoms (what else is happening when it occurs)	
*Duration not in CPT as HPI Element TOTAL	
LEVEL	

REVIEW OF SYSTEMS (ROS)	Documented
1. Constitutional (e.g., weight loss, fever)	
2. Ophthalmologic (eyes)	
3. Otolaryngologic (ears, nose, mouth, throat)	
4. Cardiovascular	
5. Respiratory	
6. Gastrointestinal	
7. Genitourinary	
8. Musculoskeletal	
9. Integumentary (skin and/or breasts)	
10. Neurological	
11. Psychiatric	
12. Endocrine	
13. Hematologic/Lymphatic	
14. Allergic/Immunologic	
TOTAL	
LEVEL	

PAST, FAMILY, AND/OR SOCIAL HISTORY (PFSH)	Documented
1. Past illness, operations, injuries, treatments, and current medications	
2. Family medical history for heredity and risk	
3. Social activities, both past and present	
TOTAL	
LEVEL	

History Level	1	2	3	4
	Problem Focused	Expanded Problem Focused	Detailed	Comprehensive
HPI	Brief 1-3	Brief 1-3	Extended 4+	Extended 4+
ROS	None	Problem Pertinent 1	Extended 2-9	Complete 10+
PFSH	None	None	Pertinent 1	Complete 2-3
			HISTORY LEVEL	

EXAMINATION ELEMENTS	Documented
CONSTITUTIONAL (OS)	
• Blood pressure, sitting	
• Blood pressure, lying	
• Pulse	
• Respirations	
• Temperature	
• Height	
• Weight	
• General appearance	
(Counts as only 1) NUMBER	

BODY AREAS (BA)	Documented
1. Head (including face)	
2. Neck	
3. Chest (including breasts and axillae)	
4. Abdomen	
5. Genitalia, groin, buttocks	
6. Back (including spine)	
7. Each extremity	
NUMBER	

ORGAN SYSTEMS (OS)	Documented
1. Ophthalmologic (eyes)	
2. Otolaryngologic (ears, nose, mouth, throat)	
3. Cardiovascular	
4. Respiratory	
5. Gastrointestinal	
6. Genitourinary	
7. Musculoskeletal	
8. Integumentary (skin)	
9. Neurologic	
10. Psychiatric	
11. Hematologic/Lymphatic/Immunologic	
NUMBER	
TOTAL BA/OS	

Exam Level	1	2	3	4
	Problem Focused	Expanded Problem Focused	Detailed	Comprehensive
	Limited to affected BA/OS	Limited to affected BA/OS & other related OS(s)	Extended of affected BA(s) & other related OS(s)	General multi-system (OSs only)
# of OS or BA	1	2-7 limited	2-7 extended	8+
			EXAMINATION LEVEL	

MDM ELEMENTS	Documented
# OF DIAGNOSIS/MANAGEMENT OPTIONS	
1. Minimal	
2. Limited	
3. Multiple	
4. Extensive	
LEVEL	

AMOUNT AND/OR COMPLEXITY OF DATA TO REVIEW	Documented
1. Minimal/None	
2. Limited	
3. Moderate	
4. Extensive	
LEVEL	

RISK OF COMPLICATION OR DEATH IF NOT TREATED	Documented
1. Minimal	
2. Low	
3. Moderate	
4. High	
LEVEL	

MDM*	1	2	3	4
	Straightforward	Low	Moderate	High
Number of DX or management options	Minimal	Limited	Multiple	Extensive
Amount and/or complexity of data	Minimal/None	Limited	Moderate	Extensive
Risks	Minimal	Low	Moderate	High
			MDM LEVEL	

*To qualify for a given type of MDM complexity, 2 of 3 elements in the table must be met or exceeded.

History:

Examination:

MDM:

Number of Key Components:

Code:

HISTORY ELEMENTS				Documented
HISTORY OF PRESENT ILLNESS (HPI)				
1. Location (site on body)				
2. Quality (characteristic: throbbing, sharp)				
3. Severity (1/10 or how intense)				
4. Duration* (how long for problem or episode)				
5. Timing (when it occurs)				
6. Context (under what circumstances does it occur)				
7. Modifying factors (what makes it better or worse)				
8. Associated signs and symptoms (what else is happening when it occurs)				
*Duration not in CPT as HPI Element			TOTAL	
			LEVEL	

REVIEW OF SYSTEMS (ROS)	Documented
1. Constitutional (e.g., weight loss, fever)	
2. Ophthalmologic (eyes)	
3. Otolaryngologic (ears, nose, mouth, throat)	
4. Cardiovascular	
5. Respiratory	
6. Gastrointestinal	
7. Genitourinary	
8. Musculoskeletal	
9. Integumentary (skin and/or breasts)	
10. Neurological	
11. Psychiatric	
12. Endocrine	
13. Hematologic/Lymphatic	
14. Allergic/Immunologic	
TOTAL	
LEVEL	

PAST, FAMILY, AND/OR SOCIAL HISTORY (PFSH)	Documented
1. Past illness, operations, injuries, treatments, and current medications	
2. Family medical history for heredity and risk	
3. Social activities, both past and present	
TOTAL	
LEVEL	

History Level	1	2	3	4
	Problem Focused	Expanded Problem Focused	Detailed	Comprehensive
HPI	Brief 1-3	Brief 1-3	Extended 4+	Extended 4+
ROS	None	Problem Pertinent 1	Extended 2-9	Complete 10+
PFSH	None	None	Pertinent 1	Complete 2-3
				HISTORY LEVEL

EXAMINATION ELEMENTS	Documented
CONSTITUTIONAL (OS)	
• Blood pressure, sitting	
• Blood pressure, lying	
• Pulse	
• Respirations	
• Temperature	
• Height	
• Weight	
• General appearance	
(Counts as only 1) NUMBER	

BODY AREAS (BA)	Documented
1. Head (including face)	
2. Neck	
3. Chest (including breasts and axillae)	
4. Abdomen	
5. Genitalia, groin, buttocks	
6. Back (including spine)	
7. Each extremity	
NUMBER	

ORGAN SYSTEMS (OS)	Documented
1. Ophthalmologic (eyes)	
2. Otolaryngologic (ears, nose, mouth, throat)	
3. Cardiovascular	
4. Respiratory	
5. Gastrointestinal	
6. Genitourinary	
7. Musculoskeletal	
8. Integumentary (skin)	
9. Neurologic	
10. Psychiatric	
11. Hematologic/Lymphatic/Immunologic	
NUMBER	
TOTAL BA/OS	

Exam Level	1	2	3	4
	Problem Focused	Expanded Problem Focused	Detailed	Comprehensive
	Limited to affected BA/OS	Limited to affected BA/OS & other related OS(s)	Extended of affected BA(s) & other related OS(s)	General multi-system (OSs only)
# of OS or BA	1	2-7 limited	2-7 extended	8+
				EXAMINATION LEVEL

MDM ELEMENTS	Documented
# OF DIAGNOSIS/MANAGEMENT OPTIONS	
1. Minimal	
2. Limited	
3. Multiple	
4. Extensive	
LEVEL	

AMOUNT AND/OR COMPLEXITY OF DATA TO REVIEW	Documented
1. Minimal/None	
2. Limited	
3. Moderate	
4. Extensive	
LEVEL	

RISK OF COMPLICATION OR DEATH IF NOT TREATED	Documented
1. Minimal	
2. Low	
3. Moderate	
4. High	
LEVEL	

MDM*	1	2	3	4
	Straightforward	Low	Moderate	High
Number of DX or management options	Minimal	Limited	Multiple	Extensive
Amount and/or complexity of data	Minimal/None	Limited	Moderate	Extensive
Risks	Minimal	Low	Moderate	High
				MDM LEVEL

*To qualify for a given type of MDM complexity, 2 of 3 elements in the table must be met or exceeded.

History:

Examination:

MDM:

Number of Key Components:

Code:

HISTORY ELEMENTS	Documented
HISTORY OF PRESENT ILLNESS (HPI)	
1. Location (site on body)	
2. Quality (characteristic: throbbing, sharp)	
3. Severity (1/10 or how intense)	
4. Duration* (how long for problem or episode)	
5. Timing (when it occurs)	
6. Context (under what circumstances does it occur)	
7. Modifying factors (what makes it better or worse)	
8. Associated signs and symptoms (what else is happening when it occurs)	
*Duration not in CPT as HPI Element TOTAL	
LEVEL	

REVIEW OF SYSTEMS (ROS)	Documented
1. Constitutional (e.g., weight loss, fever)	
2. Ophthalmologic (eyes)	
3. Otolaryngologic (ears, nose, mouth, throat)	
4. Cardiovascular	
5. Respiratory	
6. Gastrointestinal	
7. Genitourinary	
8. Musculoskeletal	
9. Integumentary (skin and/or breasts)	
10. Neurological	
11. Psychiatric	
12. Endocrine	
13. Hematologic/Lymphatic	
14. Allergic/Immunologic	
TOTAL	
LEVEL	

PAST, FAMILY, AND/OR SOCIAL HISTORY (PFSH)	Documented
1. Past illness, operations, injuries, treatments, and current medications	
2. Family medical history for heredity and risk	
3. Social activities, both past and present	
TOTAL	
LEVEL	

History Level	1	2	3	4
	Problem Focused	Expanded Problem Focused	Detailed	Comprehensive
HPI	Brief 1-3	Brief 1-3	Extended 4+	Extended 4+
ROS	None	Problem Pertinent 1	Extended 2-9	Complete 10+
PFSH	None	None	Pertinent 1	Complete 2-3
HISTORY LEVEL				

EXAMINATION ELEMENTS	Documented
CONSTITUTIONAL (OS)	
• Blood pressure, sitting	
• Blood pressure, lying	
• Pulse	
• Respirations	
• Temperature	
• Height	
• Weight	
• General appearance	
(Counts as only 1) NUMBER	

BODY AREAS (BA)	Documented
1. Head (including face)	
2. Neck	
3. Chest (including breasts and axillae)	
4. Abdomen	
5. Genitalia, groin, buttocks	
6. Back (including spine)	
7. Each extremity	
NUMBER	

ORGAN SYSTEMS (OS)	Documented
1. Ophthalmologic (eyes)	
2. Otolaryngologic (ears, nose, mouth, throat)	
3. Cardiovascular	
4. Respiratory	
5. Gastrointestinal	
6. Genitourinary	
7. Musculoskeletal	
8. Integumentary (skin)	
9. Neurologic	
10. Psychiatric	
11. Hematologic/Lymphatic/Immunologic	
NUMBER	
TOTAL BA/OS	

Exam Level	1	2	3	4
	Problem Focused	Expanded Problem Focused	Detailed	Comprehensive
	Limited to affected BA/OS	Limited to affected BA/OS & other related OS(s)	Extended of affected BA(s) & other related OS(s)	General multi-system (OSs only)
# of OS or BA	1	2-7 limited	2-7 extended	8+
EXAMINATION LEVEL				

MDM ELEMENTS	Documented
# OF DIAGNOSIS/MANAGEMENT OPTIONS	
1. Minimal	
2. Limited	
3. Multiple	
4. Extensive	
LEVEL	

AMOUNT AND/OR COMPLEXITY OF DATA TO REVIEW	Documented
1. Minimal/None	
2. Limited	
3. Moderate	
4. Extensive	
LEVEL	

RISK OF COMPLICATION OR DEATH IF NOT TREATED	Documented
1. Minimal	
2. Low	
3. Moderate	
4. High	
LEVEL	

MDM*	1	2	3	4
	Straightforward	Low	Moderate	High
Number of DX or management options	Minimal	Limited	Multiple	Extensive
Amount and/or complexity of data	Minimal/None	Limited	Moderate	Extensive
Risks	Minimal	Low	Moderate	High
MDM LEVEL				

*To qualify for a given type of MDM complexity, 2 of 3 elements in the table must be met or exceeded.

History:

Examination:

MDM:

Number of Key Components:

Code:

HISTORY ELEMENTS				Documented
HISTORY OF PRESENT ILLNESS (HPI)				
1. Location (site on body)				
2. Quality (characteristic: throbbing, sharp)				
3. Severity (1/10 or how intense)				
4. Duration* (how long for problem or episode)				
5. Timing (when it occurs)				
6. Context (under what circumstances does it occur)				
7. Modifying factors (what makes it better or worse)				
8. Associated signs and symptoms (what else is happening when it occurs)				
*Duration not in CPT as HPI Element			TOTAL	
			LEVEL	

REVIEW OF SYSTEMS (ROS)	Documented
1. Constitutional (e.g., weight loss, fever)	
2. Ophthalmologic (eyes)	
3. Otolaryngologic (ears, nose, mouth, throat)	
4. Cardiovascular	
5. Respiratory	
6. Gastrointestinal	
7. Genitourinary	
8. Musculoskeletal	
9. Integumentary (skin and/or breasts)	
10. Neurological	
11. Psychiatric	
12. Endocrine	
13. Hematologic/Lymphatic	
14. Allergic/Immunologic	
TOTAL	
LEVEL	

PAST, FAMILY, AND/OR SOCIAL HISTORY (PFSH)	Documented
1. Past illness, operations, injuries, treatments, and current medications	
2. Family medical history for heredity and risk	
3. Social activities, both past and present	
TOTAL	
LEVEL	

History Level	1	2	3	4
	Problem Focused	Expanded Problem Focused	Detailed	Comprehensive
HPI	Brief 1-3	Brief 1-3	Extended 4+	Extended 4+
ROS	None	Problem Pertinent 1	Extended 2-9	Complete 10+
PFSH	None	None	Pertinent 1	Complete 2-3
				HISTORY LEVEL

EXAMINATION ELEMENTS	Documented
CONSTITUTIONAL (OS)	
• Blood pressure, sitting	
• Blood pressure, lying	
• Pulse	
• Respirations	
• Temperature	
• Height	
• Weight	
• General appearance	
(Counts as only 1) NUMBER	

BODY AREAS (BA)	Documented
1. Head (including face)	
2. Neck	
3. Chest (including breasts and axillae)	
4. Abdomen	
5. Genitalia, groin, buttocks	
6. Back (including spine)	
7. Each extremity	
NUMBER	

ORGAN SYSTEMS (OS)	Documented
1. Ophthalmologic (eyes)	
2. Otolaryngologic (ears, nose, mouth, throat)	
3. Cardiovascular	
4. Respiratory	
5. Gastrointestinal	
6. Genitourinary	
7. Musculoskeletal	
8. Integumentary (skin)	
9. Neurologic	
10. Psychiatric	
11. Hematologic/Lymphatic/Immunologic	
NUMBER	
TOTAL BA/OS	

Exam Level	1	2	3	4
	Problem Focused	Expanded Problem Focused	Detailed	Comprehensive
	Limited to affected BA/OS	Limited to affected BA/OS & other related OS(s)	Extended of affected BA(s) & other related OS(s)	General multi-system (OSs only)
# of OS or BA	1	2-7 limited	2-7 extended	8+
				EXAMINATION LEVEL

MDM ELEMENTS	Documented
# OF DIAGNOSIS/MANAGEMENT OPTIONS	
1. Minimal	
2. Limited	
3. Multiple	
4. Extensive	
LEVEL	

AMOUNT AND/OR COMPLEXITY OF DATA TO REVIEW	Documented
1. Minimal/None	
2. Limited	
3. Moderate	
4. Extensive	
LEVEL	

RISK OF COMPLICATION OR DEATH IF NOT TREATED	Documented
1. Minimal	
2. Low	
3. Moderate	
4. High	
LEVEL	

MDM*	1	2	3	4
	Straightforward	Low	Moderate	High
Number of DX or management options	Minimal	Limited	Multiple	Extensive
Amount and/or complexity of data	Minimal/None	Limited	Moderate	Extensive
Risks	Minimal	Low	Moderate	High
				MDM LEVEL

*To qualify for a given type of MDM complexity, 2 of 3 elements in the table must be met or exceeded.

History:

Examination:

MDM:

Number of Key Components:

Code:

Abbreviations

ABG	arterial blood gases
ACLS	Advanced Cardiac Life Support
AIC	amino-imidazole carboxamide, anti-inflammatory corticoid
ALT	alanine transaminase (formerly SGPT)
ARDS	acute or adult respiratory distress syndrome
AST	aspartate amino-transferase (formerly SGOT)
ATN	acute tubular necrosis
AV	arteriovenous
b.i.d.	twice a day
BOOP	bronchiolitis obliterans organizing pneumonia
BSO	bilateral salpingo-oophorectomy
BUN	blood urea nitrogen
CABG	coronary artery bypass graft
CBC	complete blood count
CEA	carcinoembryonic antigen, carotid endarterectomy
CHF	congestive heart failure
CK	creatine kinase
COPD	chronic obstructive pulmonary disease
CPK	creatine phosphokinase
CT	computed tomography
CVA	cardiovascular accident
D	deciliter, donor
D5	dextrose 5% water
DUB	dysfunctional uterine bleeding
ENT	ear, nose, throat
EOMs	extraocular movements
FI	forced inspiration
FOB	fecal occult blood
GERD	gastroesophageal reflux disease
GI	gastrointestinal
GU	genitourinary
h	hour
H_2	histamine-2
H&H	hematocrit and hemoglobin, also stated HH
HEENT	head, ears, eyes, nose, throat
Hs	at bedtime
I&O	intake and output
IM	intramuscular
INR	International Normalized Ratio
IV	intravenous
JP	jugular process, jugular pulse
JVD	jugular vein distention

LMP	last menstrual period
MAP	mean aortic pressure, mean arterial pressure
MB	methylene blue, mesio-buccal
MDM	medical decision making
mEq	milliequivalent
mg	milligram
MI	myocardial infarction
mL	milliliter
mm	millimeter
neb	nebula, a spray, nebulin
NG	nasogastric, nitroglycerin
n.p.o.	nothing by mouth
O_2	oxygen
OBT	occult blood test
OP	outpatient
OPC	outpatient clinic
OPD	outpatient department
OPS	outpatient surgery
OPV	oral poliovirus vaccine
OR	operating room
OTC	over-the-counter
OURQ	outer upper-right quadrant
OV	office visit
PCO_2	partial pressure of carbon dioxide
PEEP	positive end expiration pressure
pH	potential of hydrogen
p.o.	by mouth
p.r.n.	as needed
PT	prothrombin time
PTH	parathyroid hormone, post-transfusional hepatitis
q	every
q.2wk	every 2 weeks
q.3h	every 3 hours
q.4h	every 4 hours
q.4wk	every 4 weeks
q.a.m.	every morning
q.d.	every day
q.d.s.	four times a day
q.h.	every hour
q.h.s.	each bedtime
q.i.d.	four times a day
q.m.	every morning
q.o.d.	every other day
q.os.	as needed
q.p.m.	every afternoon or every evening
q.q.h.	every fourth hour
q.s.	quantity sufficient
qq.	each, every
qq.h	every hour
QRS	Q-wave R-wave S-wave
RLQ	right lower quadrant
s	sans (without), sigma (sign, mark), semis (half)
S1	first heart sound
S2	second heart sound
S3	third heart sound

S4	fourth heart sound
SBE	subacute bacterial endocarditis
SIMV	synchronized intermittent mandatory ventilation
T_4	thyroxine
TMJ	temporomandibular joint
URI	upper respiratory infection

Further Text Resources

ANATOMY AND PHYSIOLOGY

Book Title	Author	Imprint	Copyright Date	ISBN-13
The Anatomy and Physiology Learning System, 4th Edition	Applegate	Saunders	2010	978-1-4377-0393-1
Gray's Anatomy for Students, 2nd Edition	Drake, Vogl, Mitchell	Churchill Livingstone	2010	978-0-443-06952-9
Anthony's Textbook of Anatomy and Physiology, 19th Edition	Thibodeau, Patton	Mosby	2010	978-0-323-05539-0

CODING

Book Title	Author	Imprint	Copyright Date	ISBN-13
Step-by-Step Medical Coding, 2013 Edition	Buck	Saunders	2013	978-1-4557-4465-7
2013 ICD-10-CM Draft Standard Edition	Buck	Saunders	2013	978-1-4457-5362-8
2013 ICD-10-PCS Draft Standard Edition	Buck	Saunders	2013	978-1-4457-5363-5
ICD-10-CM Online Training Modules	Buck	Saunders		978-1-4457-4384-1
ICD-10-PCS Online Training Modules	Buck	Saunders		978-1-4457-4603-3
2013 ICD-9-CM, Volumes 1 & 2 (Professional Edition)	Buck	Saunders	2013	978-1-4457-4572-2
2013 ICD-9-CM, Volumes 1, 2, & 3 (Professional Edition)	Buck	Saunders	2013	978-1-4557-4497-8
2013 HCPCS Level II (Professional Edition)	Buck	Saunders	2013	978-1-4557-4497-2
The Next Step, Advanced Medical Coding and Auditing, 2013 Edition	Buck	Saunders	2013	978-1-4457-4485-5
Physician Coding Exam Review 2013 with ICD-9-CM: The Certification Step	Buck	Saunders	2013	978-1-4457-4575-3

Facility Coding Exam Review 2013 with ICD-9-CM: The Certification Step	Buck	Saunders	2013	978-1-4557-2288-4
Online Internship for Medical Coding, 2013 Edition	Buck	Saunders	2013	978-1-4557-5861-6
ICD-9-CM Coding: Theory and Practice with ICD-10-CM, 2013/2014 Edition	Lovaasen, Schwerdtfeger	Saunders	2013	978-1-4557-0701-0
ICD-10-CM/PCS Coding: Theory and Practice	Lovaasen, Schwerdtfeger	Saunders	2013	978-1-4557-4249-3

PATHOPHYSIOLOGY

Book Title	Author	Imprint	Copyright Date	ISBN-13
Pathology for the Health Professions, 3rd Edition	Damjanov	Saunders	2006	978-1-4160-0031-0
Essentials of Human Diseases and Conditions, 4th Edition	Frazier, Drzymkowski	Saunders	2008	978-1-4160-4714-8
Pathophysiology for the Health Professions, 4th Edition	Gould	Saunders	2011	978-1-4377-0965-0
The Human Body in Health and Illness, 4th Edition	Herlihy	Saunders	2011	978-1-4160-6842-6
The Human Body in Health and Disease, 5th Edition	Thibodeau, Patton	Mosby	2010	978-0-323-05491-1

MEDICAL TERMINOLOGY

Book Title	Author	Imprint	Copyright Date	ISBN-13
The Language of Medicine, 9th Edition	Chabner	Saunders	2011	978-1-4377-0560-6
Jablonski's Dictionary of Medical Acronyms & Abbreviations, 6th Edition	Jablonski	Saunders	2009	978-1-4160-5899-1
Exploring Medical Language, 7th Edition	LaFleur, Brooks	Mosby	2009	978-0-323-04950-4
Building a Medical Vocabulary (with Spanish Translations), 7th Edition	Leonard	Saunders	2009	978-1-4160-5627-0
Quick & Easy Medical Terminology, 5th Edition	Leonard	Saunders	2007	978-1-4160-2494-1
Mastering Healthcare Terminology, 3rd Edition	Shiland	Mosby	2010	978-0-323-05506-2
Dorland's Illustrated Medical Dictionary, 31st Edition		Saunders	2007	978-1-4160-2364-7

INTRODUCTION TO COMPUTER

Book Title	Author	Imprint	Copyright Date	ISBN-13
Computerized Medical Office Procedures: A Worktext 3rd Edition	Larsen	Saunders	2011	978-1-4377-1608-5

BASICS OF WRITING/MEDICAL TRANSCRIPTION

Book Title	Author	Imprint	Copyright Date	ISBN-13
Medical Transcription Guide: Do's and Don'ts, 3rd Edition	Diehl	Saunders	2005	978-0-7216-0684-2
Medical Transcription: Techniques and Procedures, 7th Edition	Diehl	Saunders	2012	978-1-4377-0439-6

COMPREHENSION BUILDING/STUDY SKILLS

Book Title	Author	Imprint	Copyright Date	ISBN-13
Career Development for Health Professionals: Success in School and on the Job, 3rd Edition	Haroun	Saunders	2010	978-1-4377-0673-4

BASIC MATH

Book Title	Author	Imprint	Copyright Date	ISBN-13
Basic Mathematics for the Health-Related Professions	Doucette	Saunders	2000	978-0-7216-7938-9
Using Maths in Health Sciences	Gunn	Churchill Livingstone	2001	978-0-443-07074-7

MEDICAL BILLING/INSURANCE

Book Title	Author	Imprint	Copyright Date	ISBN-13
Health Insurance Today: A Practical Approach, 3rd Edition	Beik	Saunders	2011	978-1-4377-1770-9
Medical Insurance Made Easy: Understanding the Claim Cycle, 2nd Edition	Brown	Saunders	2006	978-0-7216-0556-2
Insurance Handbook for the Medical Office, 11th Edition	Fordney	Saunders	2010	978-1-4377-0128-9
Electronic Health Record "Booster" Kit for the Medical Office, 2nd Edition	Buck	Saunders	2012	978-1-4557-2301-0
Practice Kit for Medical Front Office Skills, 3rd Edition	Buck	Saunders	2011	978-1-4377-2201-7
ePractice Kit for Medical Front Office Skills with MedTrack Systems	Buck	Saunders	2012	978-1-4377-2722-7